Case-based Approach to Common Neurological Disorders

Krishna Kumar Oli
Gentle Sunder Shrestha
Rajeev Ojha
Pramod Kumar Pal
Sanjay Pandey · Bibhukalyani Das
Editors

Case-based Approach to Common Neurological Disorders

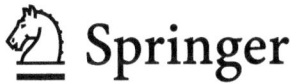 Springer

Editors
Krishna Kumar Oli
Department of Neurology
Tribhuvan University Teaching Hospital
Kathmandu, Nepal

Gentle Sunder Shrestha
Department of Anesthesiology
Tribhuvan University Teaching Hospital
Kathmandu, Nepal

Rajeev Ojha
Department of Neurology
Tribhuvan University Teaching Hospital
Kathmandu, Nepal

Pramod Kumar Pal
Department of Neurology
NIMHANS
Bangalore, India

Sanjay Pandey
Department of Neurology and Stroke
Medicine
Amrita Hospital
Faridabad, Delhi, India

Bibhukalyani Das
Neuroanaesthesia, Neurocritical Care
Institute of Neurosciences
Kolkata, India

ISBN 978-981-99-8678-1   ISBN 978-981-99-8676-7   (eBook)
https://doi.org/10.1007/978-981-99-8676-7

This Springer imprint is published by the registered company Springer Nature Singapore Pte Ltd. The registered company address is: 152 Beach Road, #21-01/04 Gateway East, Singapore 189721, Singapore

Paper in this product is recyclable

Contents

Part I CNS Infections

1 **Japanese Encephalitis** 3
Rajeev Ojha

2 **Herpes Encephalitis** 9
Rajeev Ojha

3 **Acute Bacterial Meningitis** 15
Dilli Ram Kafle and Anushka Adhikari

4 **Cryptococcal Meningoencephalitis** 19
Ghanshyam Kharel

5 **Neurocysticercosis** 25
Anushka Adhikari and Rajeev Ojha

6 **Tetanus** 35
Aamir Siddiqui

7 **Tubercular Meningitis** 43
M. Netravathi

8 **Subacute Sclerosing Panencephalitis** 51
Madhu Nagappa and Sanjib Sinha

9 **Brain Abscess** 61
A. Shobhana

Part II Cardiovascular Disorders

10 **Acute Ischemic Stroke** 71
Deependra Raj Khanal

11 **Subarachnoid Hemorrhage** 79
Prakash Kafle, S. Vignesh, Sabin Bhandari,
and Gentle Sunder Shrestha

12 **Intracerebral Hemorrhage** 97
Gopal Sedain, Sachit Sharma, and Gentle Sunder Shrestha

13   **Cerebral Sinus and Venous Thrombosis** 105
     Reema Rajbhandari and Niraj Gautam

14   **Large Hemispheric Stroke** 111
     Bikram Prasad Gajurel

Part III   Epilepsy

15   **Childhood Absence Epilepsy** 119
     Ethan Rosenberg, Janice Rodriguez Hernandez,
     and Theresa M. Czech

16   **Status Epilepticus** 125
     Laxmi Dhakal and William O. Tatum

Part IV   Neuromuscular Diseases

17   **Myasthenia Gravis** 135
     Babu Ram Pokharel

18   **Amyotrophic Lateral Sclerosis** 141
     Seena Vengalil, Saraswati Nashi, Veeramani Preethish-Kumar,
     Kiran Polavarapu, and Atchayaram Nalini

19   **Myotonic Dystrophy** 151
     Hrishikesh Kumar and Purba Basu

20   **Guillain-Barré Syndrome** 157
     Rajeev Ojha and Gaurav Nepal

21   **Inflammatory Muscle Diseases** 163
     Saraswati Nashi, Kiran Polavarapu, Seena Vengalil,
     Veeramani Preethish-Kumar, and Atchayaram Nalini

Part V   Neuroimmunology

22   **Optic Neuritis** 179
     Sanjeeta Sitaula

23   **Autoimmune Encephalitis** 187
     M. Netravathi

Part VI   Movement Disorders

24   **Progressive Supranuclear Palsy** 201
     Shweta Prasad and Pramod Kumar Pal

25   **Multiple System Atrophy** 211
     Malligurki Raghurama Rukmani, Talakad N. Sathyaprabha,
     and Ravi Yadav

26   **Lower-Body Parkinsonism** 227
     Nitish Kamble and Pramod Kumar Pal

27 **Childhood Dystonia** 237
    Anjali Chouksey and Sanjay Pandey

28 **Neurodegeneration with Brain Iron Accumulation** 249
    Roopa Rajan

29 **Frontotemporal Dementia** 257
    R. Subasree and Suvarna Alladi

30 **Parkinson's Disease** 265
    Ragesh Karn

Part VII   Others

31 **Trigeminal Neuralgia** 273
    Bibhukalyani Das and Supriyo Choudhury

32 **Hypoxic Ischemic Encephalopathy** 279
    Masoom J. Desai, Roohi Katyal, Pratik Agrawal,
    and Gentle Sunder Shrestha

33 **Coma and Vegetative State** 287
    Krishna Kumar Oli and Aashish Shrestha

34 **Metabolic Syndromes in Neurology** 297
    Anirban Ghosal

35 **Traumatic Brain Injury** 303
    Ahmed Abd Elazim and Shraddha Mainali

36 **Spinal Cord Injury** 313
    Indranil Ghosh and Subhajit Guha

37 **Alzheimer's Disease** 323
    Krishna Dhungana

38 **Intracranial Hypertension** 329
    Gentle Sunder Shrestha and Saurabh Pradhan

About the Editors

Krishna Kumar Oli is the Head of the Department of Neurology at Tribhuvan University Teaching Hospital, one of the leading tertiary-level teaching hospitals in Nepal. The department has been running the post-MD and DM course in neurology for a couple of years and has been leading in academics and training the doctors in the field of neurosciences. Prof. Oli is the current president of Nepalese Academy of Neurology.

Gentle Sunder Shrestha is a leading neurointensivist and neuroanesthesiologist at the Department of Anaesthesiology at Tribhuvan University Teaching Hospital, Kathmandu, Nepal. He has led neuroscience educational endeavors in Nepal and abroad. He has over 75 peer-reviewed publications in national and international journals and is leading book projects on "A Manual of Neuroanesthesia and Neurocritical Care" and "Practical Approach to Point-of-Care Ultrasound." He has attended multiple international neuroscience meetings as invited guest speaker and faculty. He was awarded the "Educational Day Medal" by the Ministry of Education on the occasion of the National Education Day in 2010 for his appreciable work in the education sector.

Rajeev Ojha is a dynamic young neurologist at the Department of Neurology at Tribhuvan University Teaching Hospital, Kathmandu, Nepal. He is one of the few certified neurologists in Nepal with DM in Neurology. He has a strong interest in education, training, and publications.

Pramod Kumar Pal is the Head of the Department of Neurology at NIMHANS (National Institute of Mental Health and Neuro Sciences), Bangalore, India. He has multiple publications and has special interest and expertise in movement disorders.

Sanjay Pandey is the Head of the Department of Neurology and Stroke Medicine at Amrita Institute of Medical Sciences, Faridabad, one of the leading tertiary-level teaching hospitals in India. The department is running many teaching and fellowship courses. Dr. Pandey is currently an executive committee member of the MDS-AOS section of the International Parkinson and Movement Disorders Society.

Bibhukalyani Das is the Educational Director and Director of Neuroanaesthesia, Neurocritical Care and Pain Clinic at the Institute of Neurosciences, Kolkata, India. She has multiple publications. She is the past president of the Indian Society of Neuroanaesthesiology and Critical Care (ISNACC).

Part I

CNS Infections

Japanese Encephalitis

1

Rajeev Ojha

Case Scenario

A 21-year-old patient presented with complaints of fever for 4 days, limb weakness for 3 days, and altered sensorium for 2 days. According to the patient's father, he was well 4 days back, then he developed mild fever, which was insidious in onset and not associated with chills and rigor. Same day, patient started having tingling sensation of left lower limb. Next day, patient developed weakness in left upper and lower limbs and had a high fever (104 °F). In local hospital, CT head was done, which showed no significant abnormal findings. Patient also had one episode of jerking of limbs with loss of consciousness lasting for about 1–2 min. After this episode, patient continued to have altered sensorium. Patient was then referred to our center for further management.

The patient presented to emergency department with low Glasgow Coma Scale (E2M3V2) and was intubated. On examination, his vitals were BP: 140/80 mmHg, pulse: 120/min, temperature: 103 °F. Bilateral pupils were equal and reactive to light. There was no disk edema, and movement of extraocular muscles was normal. Corneal and gag reflexes were preserved with no facial deviation. No spontaneous limb movements were observed. Muscle tone was reduced, and areflexia was elicited across all limb joints. Plantar extensor was observed in left side, while right side had flexor response. His cerebrospinal fluid was clear with total leukocytes 310/mm^3 (polymorphs: 10% and monomorphs: 90%), protein: 38 mg/dL, and sugar: 4.7 mmol/L. A provisional diagnosis of acute encephalitis syndrome was made, and the patient was then started on empirical treatment with acyclovir and ceftriaxone. Routine blood investigations with renal and hepatic function tests were normal. The MRI brain T2 fluid-attenuated inversion recovery (FLAIR) sequence showed a bilateral thalamus hyperintense lesion extending to the upper midbrain region and another hyperintense area in the right medial parietal cortex and subcortex (Fig. 1.1a–c). Herpes simplex I and II and tuberculosis polymerase chain reactions (PCRs) were negative. Japanese encephalitis serology was found to be positive. The patient's fever subsided in 3 days after admission. During his stay in the intensive care unit, the patient developed ventilation-associated pneumonia, and a tracheostomy was done on the 15th day of admission. In about 1 month of admission, mild improvement in sensorium was noted, and he was able to follow simple commands. During discharge, he was still bed bound and able to move bilateral distal fingers with no further improvement in cognitive function.

R. Ojha (✉)
Department of Neurology, Tribhuvan University Institute of Medicine, Kathmandu, Nepal

© Springer Nature Singapore Pte Ltd. 2024
K. K. Oli et al. (eds.), *Case-based Approach to Common Neurological Disorders*,
https://doi.org/10.1007/978-981-99-8676-7_1

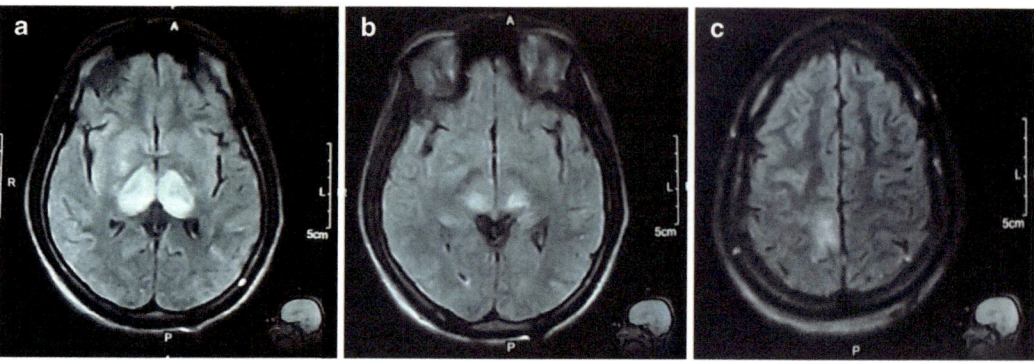

Fig. 1.1 (**a**, **b**) MRI brain T2 fluid-attenuated inversion recovery (FLAIR) sequence shows bilateral thalamus hyperintense lesion extending to upper midbrain region. (**c**) Hyperintense lesion in the right medial parietal cortex and subcortical region

1.1 Introduction

Japanese encephalitis (JE) is a mosquito-borne flavivirus encephalitis, which is one of the common encephalitides found in clinical practice in South Asian countries [1]. First outbreak of JE encephalitis was reported from Japan in 1871, followed by a severe epidemic again in 1924. The JE virus (JEV) is a single-stranded RNA virus belonging to the family Flaviviridae and the genus Flavivirus. JE virus exists in an enzootic life cycle between mosquitoes and pigs. It commonly affects children, but frequently adult cases have also been encountered. About one-third of the patients die of this disease, one-third live with severe neurological sequelae, and remaining one-third survive with mild or no sequelae [2, 3].

1.2 Epidemiology

JE virus is transmitted to humans, animals, and birds by culex mosquitoes, *C. tritaeniorhynchus*. The natural cycle of JE virus usually consists of pig-mosquito-pig or bird-mosquito-bird. Swine are the amplifying host of the JE virus, and it cannot spread directly from one person to another. There are two epidemiological patterns of transmission during the seasonal peak, like summer, and they occur sporadically throughout the year. Nepal falls under an epidemic pattern where the cases rise in the summer season. The rate of infection is more common in children aged 3–15 years, but a bimodal distribution has been found, with the elderly population being another peak. The annual incidence of the disease ranges from 30,000 to 50,000. A fatality rate of 30–40% has been reported from an Indian study [3, 4].

1.3 Pathogenesis

The incubation period of the JE virus ranges from 6 to 16 days. Infestations depend on viral and host factors. Viral factors are route of entry, titer, and neurovirulence of the inoculum, and host factors are age, general health, and immunity. After a mosquito bite, the virus replicates in the skin and then spreads to regional lymph nodes. Viral particles are then transported to connective tissue, skeletal tissue, myocardium, smooth muscle, lymphoreticular tissues, and endocrine and exocrine glands, where they amplify to cause a transient viremia. Finally, central nervous system (CNS) penetration is through hematogenous transmission. Experiments suggest that passive transfer across the endothelial cells may be an important means of crossing the blood-brain barrier. Factors that impair the blood-brain barrier are the risk factors for neuroinvasion. After the growth of the virus across vascular endothelial cells, CNS parts like the cerebral cortex, thalamus, basal ganglia, brainstem, Purkinje cells of the cerebellum, and hippocampus are involved [5, 6].

1.4 Pathology

In histopathology, leptomeninges are normal or slightly hazy with inflammatory infiltrates. In the acute stage, congestion and edema are noted around the brain parenchyma. Microscopically, meningeal inflammation, perivascular cuffing, neuronal degeneration, mononuclear and polymorphonuclear infiltration, and microglial proliferation are the features. Immunohistochemical study of lymphocytes shows cytotoxic cells such as CD4+ and CD8+. Migration of lymphocytes and monocytes toward virus-infected neurons takes place, and ultimately gliosis and apoptosis occur. In imaging, magnetic resonance imaging (MRI) will show the involvement of bilateral thalamus, basal ganglia, pons, cerebellum, and midbrain [2].

1.5 Clinical Manifestation

Patient may present with headache, fever, altered sensorium, seizure, and even coma in severe condition. Patients usually have a history of residing in an endemic area or have a travel history in that area. Early prodromal features are fever, myalgia, headache, rashes, lymphadenopathy, nausea, and vomiting followed by irritability and mild confusion [2].Some patients may spontaneously improve with mild prodromal symptoms. Altered sensorium and confusion may gradually progress to stupor and coma. Often patients present with symptoms of behavioral changes and mutism [3]. JE patients presenting with behavioral changes are frequently referred to a psychiatric clinic. Further, patients can present with features such as pulmonary oedema, hepatomegaly, splenomegaly, and thrombocytopenia [7].

Seizure and status epilepticus are common in JE and are more prevalent in children. Repeated and prolonged seizures are usually associated with poor prognosis. Seizure types are commonly focal motor, autonomic, or generalized [3]. Focal neurological deficits like hemiparesis and cranial nerve lesions, and signs like hypertonia, hyper-reflexia, and neck stiffness are also present. There can be involvement of anterior horn cells in the spinal cord, causing flaccid limb weakness, which is sometimes confused with acute poliomyelitis [8]. JE has usually been associated with Guillain-Barre syndrome with a demyelinating pattern [9]. Acute urinary retention with an atonic bladder is another feature of JE.

Movement disorders in JE are common findings. Extrapyramidal features like generalized axial and limb rigidity and tremors are seen due to the involvement of the basal ganglia [10]. Patients can manifest other features of parkinsonism like a mask face, reduced eye blink, slow activities, and impaired gait [2]. Dystonia is frequently reported in JE, especially in children and young adults [11]. Both focal and generalized, involving axial and limb dystonia, are seen. Occasional dystonic spasms may occur, leading to the requirement of mechanical ventilation [12].

1.6 Diagnosis

Diagnosis depends on the clinical manifestation correlated with living in an endemic area or a history of recent travel to such an area, serum or CSF JE virus isolation, and areas of MRI brain lesions. Blood count may show mild leukocytosis with thrombocytopenia in a few patients. Hyponatremia may be secondary to inappropriate antidiuretic hormone secretion. A CSF examination shows elevated opening pressure in about half of the patients. There may be lymphocytic pleocytosis, a normal CSF-to-plasma glucose ratio, and mildly elevated protein. The JE virus can be confirmed by IgM capture of ELISA of serum or CSF [13].

The MRI brain may show a high signal in T2 and FLAIR in the basal ganglia, thalamus, midbrain, pons, and medulla [14]. Thalamic lesions are common findings in most JE patients. Although nonspecific, an electroencephalogram (EEG) may show seizure activity, slow waves, and periodic lateralized epileptiform discharges [15].

1.7 Differential Diagnosis

1.7.1 Herpes Simplex Encephalitis

Herpes simplex encephalitis (HSE) is clinically difficult to differentiate from Japanese encephalitis. JE is usually prevalent in endemic regions or has a travel history to these regions, whereas HSE prevalence is worldwide distributed. Typical presentations are fever, headache, altered sensorium, focal neurological deficits with hemiparesis, dysarthria, ataxia, and cranial nerve involvement. CSF analysis may show RBC along with lymphocytic leukocytosis, normal or reduced sugar, and elevated protein. Herpes simplex virus PCR from CSF has a high sensitivity and specificity for the diagnosis. MRI features fluid-attenuated inversion recovery (FLAIR) or diffusion-weighted imaging (DWI) hyperintense lesions in the temporal lobe and adjacent lobes. EEG can be positive in about 80% of HSE patients, showing periodic lateralized epileptiform discharges or theta and delta waves in the temporal and frontal regions [16]. Patients usually respond well to early intravenous acyclovir treatment; however, no specific antiviral drug is available for JE.

1.7.2 Acute Disseminated Encephalomyelitis

Acute disseminated encephalomyelitis (ADEM) is an autoimmune demyelinating disease of the central nervous system with a presentation of multifocal neurological features like headache, malaise, altered sensorium, motor, sensory, and cranial nerve involvement. ADEM typically follows infection or vaccination and is common in the pediatric population. Typical MRI lesions of ADEM are bilateral, could be symmetric or asymmetric, involve deep and subcortical white matter, and are hyperintense on the FLAIR sequence. Although ADEM is usually a monophasic illness, a few percentage of similar subsets but relapsing pattern of demyelinating disorders are also reported [17]. ADEM usually responds well to high-dose corticosteroids.

1.8 Treatment

Since no specific antiviral drug is available for JE, supportive care is the major focus of management. Early administration of acyclovir is empirically given till lumbar puncture, and MRI reports and JE serology reports are available. Intravenous mannitol or 3% NaCl may be needed to control the raised intracranial pressure. Antiepileptic drugs are administered if a seizure is present. EEG monitoring is helpful to detect nonconvulsive status epilepticus if the patient is persistently unconscious. The use of intravenous immunoglobulin has been found to be effective in some studies, although more studies are needed to confirm this [16].

Prevention of JE can be done by taking protective measures against mosquito bites. Mosquito repellents, full clothing, netted windows, and the use of bed nets are the measures to be taken in endemic regions. Tourists should follow these measures while traveling to such regions. Longer-term and frequent travelers who are at risk of JEV exposure could be vaccinated.

1.9 Prognosis

Poor prognostic features are a depressed conscious level, repetitive seizures, raised intracranial pressure, secondary complications, and extended MRI lesions. Mortality occurs in up to 30% of cases due to acute cerebral edema and pulmonary complications [3]. Sequelae like limb weakness, tremor, rigidity, cognitive impairment, seizure, or behavioral disturbances are present in 30–50% of survivors [4].

References

1. Pant SD. Epidemiology of Japanese encephalitis in Nepal. J Nepal Paediatr Soc. 2009;29(1):35–7.
2. Ghosh D, Basu A. Japanese encephalitis—a pathological and clinical perspective. PLoS Negl Trop Dis. 2009;3(9):e437.
3. Solomon T, Dung NM, Kneen R, Gainsborough M, Vaughn DW, Khanh VT. Japanese encephalitis. J Neurol Neurosurg Psychiatry. 2000;68:405–15.

4. Ooi MH, Lewthwaite P, Lai BF, Mohan A, Clear D, Lim L, et al. The epidemiology, clinical features, and long-term prognosis of Japanese encephalitis in Central Sarawak, Malaysia, 1997–2005. Clin Infect Dis. 2008;47(4):458–68.

5. Solomon T, Vaughn DW. Pathogenesis and clinical features of Japanese encephalitis and West Nile virus infections. Curr Top Microbiol Immunol. 2002;267(Solomon 2000):171–94.

6. Singh SK. Molecular pathogenesis of Japanese encephalitis virus infection. In: Singh SK, editor. Vol. I, Human emerging and re-emerging infections. John Wiley & Sons; 2015. p. 113–24.

7. Turtle L, Solomon T. Japanese encephalitis—the prospects for new treatments. Nat Rev Neurol. 2018;14(5):298–313.

8. Solomon T, Kneen R, Dung NM, Khanh VC, Thuy TTN, Ha DQ, et al. Poliomyelitis-like illness due to Japanese encephalitis virus. Lancet. 1998;351(9109):1094–7.

9. Ravi V, Taly AB, Shankar SK, Shenoy PK, Desai A, Nagaraja D, et al. Association of Japanese encephalitis virus infection with Guillain-Barré syndrome in endemic areas of South India. Acta Neurol Scand. 1994;90(1):67–72.

10. Misra UK, Kalita J. Movement disorders in japanese encephalitis. J Neurol. 1997;244(5):299–303.

11. Aryal R, Shrestha S, Homagain S, Chhetri S, Shrestha K, Kharel S, et al. Clinical spectrum and management of dystonia in patients with Japanese encephalitis: a systematic review. Brain Behav. 2022;12(2):e2496.

12. Kalita J, Misra UK. Markedly severe dystonia in Japanese encephalitis. Mov Disord Off J Mov Disord Soc. 2000;15(6):1168–72.

13. Solomon T, Thao LTT, Dung NM, Kneen R, Hung NT, Nisalak A, et al. Rapid diagnosis of Japanese encephalitis by using an immunoglobulin M dot enzyme immunoassay. J Clin Microbiol. 1998;36(7):2030–4.

14. Kumar S, Misra UK, Kalita J, Salwani V, Gupta RK, Gujral R. MRI in Japanese encephalitis. Neuroradiology. 1997;39(3):180–4.

15. Kalita J, Misra UK, Pandey S, Dhole TN. A comparison of clinical and radiological findings in adults and children with Japanese encephalitis. Arch Neurol. 2003;60(12):1760–4.

16. Solomon T, Michael BD, Smith PE, Sanderson F, Davies NWS, Hart IJ, et al. Management of suspected viral encephalitis in adults—Association of British Neurologists and British Infection Association National Guidelines. J Infect. 2012;64(4):347–73.

17. Pohl D, Alper G, Van Haren K, et al. Acute disseminated encephalomyelitis: updates on an inflammatory CNS syndrome. Neurology. 2016;87:S38–45.

Herpes Encephalitis

Rajeev Ojha

Case Scenario

A 40-year-old female was admitted with the chief complaint of fever, headache, and altered sensorium for 7 days. She was well 7 days back when she felt generalized fatigue and reduced appetite. Two days later, she had a high-grade fever of 103 °F, which was associated with mild-to-moderate headache in bilateral temporal side along with nausea. Next day, patient was found to be confused and was not properly responding to commands. Patient was then taken to local hospital and admitted for 3 days. Although fever was subsided then, her sensorium further worsened and was unable to recognize own family members. Then the patient was referred to our center. Patient had one episode of generalized tonic-clonic seizure after she landed in emergency.

Patient had no significant past medical and surgical history. She was a non-smoker and non-alcoholic. On examination, vitals were blood pressure: 125/60; pulse: 78/min; respiratory rate: 18/min; and temperature: 100.2 °F. She was anxious and irritable and was not cooperative during examination; Glasgow Coma Scale was E3M6V4. Patient was not oriented to time, place, and person. Bilateral pupils were equal and reactive to light. There was no facial deviation, and gag reflex was normal. Bulk, tone, deep tendon reflexes, and power were normal in both upper and lower limbs. There were no cerebellar signs, and bilateral planters were flexor. Blood investigations were total leukocytes count: 7670/mm^3, neutrophils 70%, lymphocytes 30%, sugar: 5.2 mmol/L, urea: 5 mg/dL, creatinine: 50 mg/dL, sodium: 140 mEq/L, potassium: 3.7 mEq/L, platelet: 187,000/mm^3, chest X-ray: normal findings, and ECG: normal findings. Cerebrospinal fluid (CSF) findings: total cells: 20, lymphocytes: 90%, neutrophils: 10%, protein: 195 mg/dL, and sugar: 6.3 mmol/L. MRI brain showed asymmetric T1 low and T2 and FLAIR (Fig. 2.1) high signal intensity in the bilateral temporal, insular, and precuneus areas of the parietal lobe (left > right) with diffusion restriction. EEG showed periodic triphasic waves in frontal, parietal, and temporal areas (Fig. 2.2). CSF Herpes simplex 1 (HSV-1) PCR was found to be positive. The diagnosis of herpes encephalitis was made, and intravenous acyclovir was given for 21 days. The patient's sensorium gradually improved after 10 days of treatment and was oriented to time, place, and person during discharge.

R. Ojha (✉)
Department of Neurology, Tribhuvan University Teaching Hospital, Kathmandu, Nepal

© Springer Nature Singapore Pte Ltd. 2024
K. K. Oli et al. (eds.), *Case-based Approach to Common Neurological Disorders*,
https://doi.org/10.1007/978-981-99-8676-7_2

Fig. 2.1 Asymmetric FLAIR high signal intensity in bilateral temporal region, insular area, and precuneus area of the parietal lobe (left > right) with edema in the left medial temporal lobe, loss of left temporal horn, and compressing left midbrain suggesting uncal herniation

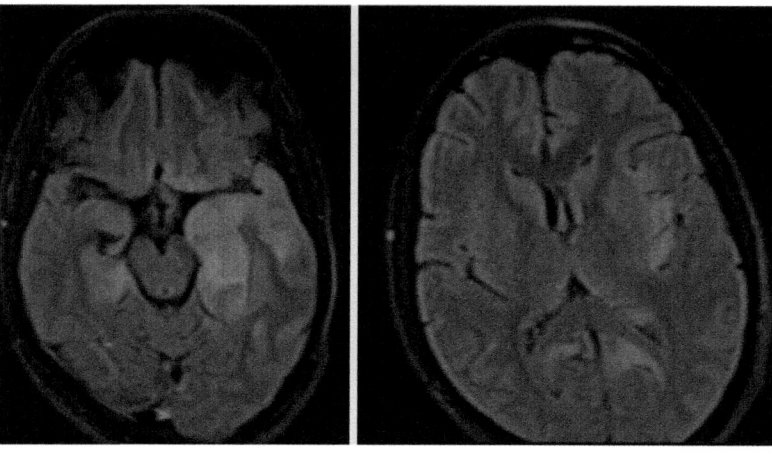

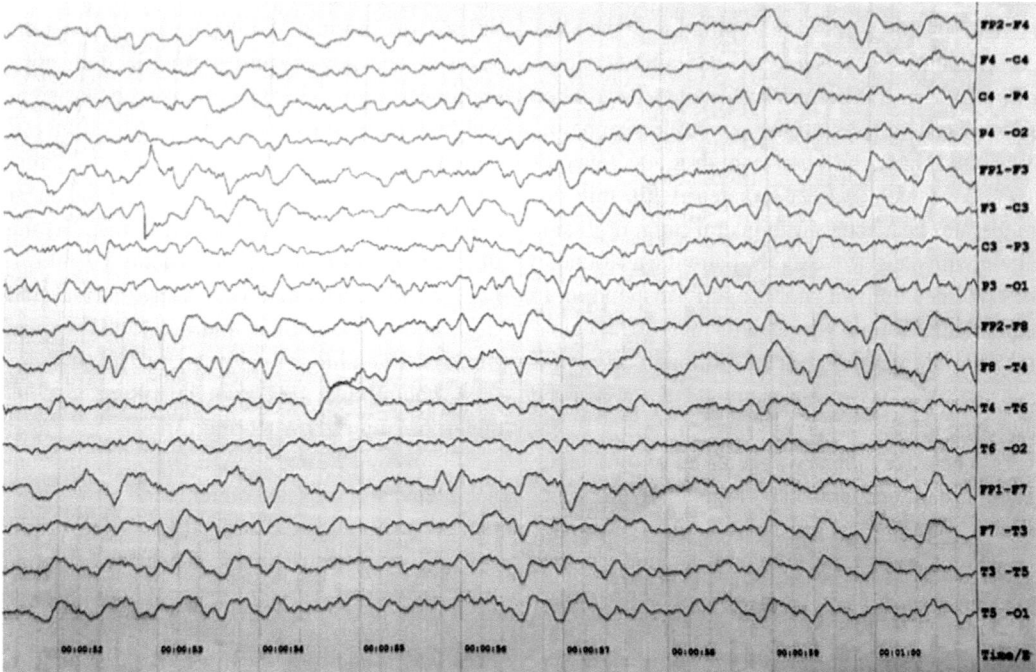

Fig. 2.2 EEG showing generalized periodic epileptiform discharges

2.1 Introduction

Encephalitis is the inflammation of the brain parenchyma resulting in neurological symptoms, with infectious etiologies being common. Herpes encephalitis is the most common cause of fatal encephalitis all around the world. Herpes viruses are the enveloped DNA viruses, out of which herpes simplex 1 has been found to be the most common sporadic cause. The clinical manifestations are usually altered sensorium, fever, headache, seizure, and focal neurologic symptoms. Despite treatment, HSV-1 encephalitis has high mortality and mortality with cognitive and other focal neurological sequelae [1].

2.2 Epidemiology

The worldwide incidence of HSE has been estimated at 1–2 per 1000,000 populations [2]. A 10-year encephalitis study in the United States found HSV to be the most common etiological pathogen [3]. Most HSE in adult patients are likely due to HSV reactivation. HSE occurs equally in males and females. Bimodal variation in age group distribution has been reported; peak incidence is under 3 years and more than 50 years. HSV-1 is common among adults and children, whereas HSV-2 is likely to cause encephalitis in infants and immunocompromised population [4]. The presence of herpes labialis along with encephalitis usually correlates with associated HSV infection.

2.3 Pathology

Brain pathology of HSE includes cytolytic viral proliferation along with immune-mediated inflammatory responses. In histopathology, necrosis involves neurons, astrocytes, oligodendrocytes in temporal lobe, infero-frontal lobe, and insular cortex of cerebral hemispheres. HSV replication is characterized by mononuclear inflammation with perivascular cuffing and focal infiltrates of inflammatory cells, along with Cowdry type A intranuclear inclusion bodies [5]. Infection further triggers the innate immune system, while adaptive immunity tries to combat the early acute infection. Toll-like receptors (TLRs), which are the pattern recognition receptors of innate system, bind to the pathogen. Then, initiation of cascades of proinflammatory cytokines like interferon, interleukins, and tissue necrosis factor takes place [6]. Finally, the development of host resistance to viral proliferation, destruction of viral cellular RNA, apoptosis of infected cells, and stopping cellular translation take place. Deficiency in immune response, both in acute and latent states, can make the host susceptible to HSE.

2.4 Pathogenesis

Out of eight human herpes virus which includes HSV-1, HSV-2, HHV3 (varicella zoster), HHV-4 (Epstein Barr), HHV-5 (Cytomegalovirus), HHV-6, HHV-7, and HHV-8, HSV-1 is the commonest pathogen for encephalitis. Mucous membrane or damaged skin is the primary access for the HSV infection. Then, retrograde axonal transport causes the transport of virus to neuronal cell body of dorsal root ganglion. Although not clear, entry to the central nervous system due to retrograde transport via olfactory or trigeminal nerves or hematogenous dissemination has been proposed [7–9]. Subsequently HSV spread to the frontal and temporal lobes, insular cortex, and rarely the brainstem occurs and can further extend to the opposite hemisphere.

2.5 Clinical Manifestation

HSE symptoms may manifest early with prodromal features like headache, myalgia, and behavioral changes [10]. Behavioral symptoms may be elevated mood, reduced sleep, hypersexuality, and hypomania, which are due to the involvement of the temporal lobe or limbic system. Extratemporal involvement is commonly seen among the pediatric population. Typical presentations are fever, headache, altered sensorium, focal neurological deficits with hemiparesis, dysarthria, ataxia, and cranial nerve involvement. Occasionally, patient can even present with quadriparesis [11]. HSV is an important cause of rhombencephalitis and brainstem encephalitis, predominantly HSV-1. The common features of brainstem encephalitis are ophthalmoplegia, dizziness, ptosis, ataxia, and limb weakness.

Seizure may be presenting complaints in about 50% of HSE patients due to involvement of the frontotemporal cortex. Seizure could usually be complex, partial, absent, or generalized [10]. Seizure in HSE can be a risk factor for postencephalitic epilepsy and a major issue for survivors [12].

Symptoms usually progress over a few days, but sometimes rapid progression in the severity of the disease occurs, and the patient may even reach the hospital in a state of loss of consciousness or comatose state. Even persistent fever may not be present and can be confused with stroke. HSE has recently been found to be associated with anti-N-methyl-D-aspartate receptor (NMDAr) autoimmune encephalitis in about 20%. So, autoimmune suspicion can be high if the patient continues worsening despite treatment or if there is a relapse in the symptoms in an improved patient [13].

2.6　Diagnosis

Lumbar puncture (LP) should be the first step to be done in suspected encephalitis after ruling out contraindication of other causes of increased intracranial pressure. Cerebrospinal fluid examination findings may include elevated protein, leukocytosis with lymphocytes predominant, and sugar usually normal or mildly reduced. Red blood cells may be seen in CSF analysis due to severe cerebral tissue necrosis. Early CSF findings with 3–5 days can be normal in HSE; repeat LP is needed in such condition.

Polymerase chain reaction (PCR) is the gold standard for the detection of herpes simplex virus DNA in CSF, which has a sensitivity of 98% and a specificity of 94–100%. This test is detectable even in the early phase, after 3 days of illness, till 2–4 weeks after the clinical onset. Even if PCR or CSF routine test is normal in early phase, acyclovir is continued if strong suspicion is present [14].

Brain computed tomography should be done to look for any signs of encephalitis and rule out other intracranial lesions. Early signs of abnormalities in brain suggest severe damage and poor prognosis. However, MRI brain with diffusion-weighted imaging (DWI) lesions in the temporal lobe is the most sensitive and specific finding for the early course [15]. Electroencephalogram (EEG) can be positive in about 80% of HSE patients, showing periodic lateralized epileptiform discharges or theta and delta waves in the temporal and frontal regions [16].

2.7　Differential Diagnosis

2.7.1　Japanese Encephalitis

Japanese encephalitis (JE) is sometimes difficult to differentiate from other encephalitis in terms of clinical manifestations. JE is a mosquito-borne transmission condition more common in endemic areas during the summer. In contrast to herpes encephalitis, routine CSF findings may not show RBC. IgM immunoassays of CSF and serum are both highly specific and sensitive tests for diagnosis of JE. Further, the MRI head shows thalamus and basal ganglia involvement, which are highly specific for JE.

2.7.2　Brain Abscess

Brain abscess can present with focal symptoms like unilateral headache or weakness, or signs like unilateral cranial nerve involvement. High-grade fever is present, but immunocompromised and elderly people may be afebrile during presentation. Papilledema is common, and lumbar puncture can be withheld till CT brain shows the size of abscess. MRI is more sensitive than CT scan, and contrast imaging is also helpful in staging the abscess [17].

2.7.3　Treatment and Prognosis

In patients with a decreased level of consciousness, management of hemodynamics and the airway should be protected. Reversible causes of encephalopathy such as hypoglycemia, hyponatremia, hypercarbia, thiamine deficiency, and alcohol withdrawal syndrome should be evaluated early for proper management. Intensive care unit monitoring may be needed for decreased sensorium, dysautonomia, and secondary infections.

Intravenous acyclovir should be started as early as possible to reduce the mortality. Doses required are 10 mg/kg every 8 h for 14–21 days. Patient should be well hydrated during acyclovir treatment to reduce the chances of nephrotoxicity. Intravenous foscarnet 90 mg/kg twice a day is used if acyclovir resistance is found. In the case of acyclovir shortage, intravenous ganciclovir 5 mg/kg twice a day is given [18].

Mortality of 20–30% has been reported in HSE, even with early treatment. Survivors may have a significant morbidity of behavioral abnormalities, cognitive impairment, epilepsy, and other residual focal neurological symptoms. HSE is also found to be associated with NMDAR autoimmune encephalitis. So, a recurrence of cognitive impairment or psychiatric behavior in recently treated HSE.

References

1. Kennedy PGE, Chaudhuri A. Herpes simplex encephalitis. J Neurol Neurosurg Psychiatry. 2002;73:237–8.
2. Hjalmarsson A, Blomqvist P, Sköldenberg B. Herpes simplex encephalitis in Sweden, 1990-2001: incidence, morbidity, and mortality. Clin Infect Dis Off Publ Infect Dis Soc Am. 2007;45(7):875–80.
3. George BP, Schneider EB, Venkatesan A. Encephalitis hospitalization rates and inpatient mortality in the United States, 2000-2010. PLoS One. 2014;9(9):e104169.
4. Berger JR, Houff S. Neurological complications of herpes simplex virus type 2 infection. Arch Neurol. 2008;65(5):596–600.
5. Dudgeon JA. Herpes encephalitis II. Pathology of herpes encephalitis. Postgrad Med J. 1969;45(524):386–91.
6. Ma Y, He B. Recognition of herpes simplex viruses: toll-like receptors and beyond. J Mol Biol. 2014;426(6):1133–47. 2013/11/19 ed.
7. Shukla ND, Tiwari V, Valyi-Nagy T. Nectin-1-specific entry of herpes simplex virus 1 is sufficient for infection of the cornea and viral spread to the trigeminal ganglia. Mol Vis. 2012;18:2711–6.
8. Mori I, Nishiyama Y, Yokochi T, Kimura Y. Olfactory transmission of neurotropic viruses. J Neurovirol. 2005;11(2):129–37.
9. Jennische E, Eriksson CE, Lange S, Trybala E, Bergström T. The anterior commissure is a pathway for contralateral spread of herpes simplex virus type 1 after olfactory tract infection. J Neurovirol. 2015;21(2):129–47.
10. Bradshaw MJ, Venkatesan A. Herpes simplex Virus-1 encephalitis in adults: pathophysiology, diagnosis, and management. Neurother J Am Soc Exp Neurother. 2016;13(3):493–508.
11. Benjamin MM, Gummelt KL, Zaki R, Afzal A, Sloan L, Shamim S. Herpes simplex virus meningitis complicated by ascending paralysis. Proc Bayl Univ Med Cent. 2013;26(3):265–7.
12. Sellner J, Trinka E. Seizures and epilepsy in herpes simplex virus encephalitis: current concepts and future directions of pathogenesis and management. J Neurol. 2012;259(10):2019–30.
13. Armangue T, Moris G, Cantarín-Extremera V, Conde CE, Rostasy K, Erro ME, et al. Autoimmune post-herpes simplex encephalitis of adults and teenagers. Neurology. 2015;85(20):1736–43. 2015/10/21 ed.
14. Steiner I, Schmutzhard E, Sellner J, Chaudhuri A, Kennedy PGE. EFNS-ENS guidelines for the use of PCR technology for the diagnosis of infections of the nervous system. Eur J Neurol. 2012;19(10):1278–91.
15. Jayaraman K, Rangasami R, Chandrasekharan A. Magnetic resonance imaging findings in viral encephalitis: a pictorial essay. J Neurosci Rural Pract. 2018;9(4):556–60.
16. Illis LS, Taylor FM. The electroencephalogram in herpes-simplex encephalitis. Lancet. 1972;1(7753):718–21.
17. Chow F. Brain and spinal epidural abscess. Contin Lifelong Learn Neurol. 2018;24(5, Neuroinfectious Disease):1327–48.
18. Tunkel AR, Glaser CA, Bloch KC, Sejvar JJ, Marra CM, Roos KL, et al. The management of encephalitis: clinical practice guidelines by the Infectious Diseases Society of America. Clin Infect Dis Off Publ Infect Dis Soc Am. 2008;47(3):303–27.

Acute Bacterial Meningitis

3

Dilli Ram Kafle and Anushka Adhikari

Case Scenario

A 37-year-old man presented to the emergency room with complaint of fever of 4 days duration. The fever was continuous, reaching a maximum of 102° Fahrenheit associated with chills but without rigor. There was nausea along with a severe headache which was sudden in onset, diffuse, constant, and exaggerated by head movement. The day before presenting to hospital, he had 5 episodes of vomiting. In the emergency room, he still had projectile vomiting. The patient was drowsy and history was taken from one of his family members. The patient was a farmer by occupation and denied any high-risk sexual behavior, blood transfusion, or intravenous blood transfusion. He also denied any past history of diabetes mellitus, tuberculosis, seizure, weakness of any parts of the body, or trauma.

On examination, the patient had a fever of 102 °F, pulse rate of 100 per minute, and respiratory rate of 20 per minute. He was drowsy and irritable. There was photophobia, neck rigidity, and positive Kernig's and Brudzinski's signs, and fundoscopic examination showed papilloedema. There was no cranial nerve involvement or focal neurological deficit. CT of the brain showed mild

cerebral edema with diffuse meningeal enhancement. On cerebral spinal fluid analysis, opening pressure was 200 mm of cerebrospinal fluid (CSF), total leukocytes count 500 (neutrophil 80% and lymphocyte 20%), protein 100 mg/dL, and glucose 30 mg/dL. His CSF gram stain and culture were negative. Blood investigation showed hemoglobin at 12 g%, a white blood cell count of 13,000/mm^3, urea 22 mg/dL, serum creatinine 1 mg/dL, and random blood glucose 90 mg/dL. The above findings were suggestive of bacterial meningitis and the patient was treated with intravenous antibiotics (ceftriaxone and vancomycin). The patient's symptoms gradually improved and he was discharged with complete recovery on the 11th day of hospital admission.

3.1 Introduction

Bacterial meningitis is a medical and neurological emergency. There is infection and inflammation of meninges along with abnormal presence of white blood cells in cerebrospinal fluid. *S. pneumoniae* and *N. Meningitidis* are the most common pathogens among the types of community acquired meningitis. Bacterial meningitis has an annual incidence of 4–6 cases per 100,000 adults [1, 2]. In developing countries, the mortality of patients with bacterial meningitis is very high with case fatality ranging from 33 to 44% [3–6].

D. R. Kafle (✉)
Department of Neurology, Nobel Medical College, Biratnagar, Nepal

A. Adhikari
Department of Medicine, District Hospital Lamjung, Lamjung, Nepal

© Springer Nature Singapore Pte Ltd. 2024
K. K. Oli et al. (eds.), *Case-based Approach to Common Neurological Disorders*,
https://doi.org/10.1007/978-981-99-8676-7_3

3.2 Epidemiology

Most cases of meningitis are caused by viruses, but are often mild and have spontaneous improvement. Viruses which commonly cause meningitis are enteroviruses, mumps, human immunodeficiency virus, Epstein–Barr virus, and herpes simplex. Common bacterial organisms associated with meningitis are *Streptococcus pneumoniae*, *Haemophilus influenza*, and *Neisseria meningitides*, which account for 75% of sporadic cases; others are *Listeria monocytogenes* and *Staphylococcus aureus*. In the neonatal group, *Escherichia coli* and Group B *streptococcus* are common organisms.

3.3 Pathogenesis

Meningitis involves inflammation of the leptomeninges, which include the arachnoid, the pia mater, and the cerebrospinal fluid. The microorganism enters the brain through the hematogenous route, with contiguous spread from otitis media, sinusitis, and congenital defects in the cranium, or is implanted directly from a penetrating injury or after a neurosurgical procedure [4]. The three most common organism for meningitis are streptococcus pneumoniae, Neisseria meningitis, Haemophilus influenzae. There is congestion of pia-arachnoid mater with polymorphs. Further, pus accumulation can promote adhesions causing complications such as cranial nerve palsies and hydrocephalus.

3.3.1 Clinical Features

Acute bacterial meningitis includes fever, headache, meningismus, and a progressive decrease in level of consciousness as classic symptoms, whereas chronic bacterial meningitis presents more subtly and symptoms last for more than 4 weeks [1, 7, 8].

1. **Neonates, infants, and children**: Lethargy, sleepiness, fussiness, jitteriness, anorexia, hypotonia, apnea, diarrhea, jaundice, and general weakness are commonly noticed by the parents of infants and neonates. Temperature instability is seen with fever or hypothermia. Children usually present with fever, severe headache, irritability, lethargy, nausea, vomiting, confusion, photophobia, stiff neck, and back pain. Some may also experience seizures.

2. **Adults**: Classic clinical features in adults include fever, headache, neck stiffness, vomiting, photophobia, and altered mental sensorium. Occasionally, they may present with focal neurological deficits and petechial rashes from either meningococcal or pneumococcal meningitis. Some patients may have cranial nerve palsies, hemiparesis, papilloedema due to raised intracranial pressure, and hydrocephalus. There may be progressive decline in consciousness with ensuing stupor and coma which may prove to be fatal due to herniation of the brain. There can be encephalitic presentation such as fever, altered sensorium, and ataxia, especially in *Listeria* infection. Partially treated bacterial meningitis can have a subacute course and is likely to be treated as tubercular meningitis. Therefore, a clear history of clinical features and treatment details is important for proper diagnosis.

3. **Patients over 65 years**: Patients over 65 years of age present with atypical symptoms. Fever, headache, and nuchal rigidity may not be present but they may present with non-specific confusion. *Streptococcus* and *Listeria* infections are common in this age group. West Nile Virus encephalitis is also prevalent in older patients and should be differentiated from bacterial meningitis.

3.4 Differential Diagnosis

Meningitis should be suspected in any patients presenting with headache, vomiting, neck stiffness, altered sensorium, and fever. However, severe headache can also be caused due to subarachnoid hemorrhage, migraine, and brain abscess. Patients with subarachnoid hemorrhage give a history of sudden onset of thunderclap headache with altered sensorium, with or without fever. CT scan of the head shows blood in the subarachnoid space. Migraine should be suspected in a young female who presents with episodic throbbing, unilateral headache associated with nausea and vomiting. Some patients may give a history of visual or sensory aura. Fever is absent in patients with migraine. When patients present with history of fever with focal neurological deficit and ring-enhancing lesion on neuroimaging, brain abscess should be suspected.

3.5   Diagnosis

On blood investigation, white blood cell counts may increase or there can even be leukopenia. Thrombocytopenia or impairment of coagulation studies can be seen in some patients. Acid fast stain, blood culture, and gram sensitivity should be sent before initiating the treatment. Lumbar puncture and CSF analysis should be done in all patients with suspected meningitis unless contraindications exist. Those contraindications where a CT scan is required before doing lumbar puncture include a history of seizure, focal neurological deficit, altered mentation, immunocompromised status, papilloedema, and a history of neurological disorder. In bacterial meningitis, the opening pressure is elevated to above 180 mm H_2O. There is pre-dominantly neutrophilic pleocytosis with cell count ranging from 250 to 10,000. The protein content is higher than 45 mg/dL in more than 90% of cases. The glucose content is diminished to concentrations below 40 mg/dL. Gram stain may show the causative organism. Culture of the CSF should also be done in all cases. Serological testing like counter-immunoelectrophoresis may be useful in cases which have received antibiotics prior to doing lumbar puncture.

The gold standard for the diagnosis of bacterial meningitis is identification of the pathogen from gram stain or culture of CSF. Culture may take about 48–72 h to be positive. Newer technology such as multiplex polymerase chain reaction helps provide a quicker and more accurate diagnosis. Laboratory facilities with various meningitis panels using PCR can identify DNA of pathogens including common bacteria such as *S. pneumonia*, *N. meningitides*, *H. influenza*, *L. monocytogens*, *E. coli*, and *S. agalactiae*. Loop-mediated isothermal amplification is a quick test which helps to amplify and detect DNA, and this method has good sensitivity for detection of *N. meningitidis*, *S. pneumoniae*, *H. influenza*, and *Mycobacterium tuberculosis* [9].

3.6   Treatment

When a patient is suspected to have bacterial meningitis, blood culture should be sent and empiric antibiotic started. The initial choice of antimicrobial therapy is dependent on the most common bacteria causing meningitis, which varies according to the patient's age and the clinical setting and also patterns of antimicrobial susceptibility. Vancomycin plus a third-generation cephalosporin is used empirically (Tables 3.1 and 3.2). Ampicillin is added to the empirical regimen in patients above the age of 50 and in those with high-risk condition like alcoholism and immunodeficiency states. After the results of culture and susceptibility testing are available, antimicrobial therapy can be modified for optimal treatment [1, 7]. Shorter courses of antibiotics have been found to be safe and effective, which could further reduce expenses and length of hospital stay, for example, 5–7 days for meningococcal infection, 10–14 for pneumococcal meningitis, and 21 days for Listeria meningitis [9].

The use of corticosteroids is associated with prevention of secondary complications including death, hearing loss, stroke, epilepsy, and learning difficulties. Dexamethasone (0.15 mg/kg every

Table 3.1 Empirical and antimicrobial therapy for bacterial meningitis

Organisms	Antibiotics
S. pneumonia, N. meningitidis, L.monocytogens	Vancomycin + ceftriaxone or cefotaxime or cefepime + ampicillin
Staphylococcus aureus, **aerobic and anaerobic streptococci**	Vancomycin + ceftriaxone or cefotaxime or cefepime + metronidazole
Staphylococcal spp., streptococcal spp., **enteric gram negative bacilli**	Vancomycin + ceftriaxone or cefotaxime or cefepime
Mycobacterium tuberculosis	Four drug therapy (isoniazid, rifampicin, ethambutol, and pyrizinamide)
Treponema pallidum	Intravenous aqueous crystalline penicillin G
Nocardia	Trimethoprim-sulfamethoxazole

Table 3.2 Commonly used drugs in bacterial meningitis and their doses in adults

Drugs	Dose (adult with normal creatinine clearance)
Vancomycin	40–60 mg/kg/day, divided into q 8–12 h dosing
Ceftriaxone	2 g, q 12 h
Cefepime	2 g, q 8 h
Cefotaxime	2 g, q 4–6 h
Ampicillin	2 g, q 4 h
Metronidazole	500 mg, q 6 h
Aqueous penicillin G	18–24 million U/day

6 h for 2–4 days) is widely used to reduce the mortality and morbidity. For maximum benefit, it is given just before or with the administration of empirical antibiotics.

3.7 Prognosis

Factors associated with poor prognosis are age, tachycardia, reduced platelet counts, drowsiness and CSF leukocyte count $<1000 \times 10^9$ cells per mL [9]. Early initiation of antibiotics and steroid are associated with good prognosis. Although there has been a declining trend in the case fatality rate following a bacterial meningitis, the occurrence of neurological sequel has remained almost the same [10] Sequel rate of 22–26% has been found including mental retardation, seizure, hydrocephalus, hemiparesis, paraparesis and headache [6, 11].

References

1. Van de Beek D, de Gans J, Spanjaard L, Weisfelt M, Reitsma JB, Vermeulen M. Clinical features and prognostic factors in adults with bacterial meningitis. N Engl J Med. 2004;351:1849–59.
2. Schuchat A, Robinson K, Wenger JD, et al. Bacterial meningitis in the United States in 1995. N Engl J Med. 1997;337:970–6.
3. Bryan JP, de Silva HR, Tavares A, Rocha H, Scheld WM. Etiology and mortality of bacterial meningitis in northeastern Brazil. Rev Inf Dis. 1990;12:128–35.
4. Hoffman O, Weber RJ. Pathophysiology and treatment of bacterial meningitis. Ther Adv Neurol Disord. 2009;2(6):1–7.
5. Guirguis N, Hafez K, Kholy MA, Robbins JB, Gotschlich EC. Bacterial meningitis in Egypt: analysis of CSF isolates from hospital patients in Cairo, 1977–78. Bull WHO. 1983;61:517–24.
6. Ford H, Wright J. The impact of bacterial meningitis in Swaziland: an 18 month prospective study. J Epidemiol Commun Hlth. 1994;48:276–80.
7. Durand ML, Calderwood SB, Weber DJ, et al. Acute bacterial meningitis in adults. A review of 493 episodes. N Engl J Med. 1993;328(1):21–8.
8. Thomas KE, Hasbun R, Jekel J, Quagliarello VJ. The diagnostic accuracy of Kernig's sign, Brudzinski's sign, and nuchal rigidity in adults with suspected meningitis. Clin Infect Dis. 2002;35(1):46–52. https://doi.org/10.1086/340979.
9. McGill F, Heyderman RS, Panagiotou S, Tunkel AR, Solomon T. Acute bacterial meningitis in adults. Lancet. 2016;388(10063):3036–47.
10. Tunkel AR, Hartman BJ, Kaplan SL, et al. Practice guidelines for the management of bacterial meningitis. Clin Infect Dis. 2004;39:1267–84.
11. Smith AL. Neurological sequelae of meningitis. N Engl J Med. 1988;319:1012–3.

Cryptococcal Meningoencephalitis

Ghanshyam Kharel

Case Scenario

A 47-year female presented with 6 months of episodic fever. She was evaluated by a paramedic in a local clinic and was treated with some antibiotics. Her symptoms improved transiently, but fever was persistent. Fever pattern was on and off type, with a maximum temperature of 102 °F, once or twice a month. She also had frequent headache, nausea, non-projectile vomiting, and pain around the nape of her neck for the last 4 months. There was no associated cough, shortness of breath, skin rashes, lumps, and nodes in axilla, neck, and groin, altered sensorium, abnormal body movements, or urinary symptoms. She had a history of hysterectomy 11 years back and was needed blood transfusion then. She consumes a mixed diet, is non-alcoholic, and neither smokes nor chews tobacco.

On examination, her blood pressure was 120/80 mmHg; pulse was 96/min (regular); respiratory rate was 20/min; temperature was 98.2 °F, and SPO_2 was 99% in room air. On general examination, she was pale, but no jaundice, clubbing, dehydration, lymphadenopathy, cyanosis, or edema was present. On systemic examination, she had basal crepitation on bilateral lungs. Her cardiovascular system and gastrointestinal system examinations were normal. On neurological

examination, there was no altered sensorium or meningeal signs. Bilateral features of disk edema were noted, and the rest of the other neurological examinations were normal.

During evaluation, patient was found to have anemia (hemoglobulin: 8.1 g/dL), stool occult blood was positive, and upper gastrointestinal endoscopy revealed antral gastritis. Her blood investigations such as renal function test, liver function test, and random sugar were in normal range. The serology of leptospirosis, scrub typhus, dengue, malaria, hepatitis, and kala-azar was negative. Human acquired immunodeficiency virus (HIV) serology was found to be positive and was again confirmed with ELISA test. CD-4 count was 10 cells/μL. Her chest X-ray and CT head were normal. Echocardiography revealed global hypokinesia of left ventricle with moderate mitral regurgitations, dilated left atrium, and moderate left ventricular systolic dysfunction with ejection fraction of 30–35%. Ultrasonography chest and abdomen revealed bilateral mild pleural effusion. The cerebrospinal fluid (CSF) analysis was done, which revealed 20 cells/cmm³ with all lymphocytes, sugar 2.5 mmol/L, and protein 13.8 mg/dL. India ink examination in cerebrospinal fluid (CSF) showed *Cryptococcus neoformans*, and CSF cryptococcal antigen was also positive. She was given amphotericin deoxycholate (0.7 mg/kg daily) and fluconazole (400 mg twice daily). During hospital stay, she received multiple blood transfusion.

G. Kharel (✉)
Department of Neurology, National Institute of Neurological and Allied Sciences, Kathmandu, Nepal

© Springer Nature Singapore Pte Ltd. 2024
K. K. Oli et al. (eds.), *Case-based Approach to Common Neurological Disorders*,
https://doi.org/10.1007/978-981-99-8676-7_4

After 2 weeks, amphotericin was stopped, and fluconazole was continued (200 mg twice daily) along with antiretroviral therapy. She was discharged in improved condition and was advised to review in a regular outpatient clinic.

4.1 Introduction

Cryptococcosis is a fungal infection due to *Cryptococcus gattii or Cryptococcus neoformans. Cryptococcus neoformans* meningoencephalitis is the most frequently encountered central nervous system manifestation of cryptococcosis [1]. Pigeon excreta is the main source of this organism, and other avian species excreta are also implicated. This infection has become increasingly prevalent in immunocompromised patients and belongs to basidiomycetous, encapsulated yeasts.

4.2 Epidemiology

Incidence of cryptococcal meningoencephalitis does not much differ in relation to age, occupation, or ethnicity. The majority of patient suffering from cryptococcal infection is immunocompromised, and AIDS accounts for most of them and is prevalent worldwide. Malignancy, sarcoidosis, prolonged steroid therapy, liver disease, and the use of immunosuppressive drugs are the other conditions that are associated with this infection [1–3]. Cryptococcosis is a common AIDS-presenting illness and is the fourth most common opportunistic infection in people living with HIV AIDS. It has been estimated that there are approximately 1 million new cases of cryptococcal CNS infection worldwide each year, with over 600,000 deaths; however, with the availability of highly effective antiretroviral drugs, the incidence has dropped [4, 5]. In low-income countries, there are relatively few studies about cryptococcal meningoencephalitis as opportunistic infection in patients living with HIV AIDS and very rare studies done in patient without HIV infection [6–9].

4.3 Pathophysiology

Cryptococcosis can develop in any animal including human being. The organism is generally transmitted via the respiratory route by inhalation of airborne fungi or via hematogenous dissemination. It also has a tendency to localize to the central nervous system of the patient. Patients usually present symptoms of chronic meningitis as the inflammatory response in the brain is generally milder. CSF shows the infiltrated inflammatory cells which predominantly comprise mononuclear cells with occasional polymorphonuclear leukocytes. Diffuse involvement of the brain is frequently encountered. Some case may present as localized cryptococcoma infection.

4.4 Clinical Manifestations

The central nervous system is the common site of cryptococcosis in both immunocompromised and immunocompetent patients. The infection generally involves both the brain parenchyma and meninges, causing cryptococcal meningoencephalitis of subacute to chronic duration. The most common symptoms of cryptococcal meningoencephalitis include malaise, headache, fever, visual disturbances, personality change, and impaired sensorium. Fever may be observed in less than half of the cases often delaying the presentation to healthcare [9, 10]. Patients may have stiff neck, photophobia, and vomiting in 25–33% [10]. Disk edema and visual involvement occur in 40% of the patients [11]. Coma is a rare presenting symptom. Patients with cryptococcoma may present with weakness, sensory loss, aphasia, or ataxia, and symptoms depend upon the cerebral location of the cryptococcoma [9]. Patients may also present with features of disseminated disease, including cough, dyspnea, and skin rash. Patients with HIV infection or any other condition with reduced immune status, high index of suspicion of cryptococcal central nervous system (CNS) infection should be sought. Patients are frequently misdiagnosed with tubercular meningitis as the cerebrospinal fluid (CSF) picture and symptoms closely mimic each other.

4.5 Diagnosis

cryptococcal meningoencephalitis usually has subacute onset of symptoms, and presentations can be nonspecific, making the diagnosis often challenging. It should be suspected in any immunocompromised patient with headache, fever, or any signs or symptoms referable to the central nervous system. As the delayed treatment consequence is grave, cryptococcal meningitis should also be considered in immunocompetent patients presenting with symptoms and signs of subacute to chronic meningitis.

CSF analysis with a measurement of opening pressure is helpful in the diagnosis of cryptococcal meningoencephalitis. Opening pressure is markedly elevated in patients with cryptococcal meningoencephalitis with HIV infection than without HIV infection. Removal of CSF may be beneficial for both diagnostic and therapeutic purposes. The CSF examination with India ink shows encapsulated organism in approximately 50% of non-HIV infected patients and 75% in HIV-infected patients. Cell counts of the CSF usually show less than 200 cells/mm^3 with lymphocytic predominance [12]. CSF sugar and protein are usually elevated but may be normal in some cases. The diagnosis of cryptococcal meningoencephalitis can be confirmed by detecting the organism in CSF culture. CSF for cryptococcal antigen is an alternative test and is highly sensitive and specific for the diagnosis of cryptococcal meningoencephalitis. This test can be obtained in serum or even immediately after the lumbar puncture.

Neuroimaging of the brain with a CT scan or MRI scan prior to lumbar puncture is required in the presence of papilledema, impaired sensorium, or any focal neurologic signs. MRI of the brain is preferred as it is more sensitive than CT for identifying CNS cryptococcal lesions. There may be a bilateral T2 punctate hyperintense lesion in Virchow-Robin spaces in MRI, also termed a pseudocyst, suggesting the space is filled with cryptococci and their mucoid exudates [7]. These pseudocysts don't enhance on contrast MRI imaging. However, neuroimaging frequently shows no abnormality, nonspecific changes, or mild cerebral atrophy without obstruction. In some patients, hydrocephalus may be seen, and a few patients may demonstrate mass lesions.

4.6 Differential Diagnosis

The differential diagnosis of cryptococcal meningoencephalitis includes all conditions with fever and headache of subacute to chronic duration. This includes tuberculosis meningitis, toxoplasmosis, lymphoma, and syphilis. Patients with tuberculosis meningitis may have lesions in the lung with related finding and lesions in the chest X-ray.

Patients with toxoplasmosis may have a focal neurological deficit with abnormal neuroimaging. An MRI of the brain frequently shows ring-enhancing lesions around the basal ganglia. Toxoplasmosis is also associated with constitutional symptoms, such as fever, chills, and sweats, bilateral, symmetrical, non-tender adenopathy, and chorioretinitis.

An MRI of CNS lymphoma also had a single, ring-enhancing lesion with a focal deficit clinically. It may be associated generalized lymphadenopathy. Patients with syphilitic meningitis usually have normal mental status and maculopapular rashes. There is a history of sexual exposure with an infected partner, which can occur with HIV-associated cryptococcal meningoencephalitis too.

4.7 Treatment

Amphotericin B, fluconazole, and flucytosine are the major drugs in combination for the treatment of cryptococcal meningoencephalitis, which requires three phases of treatment: induction, consolidation, and maintenance. Induction phase includes parental liposomal amphotericin at a dose of 3–4 mg/kg once daily and flucytosine at a dose of 100 mg/kg/day in four divided doses. In resource-limited settings, amphotericin B deoxycholate at a dose of 0.7 mg/kg once daily and fluconazole 400 mg twice can be given [13, 14].

However, due to the higher side effect profile and slightly lower efficacy with the second regime, the first regime is preferred. The induction phase is given a minimum of 2 weeks. After 2 weeks of induction, a CSF culture is required to check the sterilization of the CSF. Patients may require longer induction period if CSF sterilization is not achieved. Patients whose CSF cultures remain positive should continue the induction regimen with serial lumbar punctures every 2 weeks until the CSF becomes sterile [15].

In the consolidation phase, fluconazole at a dose of 800 mg daily is given for the next 8 weeks. The maintenance phase includes therapy with fluconazole (200–400 mg orally daily) for 1 year after diagnosis. Long-duration therapy may be warranted for those receiving very high doses of immunosuppressive agents. Maintenance therapy can be discontinued in patients with HIV infection on antiretroviral therapy (ART) who have a CD4 cell count more than 100 cells/microL and have an undetectable viral load on ART for more than 3 months [15].

Patients receiving antifungals for cryptococcal meningoencephalitis should be monitored for drug-related adverse effects. Amphotericin B deoxycholate is more nephrotoxic and can cause disturbance of electrolytes and blood counts than liposomal formulation. Serial monitoring of renal function, electrolytes, and blood counts is routinely required. Pre- and post-hydration of the patient is required for reducing the risk of nephrotoxicity. Flucytosine has been usually associated with gastrointestinal problems, increased liver enzymes, and anemia. Fluconazole can cause an increase in liver enzymes and should be regularly monitored.

The intracranial pressure is usually high in cryptococcal meningoencephalitis and should be measured at the time of the initial lumbar puncture. If the CSF opening pressure is ≥25 cm of CSF or there are symptoms or signs of raised intracranial pressure during induction therapy, CSF drainage should be done to decrease the pressure to a normal pressure of ≤20 cm. Therapeutic lumbar drainage should be repeated daily in the setting of clinical symptoms or signs and persistent pressure elevations of ≥25 cm of CSF. Mannitol, acetazolamide, and steroids are not useful for the control of elevated intracranial pressure [16].

4.8　Prognosis

The prognosis of patients with cryptococcal meningoencephalitis depends on the nature of the underlying immunosuppression. Mortality is higher in patients with malignancy, and relapse is higher in patients with cirrhosis [17, 18]. Patients with a positive India ink examination of the CSF, a CSF white blood cell count <20/microL, an initial CSF or serum cryptococcal antigen titer >1:32, and/or a high opening pressure on lumbar puncture also have a poorer prognosis.

References

1. Vilchez RA, Fung J, Kusne S. Cryptococcosis in organ transplant recipients: an overview. Am J Transplant. 2002;2:575.
2. Spec A, Raval K, Powderly WG. End-stage liver disease is a strong predictor of early mortality in Cryptococcosis. Open Forum Infect Dis. 2016;3:ofv197.
3. Bernard C, Maucort-Boulch D, Varron L, et al. Cryptococcosis in sarcoidosis: cryptOsarc, a comparative study of 18 cases. QJM. 2013;106:523.
4. Desalermos A, Kourkoumpetis TK, Mylonakis E. Update 4. On the epidemiology and management of cryptococcal meningitis. Expert Opin Pharmacother. 2012;13:783.
5. Rajasingham R, et al. Global burden of disease of HIV-associated cryptococcal meningitis: an updated analysis. Lancet Infect Dis. 2017;17(8):873–81. https://doi.org/10.1016/S1473-3099(17)30243-8. Epub 2017 May 5.
6. Dhungel BA, Dhungel KU, Easow JM, Singh YI. Opportunistic infection among HIV seropositive cases in Manipal Teaching Hospital, Pokhara, Nepal. Kathmandu Univ Med J. 2008;6(23):335–9.
7. Satishchandra P, Mathew T, Gadre G, Nagarathna S, Chandramukhi A, Mahadevan A, Shankar SK. Cryptococcal meningitis: clinical, diagnostic and therapeutic overviews. Neurol India. 2007;55(3):226.
8. Rodriguez-Tudela JL, Alastruey-Izquierdo A, Gago S, Cuenca-Estrella M, León C, Miro JM, et al. Burden of serious fungal infections in Spain. Clin Microbiol Infect. 2015;21(2):183–9. [Internet]. Elsevier BV.
9. Kharel G, Karn R, Rajbhandari R, Ojha R, Agrawal JP. Spectrum of cryptococcal meningoencephalitis in Tertiary Hospital in Nepal. J Inst Med. 2018;40:2.

10. Cox GM, Perfect JR. Cryptococcus 10. neoformans and gattii and Trichosporon species. In: Edward LA, editor. Topley and Wilson's microbiology and microbial infections. 9th ed. London: Arnold Press; 1997.

11. Kestelyn P, Taelman H, Bogaerts J, Kagame A, Abdel Aziz M, Batungwanayo J, Stevens AM, Van de Perre P. Ophthalmic manifestations of infections with Cryptococcus neoformans in patients with the acquired immunodeficiency syndrome. Am J Ophthalmol. 1993;116:721–7.

12. Brouwer AE, Rajanuwong A, Chierakul W, et al. 13. Combination antifungal therapies for HIV-associated cryptococcal meningitis: a randomized trial. Lancet. 2004;363:1764.

13. Loyse A, Wilson D, Meintjes G, et al. Comparison of 22. The early fungicidal activity of high-dose fluconazole, voriconazole, and flucytosine as second-line drugs given in combination with amphotericin B for the treatment of HIV-associated cryptococcal meningitis. Clin Infect Dis. 2012;54:121.

14. Pappas PG, Chetchotisakd P, Larsen RA, et al. A phase 23. II randomized trial of amphotericin B alone or combined with fluconazole in the treatment of HIV-associated cryptococcal meningitis. Clin Infect Dis. 2009;48:1775.

15. Perfect JR, et al. Clinical practice guidelines for the management of cryptococcal disease: 2010 update by the infectious diseases society of America. Clin Infect Dis. 2010;50(3):291–322. https://doi.org/10.1086/649858.

16. Newton PN, et al. A randomized, double-blind, placebo-controlled trial of acetazolamide for the treatment of elevated intracranial pressure in cryptococcal meningitis. Clin Infect Dis. 2002;35(6):769–72. https://doi.org/10.1086/342299. Epub 2002 Aug 26.

17. Jarvis JN, Bicanic T, Loyse A, et al. Determinants of 24. Mortality in a combined cohort of 501 patients with HIV-associated Cryptococcal meningitis: implications for improving outcomes. Clin Infect Dis. 2014;58(5):736–45.

18. Chau TT, Mai NH, Phu NH, et al. A prospective 25. Descriptive study of cryptococcal meningitis in HIV uninfected patients in Vietnam - high prevalence of *Cryptococcus neoformans vargrubii* in the absence of underlying disease. BMC Infect Dis. 2010;10:199.

Neurocysticercosis

5

Anushka Adhikari and Rajeev Ojha

Case Scenario

A 55-year-old woman presented with multiple episodes of tingling sensation in the right leg and right hand for 3 days. Such episodes lasted for about 1 min, and recurred 5–6 times per day. There was one episode of burning pain around the neck followed by sudden fainting 1 day before. Her husband noticed that there was tightening of her limbs, her head was deviated to the right side, and there was uprolling of the eyes and frothing from the mouth. This episode lasted for about 1–2 min and the patient was then sleepy and only responsive to loud noise for 10–15 min before she was fully aroused. There was no incontinence, postictal headache, or trauma during the episode. On examination, her general condition was fair and vitals were stable: blood pressure was 130/80 mmHg, pulse 68/min, temperature 98 °F, and respiratory rate 15/min. On general examination, she was alert and oriented to time, place, and person. There were no signs of pallor, jaundice, clubbing, cyanosis, lymphadenopathy, dehydration, or edema. Bilateral chests were clear, heart sounds were normal without murmur, and abdomen was non-tender with no organomegaly palpation. On neurological exami-nation, higher mental functions were intact with normal cranial nerves, coordination, and gait examination. Her limb power was normal without any sensory involvement. Deep tendon reflexes were normal without any pyramidal signs.

On routine investigation, complete blood count, renal function test, calcium, random blood sugar, urine routine, and ECG were normal. Her CT scan of the head showed a single calcification in the right occipital region (Fig. 5.1). MRI of the brain showed a hyperintense lesion in the bilateral frontal lobe with multiple cysts with and without dot-like structure in the middle, and contrast T1 image showed multiple ring-like structures with and without dot-like structure suggestive of NCC in multiple stages (Figs. 5.2 and 5.3). Ocular NCC was ruled out and the patient was then treated with oral prednisolone with levetiracetam. Twenty-four hours after initiation of prednisolone, albendazole was started and given for 10 days. Prednisolone was tapered and stopped after 10 days whereas levetiracetam was continued. On 3-month follow-up, the patient had no repeated seizure episodes.

A. Adhikari
Department of Medicine, District Hospital Lamjung, Lamjung, Nepal

R. Ojha (✉)
Department of Neurology, Tribhuvan University Teaching Hospital, Kathmandu, Nepal

© Springer Nature Singapore Pte Ltd. 2024
K. K. Oli et al. (eds.), *Case-based Approach to Common Neurological Disorders*,
https://doi.org/10.1007/978-981-99-8676-7_5

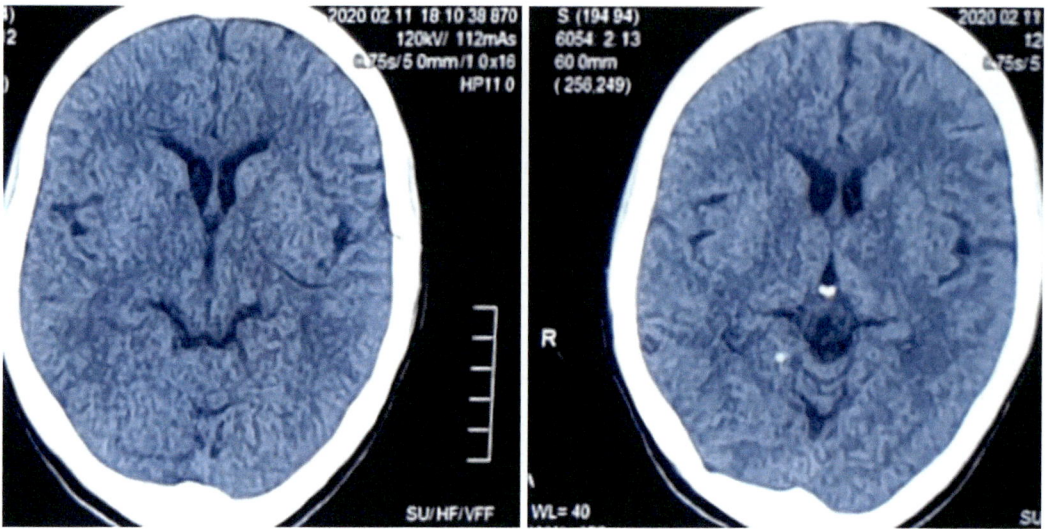

Fig. 5.1 Plain CT scan of head showed a calcification in right occipital region (Figs. 5.2 and 5.3)

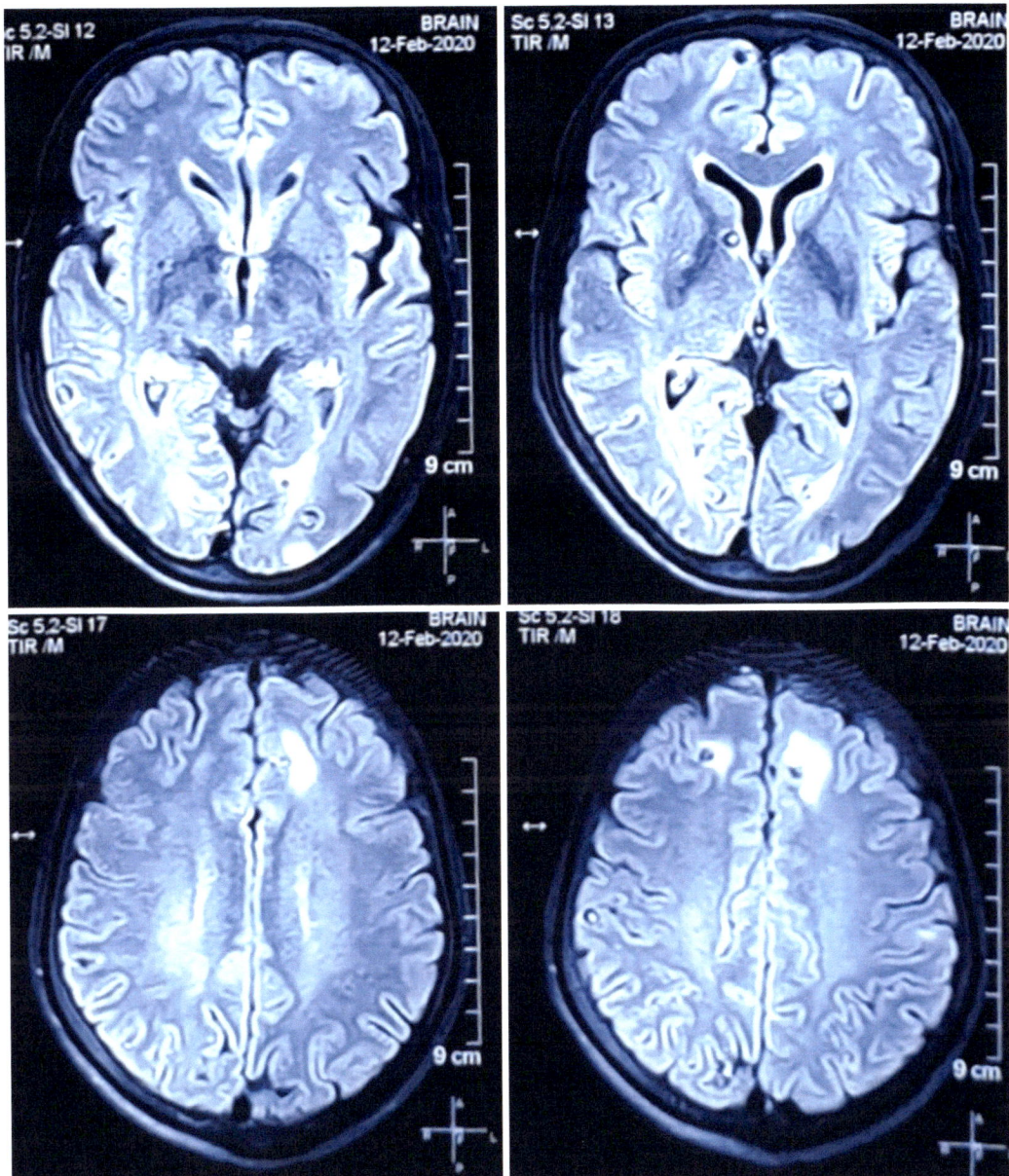

Fig. 5.2 FLAIR MRI of brain showed multiple cysts with central scolex in bilateral frontal, parietal, and basal ganglia region

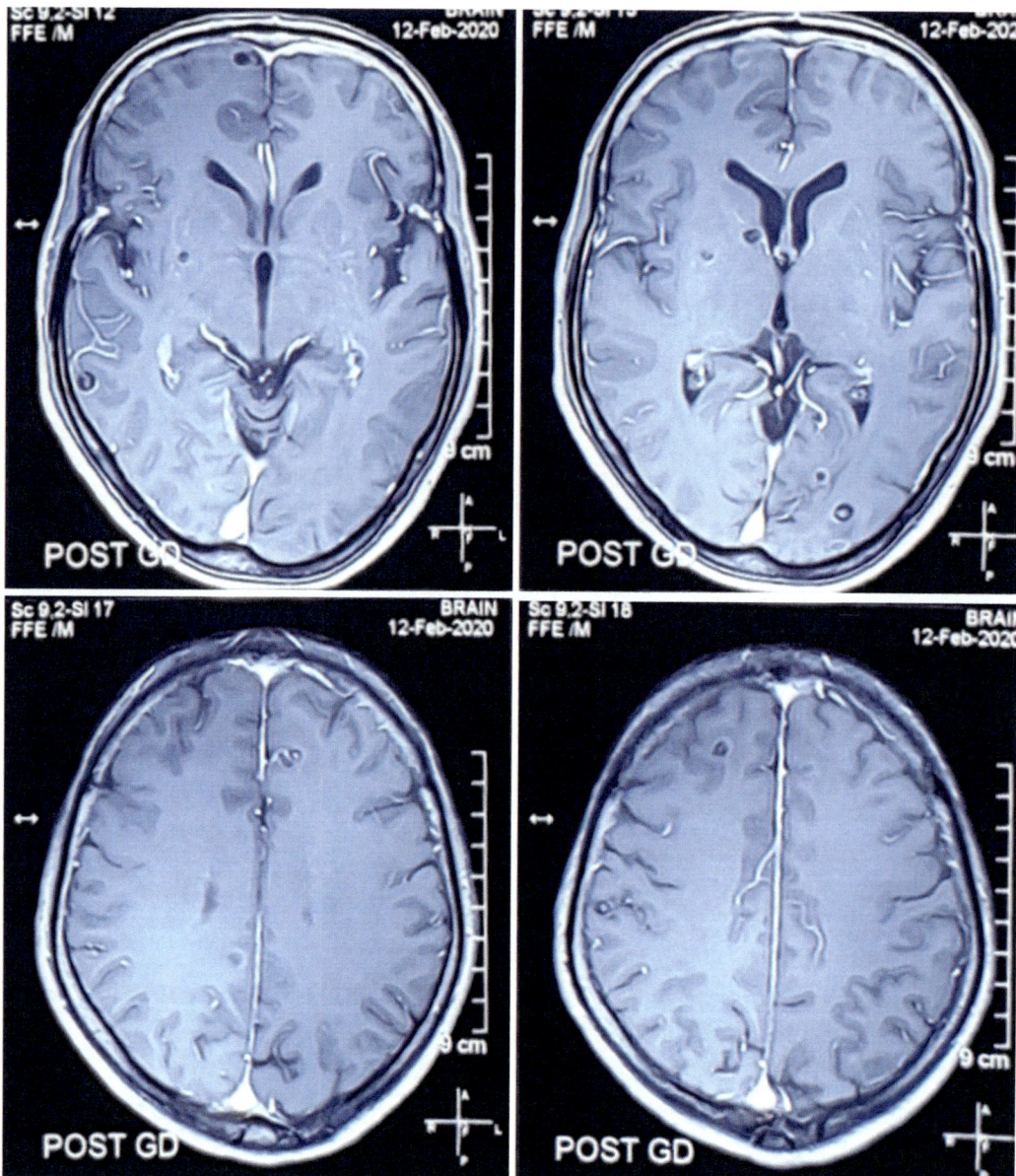

Fig. 5.3 T1 contrast MRI showed multiple cysts with and without central scolex in bilateral frontal, parietal, and basal ganglia region suggestive of NCC in multiple stages

5.1 Introduction

Neurocysticercosis (NCC) is a parasitic infection of the nervous system and is caused by the ingestion of eggs of pork tapeworm (*Taenia solium*) by contaminated hands, food, and water. In most low-income nations with subpar sanitation where pigs are reared, this tapeworm is endemic [1].

Rather than local transmission, instances of NCC in industrialized countries are primarily attributable to immigration from endemic areas. The numbers of patients with NCC are increasing with increase in immigration from endemic regions. It is one of the most significant causes of seizures in such endemic regions. Due to lower incomes,, the majority of people being illiterate, practice of open defecation, and improper sanitation and poor management of meat and meat products, the prevalence of NCC is higher in South Asian countries [2].

The combination of sophisticated diagnostic testing, anthelminthic and corticosteroid therapy, and minimally invasive neurosurgery has improved the prognosis of this disease over the last decade. Despite this advancement, however, it is one of the major public health problems in the developing world. However, the numbers of NCC-producing causes are decreasing in some endemic areas where improvements in sanitation, planned urbanization and widespread use of antiparasitic therapy have played a major role.

5.2 Epidemiology

Due to migration from rural areas, NCC has been increasing recently in its prevalence in urban areas as well. There are about 2.5 million people carrying the adult tapeworm worldwide and most of them are infected with cysticerci. *T. solium* is endemic in Latin America, India, China, Nepal and sub-Saharan Africa. It is widely prevalent in urban middle-class areas in countries where it is endemic. Most *T. solium* cases have been reported among Hispanic populations. It is rare in Eastern and Central Europe, Australia, Japan, New Zealand, Israel, and Muslim countries of Asia and Africa [3].

Usually both sexes are affected by NCC. One of the more severe forms of NCC, cysticercal encephalitis, is more commonly seen in women than in men. This disease has been reported in all age groups. However, it is most commonly seen in the third and fourth decades of life. Cysticercosis is uncommon in children younger than 2 years because of the long incubation period of *T. solium*.

5.3 Lifecycle of the Parasite

The definitive host of *T. Solium* is the human being, and the intermediate host is the pig. Sometimes both pigs and humans can be the intermediate hosts. The larval form of *T. Solium* (cysticercus) is the infective form. These tapeworms are 2–3 m long, segmented, tape-like, and belong to the class Cestoda. The head end known as scolex contains suckers with hooks and rostellum. The rostellum resembles a sun, and is hence called "solium." The body of the tapeworm is called the strobili and is divided into segments called proglottids (800–900 in number). The proglottid contains both male and female reproductive organs, and is devoid of an alimentary system.

Normally, the larvae are cystic. When a human host swallows infected pork, the larvae stick to the gut wall via suckers and hooks, and mature into adult tape worms. Gravid proglottids and fertile eggs containing an oncosphere (embryo) are discharged into the environment. Pigs and other free-roaming animals have access to human feces. Pigs unintentionally consume human feces. Following ingestion, embryos are liberated from the eggs in the intestine and enter the bloodstream, where they travel to the peripheral tissues, including the CNS, and develop as cysticerci. Pigs thus serve as intermediate hosts. When humans consume undercooked pork meat laced with cysts, the lifecycle of *T. solium* is completed. Similarly, after consuming T. solium eggs, humans can acquire cysticercosis, which usually develops via the faeco-oral route from close contact with the carriers (Fig. 5.4) [4].

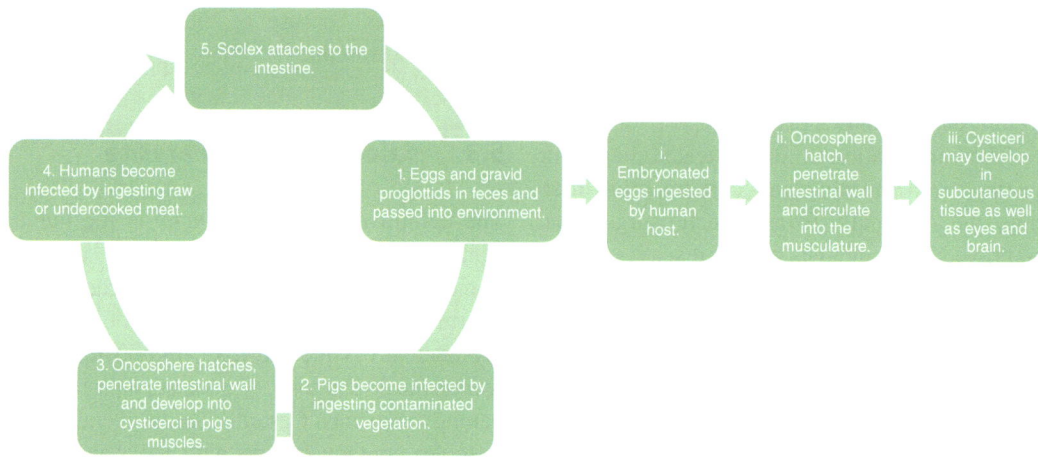

Fig. 5.4 Life Cycle of *Taenia solium*

5.4 Clinical Manifestations

According to the location of cysts, neurocysticercosis can be: (a) parenchymal: occurring in the brain predominantly at the grey–white junction and (b) extraparenchymal: occurring in meninges, ventricles, basilar cisterns, subarachnoid space, and spinal cord. Clinical manifestation of NCC depends on various factors: number, location, size, stages of the cysticercosis, and the intensity of the immune response to degenerating cysts. Carriers may be completely asymptomatic or the disease can lead to severe morbidity and death.

1. Epilepsy
2. Focal neurological deficit
3. Raised intracranial pressure
4. Cognitive decline
5. Other manifestations: any neurological symptoms, headache, stroke, involuntary movements, hydrocephalus, chronic meningitis, and cranial nerve abnormalities

5.4.1 Epilepsy/Seizures

In most endemic countries, about 30% of patients reported with epilepsy are diagnosed with NCC. According to research findings, patients with NCC-related epilepsy typically suffer generalized seizures. When the cysts disintegrate, there is an immediate inflammatory reaction that leads to the release of parasitic antigens. Degenerating cysts elicit a strong host reaction and are a common cause of seizures. However, seizures have been seen in patients with only vesicular cysts and no contrast enhancement or edema [5].

5.4.2 Focal Neurological Deficits

The of parenchymal brain cysts or edema around the cyst might cause focal deficits in NCC patients. Symptoms like limb weakness, sensory loss, ataxia, aphasia, and altered sensorium are common [4]. Ischemic stroke has also been associated with NCC due to occlusion of intracranial arteries, mainly medium and small arteries [6, 7]. If cranial nerves are entrapped patients might present with extraocular muscle paralysis, facial nerve palsy, hearing loss, or trigeminal neuralgia.

5.4.3 Raised Intracranial Pressure

This could be due to a variety of pathologic processes in NCC patients. Hydrocephalus can be caused by cysts or inflammation causing mechanical restriction to CSF drainage from any ventricle, Sylvius aqueduct, Luschka's foramina, Magendie's foramina, or Monroe's foramina [8]. Hydrocephalus and increased intracranial pressure can have a subacute or chronic clinical history. However, hydrocephalus caused by a fourth ventricle cyst can cause Burns' syndrome, which can be described by a sudden loss of consciousness caused by head movements. If neurosurgical care is not accessible, hydrocephalus with neurocysticercosis has a high mortality rate [9, 10]. Cysticercotic encephalitis is a serious form of parenchymal neurocysticercosis usually reported in young women which manifests with features of raised intracranial pressure, altered sensorium and seizure [11].

5.4.4 Cognitive Decline

Subclinical deficits to dementia might occur in a patient with neurocysticercosis [12, 13]. Before the development of neuroimaging technologies, patients with neurocysticercosis were treated in psychiatric hospitals. Psychomotor epilepsy or post-ictal psychoses were represented by psychotic episodes in parenchymal neurocysticercosis.

5.5 Diagnosis

Diagnosis typically requires neuroimaging and serological testing as histological confirmation of the parasite is not possible. However, diagnosing neurocysticercosis remains difficult. A careful history-taking including questions regarding residence, whether living in high-risk area or not, and extended travel in developing countries is useful.

5.6 Neuroimaging

The morphology and localization of the cysts, burden of infection, and presence of surrounding inflammation are commonly evaluated by CT scan and MRI. How the parenchymal lesion looks on neuroimaging signifies the stage of involution [14]. Live vesicular cysts are small and spherical, and imaging often shows the scolex, which is a cystic structure with a dot. Scolexes on single or numerous cysts confirm

the diagnosis. After the degenerative process, the cysts have poorly defined edges with edema and a prominent ring or nodular contrast enhancement. Nodular lesions correlate to the granular stage and are surrounded by hyperintense rims which are characteristic of gliosis. On a CT scan, calcified cysticerci appear as non-enhancing hyperdense nodules with no peripheral edema. Cysticerci within cortical sulci remain cystic, do not develop, and eventually deteriorate, vanish, or turn into residual calcified scars. On the other hand, cystic lesions on the basal CSF cisterns and Sylvian fissures displace the neighboring structures. Basal subarachnoid cysticercosis affects the spinal cord in around 60% of cases, and cysts without a recognizable scolex can be mistaken for spinal tumors [6].

MRI shows intraventricular and cisternal cysts more clearly when FLAIR (Fluid Attenuated Inversion Recovery), FIESTA (Fast Imaging Employing Steady State Acquisition Sequence), CISS (Constructive Interference in Steady State), and BFFE (Balanced Fast Field Echo) are used [14–16]. As MRI provides better clarity of NCC lesions, it is the ideal technology for imaging cysticercosis of the spinal cord and spinal subarachnoid space.

5.7 Laboratory and Immunological Diagnosis

Enzyme-linked immunoelectrotransfer blot (EITB) is the best serological test that uses lentil lectin purified glycoprotein antigens which detect antibodies to *T. solium* in serum. In patients with two or more live cysts in the nervous system, EITB is 98% sensitive. CSF antibody detection is slightly lower than serum [17]. The sensitivity is even poorer in patients with calcified cysticerci [18]. Enzyme-linked immunosorbent assay (ELISA) has 89% sensitivity in detection of antibodies to *T. solium* in CSF. It is still used when EITB is not available [19]. Sometimes ELISA is useful in determining the response to treatment in subarachnoid neurocysticercosis.

CSF examination is usually not necessary for the diagnosis of NCC, but it might be useful sometimes to rule out other cerebral infections. Stool examination can confirm taeniasis in about 10–15% of NCC patients. Brain biopsy with histopathological evaluation may be necessary in rare cases.

5.8 Diagnostic Criteria

Diagnostic criteria for neurocysticercosis were published in 2001, and include absolute, major, minor, and epidemiological criteria which were last revised in 2017 [20]. The interpretation of these categories allows for a diagnosis of either definitive or probable neurocysticercosis.

Absolute Criteria
  (a) Histological demonstration of the parasite from biopsy of a brain or spinal cord lesion
  (b) Visualization of subretinal cysticercus
  (b) Neuroradiologic demonstration of cystic lesions containing a scolex
Neuroimaging Criteria
  Major Neuroimaging Criteria
    (a) Cystic lesions without a discernible scolex
    (b) Enhancing lesions
    (c) Multilobulated cystic lesions in the subarachnoid space
    (d) Typical parenchymal brain calcifications
  Confirmative Neuroimaging Criteria
    (a) Resolution of cystic lesions after cysticidal drug therapy
    (b) Spontaneous resolution of single small enhancing lesions
    (c) Migration of ventricular cysts documented on sequential neuroimaging studies
  Minor Neuroimaging Criteria
    Obstructive hydrocephalus (symmetric or asymmetric) or abnormal enhancement of basal leptomeninges
Clinical/Exposure Criteria
  Major Clinical/Exposure
    (a) Detection of specific anticysticercal antibodies or cysticercal antigens by well-standardized immunodiagnostic tests
    (b) Cysticercosis outside the central nervous system
    (c) Evidence of a household contact with *T. Solium* infection
  Minor Clinical/Exposure
    (a) Clinical manifestations suggestive of neurocysticercosis
    (b) Individuals coming from or living in an area where cysticercosis is endemic

5.9 Degrees of Diagnostic Certainty

Definitive
– One absolute criterion
– Two major neuroimaging criteria plus any clinical/exposure criteria
– One major criterion and one confirmative neuroimaging criterion plus any clinical/exposure criteria
– One major neuroimaging criterion plus two clinical/exposure criteria (including at least one major clinical/exposure criterion), together with the exclusion of other pathologies producing similar neuroimaging findings

Probable
– One major neuroimaging criterion plus two clinical/exposure criteria
– One minor neuroimaging criterion plus at least one major clinical/exposure criterion

5.10 Treatment

Treatment of parenchymal neurocysticercosis includes symptomatic therapy, anti-parasitic treatment, and surgery. Patients with NCC and epilepsy respond better to anti-parasitic and anti-epileptic drugs. Anti-epileptic drugs should be continued for at least 2 years after the last seizure. However, once the granuloma resolves on imaging, antiepileptic drugs can be safely titrated and stopped in more than 85% of cases [21]. Dexamethasone (0.1 mg/kg/day) is given 1 day before anti-parasitic therapy and maintained for 1–2 weeks and can be slowly tapered [22]. Anti-parasitic drugs can usually destroy about 60–80% of cysts. Albendazole (15 mg/kg/day for 2 weeks) and praziquantel (50 mg/kg/day for 2 weeks) are frequently used anti-parasitic drugs [23]. Combinations of two anti-parasitic drugs increase the cysticidal efficacy and damage the parasite by different mechanisms [24]. A combination of albendazole and praziquantel is relatively safe and helps resolve the cysts in a patient with three or more cysts. Patients with seizures and calcified inactive lesions on CT do not require specific therapy other than anti-convulsant medications.

5.11 Treatment of Extraparenchymal Neurocysticercosis

Small subarachnoid cysts are treated in the same manner as parenchymal brain cysts. Routine corticosteroid administration is required in patients with subarachnoid cysts to avoid the risk of stroke [25]. Methotrexate has also been demonstrated in some tests to be effective as a substitute for steroids. In cases of massive cysts in the Sylvian fissure, medical therapy with albendazole and corticosteroids is similarly effective [26]. Most cases of hydrocephalus require immediate CSF draining or shunt implantation. However, a large dose of dexamethasone (16 mg/kg/day or more) may provide temporary relief from hydrocephalus. Ventricular cysts are surgically treated with excision or with anti-parasitic medication. A ventriculoscope is used for endoscopic cyst removal in the third and lateral ventricles. Cysts in the fourth ventricle are removed using neuroendoscopy through the aqueduct via the suboccipital route, or with open microsurgical dissection.

5.12 Prevention and Control of Parasites

Neurocysticercosis is a global public health problem. Certain measures should be made in practice to prevent and control this disease. There is a need for improvement in sanitation and access to clean drinking water. Every country should step forward to achieve Universal Health Coverage, and investments in quality health care should be increased for infrastructure. Awareness programs in all schools and deprived communities should also be conducted properly. The drug of choice cysticercosis must be available at health outlets at all levels with periodic review and assessments.

References

1. Ojha R, Shah D, Shrestha A, Koirala S, Dahal A, Adhikari K, et al. Neurocysticercosis in Nepal: a retrospective clinical analysis. Neuroimmunol Neuroinflam. 2015;2(3)
2. Nash TE, Garcia HH. Diagnosis and treatment of neurocysticercosis. Nat Rev Neurol. 2011;7(10):584–94.
3. Ndimubanzi PC, Carabin H, Budke CM, Nguyen H, Qian YJ, Rainwater E, et al. A systematic review of the frequency of neurocyticercosis with a focus on people with epilepsy. PLoS Negl Trop Dis. 2010;4(11):e870.
4. Del Brutto OH. Neurocysticercosis. Semin Neurol. 2005;25(3):243–51.
5. Garcia HH, Pretell EJ, Gilman RH, Martinez SM, Moulton LH, Del Brutto OH, et al. A trial of antiparasitic treatment to reduce the rate of seizures due to cerebral cysticercosis. N Engl J Med. 2004;350(3):249–58.
6. Callacondo D, Garcia HH, Gonzales I, Escalante D, Nash TE. Cysticercosis Working Group in P. High frequency of spinal involvement in patients with basal subarachnoid neurocysticercosis. Neurology. 2012;78(18):1394–400.
7. Cantu C, Barinagarrementeria F. Cerebrovascular complications of neurocysticercosis. Clinical and neuroimaging spectrum. Arch Neurol. 1996;53(3):233–9.
8. Lobato RD, Lamas E, Portillo JM, Roger R, Esparza J, Rivas JJ, et al. Hydrocephalus in cerebral cysticercosis. Pathogenic and therapeutic considerations. J Neurosurg. 1981;55(5):786–93.
9. Santo AH. Cysticercosis-related mortality in the state of Sao Paulo, Brazil, 1985-2004: a study using multiple causes of death. Cad Saude Publica. 2007;23(12):2917–27.
10. Torres-Corzo JG, Tapia-Perez JH, Vecchia RR, Chalita-Williams JC, Sanchez-Aguilar M, Sanchez-Rodriguez JJ. Endoscopic management of hydrocephalus due to neurocysticercosis. Clin Neurol Neurosurg. 2010;112(1):11–6.
11. Rangel R, Torres B, Del Bruto O, Sotelo J. Cysticercotic encephalitis: a severe form in young females. Am J Trop Med Hyg. 1987;36(2):387–92.
12. Bianchin MM, Dal Pizzol A, Scotta Cabral L, Martin KC, de Mello Rieder CR, de Andrade DC, et al. Cognitive impairment and dementia in neurocysticercosis: a cross-sectional controlled study. Neurology. 2010;75(11):1028; author reply -9.
13. Rodrigues CL, de Andrade DC, Livramento JA, Machado LR, Abraham R, Massaroppe L, et al. Spectrum of cognitive impairment in neurocysticercosis: differences according to disease phase. Neurology. 2012;78(12):861–6.
14. Lerner A, Shiroishi MS, Zee CS, Law M, Go JL. Imaging of neurocysticercosis. Neuroimaging Clin N Am. 2012;22(4):659–76.
15. Govindappa SS, Narayanan JP, Krishnamoorthy VM, Shastry CH, Balasubramaniam A, Krishna

SS. Improved detection of intraventricular cysticercal cysts with the use of three-dimensional constructive interference in steady state MR sequences. AJNR Am J Neuroradiol. 2000;21(4):679–84.

16. Mont'Alverne Filho FE, Machado Ldos R, Lucato LT, Leite CC. The role of 3D volumetric MR sequences in diagnosing intraventricular neurocysticercosis: preliminar results. Arq Neuropsiquiatr. 2011;69(1):74–8.

17. Rodriguez S, Dorny P, Tsang VC, Pretell EJ, Brandt J, Lescano AG, et al. Detection of Taenia solium antigens and anti-T. Solium antibodies in paired serum and cerebrospinal fluid samples from patients with intraparenchymal or extraparenchymal neurocysticercosis. J Infect Dis. 2009;199(9):1345–52.

18. Rodriguez S, Wilkins P, Dorny P. Immunological and molecular diagnosis of cysticercosis. Pathog Glob Health. 2012;106(5):286–98.

19. Odashima NS, Takayanagui OM, Figueiredo JF. Enzyme linked immunosorbent assay (ELISA) for the detection of IgG, IgM, IgE and IgA against Cysticercus cellulosae in cerebrospinal fluid of patients with neurocysticercosis. Arq Neuropsiquiatr. 2002;60(2-B):400–5.

20. Del Brutto OH, Nash TE, White AC Jr, Rajshekhar V, Wilkins PP, Singh G, et al. Revised diagnostic criteria for neurocysticercosis. J Neurol Sci. 2017;372:202–10.

21. Rajshekhar V, Jeyaseelan L. Seizure outcome in patients with a solitary cerebral cysticercus granuloma. Neurology. 2004;62(12):2236–40.

22. Nash TE, Mahanty S, Garcia HH, Cysticercosis Group in P. Corticosteroid use in neurocysticercosis. Expert Rev Neurother. 2011;11(8):1175–83.

23. Sotelo J, del Brutto OH, Penagos P, Escobedo F, Torres B, Rodriguez-Carbajal J, et al. Comparison of therapeutic regimen of anticysticercal drugs for parenchymal brain cysticercosis. J Neurol. 1990;237(2):69–72.

24. Garcia HH, Gonzales I, Lescano AG, Bustos JA, Zimic M, Escalante D, et al. Efficacy of combined antiparasitic therapy with praziquantel and albendazole for neurocysticercosis: a double-blind, randomised controlled trial. Lancet Infect Dis. 2014;14(8):687–95.

25. Bang OY, Heo JH, Choi SA, Kim DI. Large cerebral infarction during praziquantel therapy in neurocysticercosis. Stroke. 1997;28(1):211–3.

26. Proano JV, Madrazo I, Avelar F, Lopez-Felix B, Diaz G, Grijalva I. Medical treatment for neurocysticercosis characterized by giant subarachnoid cysts. N Engl J Med. 2001;345(12):879–85.

Tetanus

Aamir Siddiqui

Case Scenario

A 37-year old male farmer was referred with clinical suspicion of meningitis. He was brought to the emergency department with history of fever, jaw and neck pain, and generalized body stiffness. Escorting relatives reported that the symptoms had started approximately 5 days earlier, when he started to develop "low-grade fever." Fever was associated with progressively worsening body aches, difficulty in opening his mouth, and difficulty in moving his neck. They denied any history of sore throat or toothache or any known preexisting medical conditions. They also reported an alteration in conscious level that had gradually worsened over the last 24 h that alarmed them enough to seek urgent medical assistance. During initial evaluation, the patient was found to be dehydrated and febrile with a temperature of 99 °F, while other vital signs were normal. Physical examination showed restricted movements at the temporomandibular joint and neck, and no enlarged lymph nodes were evident. A 3–4 cm in diameter wound was seen in the right foot, and on inquiry, his relatives reported that he had hurt himself during farming and the wound had been there for the last 10 days. The wound was clean, without any redness (erythema), discharge, or necrosis. In lab data, WBC (white blood count) was 12,000/μL; otherwise all other basic hematological and biochemical results were within normal range. A brain and maxillofacial CT scan was performed which yielded insignificant findings. On grounds of clinical history and available test results, the patient was admitted with a provisional diagnosis of meningitis.

On the medical ward, a feeding nasogastric tube was placed by the attending physician, on grounds of jaw restrictions and altered conscious level. During close observation during hospital stay, it was noticed that the alleged seizures were severe spasms of neck and back muscles, accompanied by clenching of the jaw. Diazepam, followed by midazolam, was used to control muscle spasms, and it was repeated when required. With the current clinical findings and considering the history of recent injury to the foot and unreliable vaccination history, provisional diagnosis was reviewed and a differential diagnosis of tetanus was included.

While standard antimicrobial therapy was continued, therapeutic trials with tetanus immunoglobulin 500 IU were given intramuscularly, followed by tetanus toxoid. Meningitis was ruled out through lumbar puncture and microbiologist analysis of cerebrospinal fluid. By the fourth day of admission, the spasms had fully ceased, and the patient was able to slightly open his mouth when compared to previous days, and his neck was also found to be suppler. An oral liquid diet

A. Siddiqui (✉)
Pacific International Hospital,
Port Moresby, Papua New Guinea
e-mail: draamir@pihpng.com

© Springer Nature Singapore Pte Ltd. 2024
K. K. Oli et al. (eds.), *Case-based Approach to Common Neurological Disorders*,
https://doi.org/10.1007/978-981-99-8676-7_6

was then started, followed by a soft semi-solid diet over later days. On the sixth day, the patient was commenced on oral medications. With successful recovery, and absence of any further trismus or drooling, he was discharged on day 11.

6.1 Introduction

Tetanus is a non-communicable disease caused by bacteria called *Clostridium tetani*, which are obligate anaerobic gram-positive organisms. While the incidence of tetanus is low in developed countries, it still remains one of the most common causes of death worldwide. In the developing world, it has been reported to be associated with high mortality rates, especially involving neonates (nearly 50%). Acute respiratory failure and cardiovascular complications due to autonomic instability have frequently been found to be associated with tetanus deaths. Currently, with effective immunization programs and increasing coverage of medical services including acute and intensive care, tetanus-associated deaths have been significantly reduced [1].

6.2 Epidemiology

Despite the efforts of the World Health Organization to eradicate tetanus, it remains endemic in developing countries. A 2016 WHO report estimated approximately 13,502 reported cases and 72,600 deaths in <5 years [2]. The majority of reported tetanus cases have been found to be birth associated and occurring in low-income countries. The majority of cases were found among unvaccinated mothers and their newborns, and especially where proper hygiene couldn't be ascertained during the peripartum period, including unsterile deliveries and poor cord care [3, 4]. This has been depicted in the World Health Organization's Global Burden of Disease study of 2015, where a higher rate of neonatal mortality was observed to be related to tetanus [5].

Mostly due to good health coverage and efficient immunization programs, tetanus is rela-tively uncommon in developed countries [6]. In such countries, the disease has been found to be prevalent in the elderly population, mostly due to inefficient vaccination [7, 8]. Similarly, reports of neonatal tetanus are rare, and cases mostly occur among children of unimmunized mothers following poor hygiene and cord care [9, 10].

6.3 Microbiology

Tetanus is caused by *Clostridium tetani*, a gram-positive bacillus, commonly found in soil. However, it has also been isolated from feces of humans and domesticated animals [11]. It is a mobile, spore-forming obligate anaerobe, which is not destroyed simply by boiling. It can be eliminated through autoclaving at 120 °C for 15 min under atmospheric pressure. In-vitro growth is rare; hence culture is rarely successful in growing the bacteria, and very few details are available on its antimicrobial sensitivity. Tetanus diagnosis generally revolves around clinical assessment. Most of the symptoms and signs related to tetanus are secondary to the effects of its potent exotoxin. The coding DNA to this exotoxin is embedded in a plasmid, and not all the strains possess the plasmid. Hence mere detection of bacteria is not diagnostic of infection. The role of the toxin as such within the organism is yet unknown [12].

6.4 Natural History of Disease

The incubation period of tetatus is about 7–10 days, but can range between 1 and60 days. The time from onset of the first symptom to development of spasm can vary between one day and one week. These periods have been found to be associated with the severity of disease: the shorter the period the more severe the disease. Muscle rigidity and spasms are early signs, which gradually become severe. Autonomic instability has been found to follow spasms and persist over weeks. Spasms usually last for the first 2–3 weeks and gradually reduce, whereas stiffness may persist for a considerably longer period. Recovery is expected with destruction of the exotoxins and regeneration of axon terminals [13].

6.5 Pathophysiology

The tetanus bacillus secretes toxins, namely tetanospasmin and tetanolysin. Tetanolysin destroys the healthy tissues surrounding infected or necrotic tissues, and provides optimal anaerobic conditions for bacterial growth [14], whereas tetanospasmin is responsible for most of the clinical syndrome. Once internalization of toxin starts, it is transported within the axon to its cell body [15]. This initially involves motor nerve fibers, followed by sensory and autonomic nerves. Once the toxins have reached the cell body, they easily diffuse out, affecting nearby neurons. Tetanus symptoms start to appear once these toxins involve spinal inhibitory interneurons. This occasionally involves medullary and hypothalamic centers.

The effects of the tetanospasmin result from preventing release of neurotransmitters [16]. Tetanospasmin has been associated with cortical convulsion in animal studies [17]. However, whether this mechanism is involved in developing periodic spasm and autonomic instability in humans remains unclear. Its pre-junctional effect at the neuromuscular junction has been associated with weakness between spasms. This could be associated with cranial nerve paralysis, which is evident in cephalic tetanus and the myopathies observed following recovery [18].

Disinhibited autonomic discharges can lead to dysregulated autonomic nervous system, resulting in sympathetic overactivity and excessive discharge of catecholamine in plasma. Similarly, uncontrolled discharge from efferent motor neurons, situated in the spinal cord and brainstem, leads to spasms and muscular rigidity. Muscle spasms can be intense and painful, and sometimes powerful enough to lead to tendon rupture and fractures. Due to the short axonal pathway, muscles of the jaw, face, and head and neck are often the first to be involved, followed by the trunk and limbs. Other axial muscles such as the hands and feet are often spared. With loss of reflex inhibition of antagonist muscle groups, and simultaneous agonist and antagonist muscle contraction, tetany sometimes may be mistaken for convulsions.

The toxins irreversibly bind to surrounding tissues, and once bound cannot be neutralized by tetanus immunoglobulin (TIG). In such scenarios, administration of TIG may be beneficial in preventing axonal binding in the central nervous system (CNS), or when toxin binding is still limited to peripheries and has not yet progressed to the CNS [18].

6.6 Clinical Manifestation

Tetanus is usually associated with an injury that is often contaminated with soil, manure, or a piece of rusted metal. Wounds from burns, ulcers, gangrene, septic abortions, child-birth, or surgery can be complicated by tetanus.

C. tetani infection is usually associated with three clinical syndromes, (1) localized, (2) generalized, and (3) cephalic. Localized tetanus is relatively uncommon, and as the name suggests the sustained muscle contractions are localized at the injury site. It is seen in peripheral injuries or when toxin load is low, and has low mortality rates [19]. Cephalic tetanus where localized tetanus from an infected head wound or ear infections leads to paralysis of cranial nerves, followed by generalized tetanus, has exceptionally high mortality rates [20]. During initial presentation, cephalic tetanus can often be mistaken for Bell's palsy or trigeminal neuritis.

On the other hand, generalized tetanus is more frequently seen in clinical setups, and is associated with more generalized spasms. It first involves the head and neck, followed by rigidity and spasms spread over the whole body. Symptoms of generalized tetanus may be confused with those of strychnine poisoning, hypocalcemia, dystonic drug reactions, and hysteria.

Neck stiffness, throat pain, and inability to open the mouth are early symptoms of generalized tetanus [21], followed by masseter spasms leading to more classical **trismus** or **lockjaw**. Progressive extension and involvement of other facial muscles can cause the typical tetanus facial expression, called *risus sardonicus*, and dysphagia, once the pharyngeal muscles are affected. Laryngeal spasms soon follow the pharyngeal muscle spasms, and have been associated with episodes of aspiration and other life-threatening airway obstructions. The rigidity of the neck muscles can contribute to head retraction, and truncal rigidity may lead to **opisthotonos**. It may also be associated with reduced chest wall compliance leading to difficulty breathing, and if they continue, such spasms can lead to respiratory failure [22]. Rigidity, muscle spasms, and autonomic dysfunction make up the tetanus triad that is often witnessed in such critically ill patients. Besides tetanus-related spasticity, episodic agonist and antagonist muscle group spasm can give a convulsion-like appearance, adding confusion for young clinicians. Tetanus spasms are both spontaneous and can be triggered by emotional, physical, or visual and auditory stimuli.

6.6.1 Severity Grading

Various severity grading systems have been proposed, among which Ablett classification (Table 6.1) is most commonly used [23].

Table 6.1 Ablett classification of severity

Grade	Clinical features
I (mild)	Mild trismus, general spasticity, no respiratory embarrassment, no spasms, no dysphagia
II (moderate)	Moderate trismus, rigidity, short spasms, mild dysphagia, moderate respiratory involvement, respiratory rate >30, mild dysphagia
III (severe)	Severe trismus, generalized spasticity, prolonged spasms, respiratory rate >40, severe dysphagia, apnoeic spells, pulse >120
IV (very severe)	Grade 3 plus severe autonomic disturbances involving the cardiovascular system

6.7 Diagnosis

Tetanus is primarily diagnosed on clinical grounds, supported by history of contaminated wound infection and epidemiological details [7]. Blood counts are often normal, but sometimes moderate leucocytosis may be present. Though laboratory studies have limited value in diagnosing tetanus, it may be helpful to exclude other differential diagnoses. Similarly, lumbar puncture is often not necessary in diagnosing tetanus but may help to rule out meningitis.

Wound swab could be cultured in suspected cases of tetanus; however, it cannot be ruled out in absence of growth of *C. tetani* species. This is secondary to the observations that this organism is often non-recoverable from tetanus-infected people, and in some cases may be isolated in otherwise healthy people.

6.8 Differential Diagnosis

Strychnine poisoning closely mimics tetanus. However, a number of conditions like dental or other local infections, encephalitis, seizure disorders, mandible dislocation, hysteria, and neoplasm may also cause trismus, and need to be differentiated from tetanus.

6.9 Treatment

Tetanus is a medical emergency that requires management at an intensive care unit. Its management is targeted toward three major goals:

1. Neutralize unbound toxin (i.e., outside the CNS)
   (a) Human tetanus immunoglobulin (TIG) has been associated with improved survival and considered the standard of care. Once administered intramuscularly it helps in neutralizing the unbound toxins but has limited to no effect on toxins

which have already bound to nerves [6]. The optimal dose regimen of immunoglobulin has yet to be established, but a single intramuscular dose of 500 units has recently been recommended both for children and adults [6, 7, 24]. The previous recommendation of 3000–6000 units is still practiced by some clinicians, part of which was used to infiltrate around the wound [7]. Perilesional and intrathecal immunoglobulin use remains controversial and is often not recommended [25]. TIG and tetanus toxoid are recommended to be administered at different sites.

2. Prevent further release of toxins
   (a) Early wound debridement helps in eradicating spores and removing necrotic tissues that might harbor toxins. Appropriate timing for debridement is not established, but it is suggested to be performed 1–6 h after immunoglobulin therapy [25].
   (b) Antimicrobial therapy may not be sufficient or may have a limited role in treatment of tetanus, yet it is universally recommended. Intravenous metronidazole at doses of 30 mg/kg per day (max 4gm/day) given at 6–8-h intervals is the preferred antimicrobial of choice [24]. Alternatively, penicillin G at doses of 100,000 U/kg per day (maximum 12 million units per day) can be administered at an interval of 4–6 h. Antimicrobial therapy is recommended for 10–14 days [24]. In suspected mixed infections, ceftriaxone, erythromycin, clindamycin, tetracycline, and chloramphenicol are acceptable antimicrobial choices.

3. Minimize the effects of the CNS-bound toxin
   (a) This mostly includes use of sedation/muscle relaxants to control rigidity and spasms, provide respiratory/ventilatory support (where required) and manage autonomic dysfunction.

6.9.1 Intensive Care

Intensive care is required in management of patients with respiratory and/or autonomic dysfunctions.

1. Sedation and avoidance of stimulants like light and sound is the primary line of treatment to manage muscle spasms and autonomic dysfunction. Preferable agents include benzodiazepines like diazepam or midazolam given intravenously or intramuscularly at doses of 0.1 mg/kg that can be repeated every 1–4 h. Midazolam can be given as a continuous infusion at rates of 2 to 10 mg/h.

   Parenteral opioids like morphine (at doses of 0.1 mg/kg given every 2–6 h) or pethidine (1 mg/kg as frequently as 2–6 hourly) can help maintain adequate sedation in combination with benzodiazepines. Morphine can also be used in continuous infusion at rates of 1–10 mg/h. Alternatively, propofol can also be used, and is currently popular due to its early reversibility [25].

2. Addition of muscle relaxants like vecuronium or atracurium is often indicated when the above sedatives alone or in combination are inadequate. In contrast, pancuronium, a long-acting agent, should be avoided as it has been found to worsen autonomic instability through inhibiting catecholamine reuptake [25].

   Other drugs like dantrolene and intrathecal baclofen have been used in some studies [26], but their role is unproven.

3. **Treatment of autonomic dysfunction.** Fluid resuscitations have been useful to minimize the effects of autonomic instability. Some researchers have also used opioid infusion of morphine and fentanyl, as the first-line treatment for dysautonomia [25]. Magnesium sulfate use has also been advocated in randomized clinical trials both for control of autonomic dysfunction [27] and as an adjunct treatment to control spasms.

6.9.2 Other Adjunct Therapies

- Magnesium sulfate through its action as a pre-synaptic neuromuscular blocker can be used as an effective adjunct to improve relaxation and sedation and in controlling the autonomic disturbance in tetanus. It reduces catecholamine release from both the nerves and adrenal glands, as well as having been associated with reduction of catecholamines receptor responsiveness. A loading dose of 40 mg/kg body weight administered over 30 min, followed by a continuous infusion of 2gm/h, has been observed to reduce the requirements of muscle relaxants or other medications used to reduce spasms [27].
- Alpha-2 agonists, such as clonidine, may have a role by inhibiting the norepinephrine release from pre-junctional nerve endings.
- Tetanus toxoid should be administered in all patients with tetanus, commencing immediately upon diagnosis. This is important as acute illness doesn't confer immunity [28].

6.9.3 Other Supportive Care

Enteral feeding should be started during the early phase of in-hospital treatment in order to prevent malnutrition associated with dysphagia, autonomic dysfunction involving the gastrointestinal tract, etc.

Endotracheal intubation should not be delayed, and early tracheostomy should be facilitated in patients requiring artificial ventilation. Respiratory complications can be prevented by appropriate chest physiotherapy and oral and respiratory tract care due to increased secretions. Severely ill patients remain immobile for a significantly longer period; hence, measures to minimize the risks of decubitus ulcers, venous thromboembolism, and gastrointestinal hemorrhage should be considered earliest [25].

6.10 Vaccination

Prophylactic vaccination against tetanus has been available since 1923. Three injections each at one-month intervals are recommended and can be started as early as at 2 months of age [28]. The second dose provides immunity whereas the third injection prolongs the duration of immunity [29]. A booster dose is often advised before the fifth birthday [28, 30]. Though neonates receive immunity through transplacental transfer of immunoglobulin following maternal vaccination, this may be impaired in the immunocompromised states and in the presence of maternal HIV infection. Immunity conferred by vaccines is not life-long, and hence revaccination is recommended at 10-year intervals.

Post-exposure prophylaxis, i.e., in management of wounds that have the potential for tetanus contamination, is depicted in Table 6.2 [31].

Table 6.2 Guide to tetanus prophylaxis in wound management

History of tetanus immunization	Clean, minor wounds		All other wounds	
	Tetanus toxoid-containing vaccine	TIG (tetanus immuno-globulin)	Tetanus toxoid-containing vaccine	TIG (tetanus immuno-globulin)
Unknown or fewer than 3 doses in a vaccine series	Yes	No	Yes	Yes
3 or more doses in a vaccine series and less than 5 years since the last booster dose	No	No	No	No
3 or more doses in a vaccine series and more than 5 years but less than 10 years since the last booster dose	No	No	Yes	No
3 or more doses in a vaccine series and more than 10 years since the last booster dose	Yes	No	Yes	No

6.11 Complications

Complications are listed in Table 6.3 [30]. These may occur as a result of the disease, for example laryngospasm; as a consequence of simple treatment, for example sedation leading to coma, aspiration, or apnea; or as a result of intensive treatment, for example ventilator-associated pneumonia.

Table 6.3 Complications from tetanus

Body system	Complications
Airway	Aspiration Laryngospasm/obstruction Sedative-associated obstruction
Respiratory	Apnea Hypoxia Type I (atelectasis, aspiration, pneumonia) and type II respiratory failure (laryngeal spasm, prolonged truncal spasm, excessive sedation) acute respiratory distress syndrome Complications of prolonged assisted ventilation (e.g., pneumonia) Tracheostomy complications (e.g., tracheal stenosis)
Cardiovascular	Tachycardia, hypertension, ischemia Hypotension, bradycardia Tachyarrhythmias, bradyarrhythmia Asystole Cardiac failure
Renal	High-output renal failure Oliguric renal failure Urinary stasis and infection
Gastrointestinal	Gastric stasis Ileus Diarrhea Hemorrhage
Miscellaneous	Weight loss Thromboembolism Sepsis with multiple organ failure Fracture of vertebrae during spasms Tendon avulsions during spasms

6.11.1 Prognosis

Case fatality rate and causes of death vary from country to country based on availability of resources and healthcare facilities. Availability and introduction of intensive care support has been associated with a reduction in case mortality from 44 to 15% [1]. In resource-limited developing countries which lack facilities to support prolonged ventilation and intensive care, deaths from severe tetanus have been higher and often above 50%. These deaths are primarily secondary to airway obstruction and organ failure (respiratory, renal, etc.). In contrast, in developed countries, a mortality rate of below 10% is often taken as an acceptable goal [29].

Neonatal tetanus carries poorer prognosis and higher fatality when compared to adult tetanus. Patients with severe tetanus generally require intensive care treatment over 3–5 weeks. Among survivors, recovery is often complete and they are expected to return to normal functions. However, in several studies some persisting physical and psychological problems secondary to neurological and electroencephalographic sequel of tetanus have been evident including irritability, insomnia, seizures, decreased libido, postural hypotension, and electroencephalogram changes [32].

References

1. Trujilo MH. Impact of intensive care management on the prognosis of tetanus. Chest. 1987;92:63–5.
2. World Health Organization. WHO Tetanus Global Report. https://www.who.int/immunization/monitoring_surveillance/burden/vpd/surveillance_type/passive/tetanus/en/
3. World Health Organization. Tetanus vaccines: WHO position paper—February 2017. Wkly Epidemiol Rec. 2017;6(92):53–76.
4. Hodowanec A, Bleck TP. Tetanus (*Clostridium tetani*). In: Mandell, Douglas, Bennett, editors. Principles and practice of infectious diseases. 8th ed. Philadelphia: Elsevier; 2015.

5. Kyu HH, Mumford JE, Stanaway JD, et al. Mortality from tetanus between 1990 and 2015: findings from the global burden of disease study 2015. BMC Public Health. 2017;17:179.
6. Government of Canada. Tetanus toxoid. In: Canadian immunization guide 2016. https://www.canada.ca/en/publichealth/services/publications/healthy-living/canadianimmunization-guide-part-4-active-vaccines/page-22-tetanus-toxoid.html.
7. Roper MH, Wassilak SGF, Tiwari TSP, Orenstein WA. Tetanus toxoid. In: Plotkin SA, Orenstein WA, Offit PA, editors. Vaccines. 6th ed. China: Elsevier Saunders Inc.; 2013. p. 746–72.
8. Tosun S, Batirel A, Oluk AI, et al. Tetanus in adults: results of the multicenter ID-IRI study. Eur J Clin Microbiol Infect Dis. 2017;36:1455.
9. Centers for Disease Control and Prevention. Neonatal tetanus—Montana, 1998. Morb Mortal Wkly Rep (MMWR). 1998;47(43):928–30.
10. Yaffee AQ, Day DL, Bastin G, et al. Notes from the field: obstetric tetanus in an unvaccinated woman after a home birth delivery—Kentucky, 2016. Morb Mortal Wkly Rep (MMWR). 2017;66(11):307–8.
11. Wilkins CA, Richter MB, Hobbs WB. Occurrence of clostridium tetani in soil and horses. S Afr Med J. 1988;73:718–20.
12. Mellanby J, Green J. How does tetanus toxin work? Neuroscience. 1981;6:281–300.
13. Mellanby J.Green J. How does tetanus toxin work? Neuroscience. 1981;6:281–300
14. Dance M, Lipman J. Tetanus: an intesivist's view. Int J Intensive Care. 1994;1:56–60.
15. Pinder M. Controversies in the management of severe tetanus. Intensive Care Med. 1997;14:129–43.
16. Kerr J. Current topics in tetanus. Intensive Care Med. 1979;5:105–10.
17. Curtis DR, De Groat WC. Tetanus toxin and spinal inhibition. Brain Res. 1968;10:208–12.
18. Carresa R, Lanari A. Chronic effects of tetanus toxin applied locally to the cerebral cortex of the dog. Science. 1962;137:342–3.
19. Brook I. Current concepts in the management of clostridium tetani infection. Expert Rev Anti Infec Ther. 2008;6:327–36.
20. Dutta TK. Localised tetanus mimicking incomplete transverse myelitis. Lancet. 1994;343:983–4.
21. Jagoda A, Riggio. Cephalic tetanus: a case report and review of the literature. Am J Emerg Med. 1988;6:6; 128-30.
22. Edmondson RS, Flowers MW. Intensive care in tetanus: management, complications and mortality in 100 cases. BMJ. 1979;1:1401–4.
23. Kokal KC. Disordered pulmonary function in tetanus. J Assoc Physicians India. 1984;32:691–5.
24. Ablett JJL. Analysis and main experiences in 82 patients treated in the Leeds Tetanus unit. In: Ellis M, editor. Symposium on tetanus in Great Britain. Boston Spa: National Lending Library; 1967. p. 1–10American Academy of Pediatrics. Tetanus (Lockjaw). In: Pickering LK ed. Redbook 2012 *Report of the Committee on Infectious Diseases 29th ed.* Elk Grove Village, IL: American Academy of Pediatrics, 2012; 707–712.
25. Centers for Disease Control and Prevention. Chapter 21—Tetanus. Epidemiology and prevention of vaccine-preventable diseases, The pink book: updated 13th edition 2015:341–352.
26. Engrand N, Guerot E, Rouamba A, Vilain G. The efficacy of intrathecal baclofen in severe tetanus. Anesthesiology. 1999;90:1773.
27. Thwaites CL, Yen LM, Loan HT, et al. Magnesium sulphate for treatment of severe tetanus: a randomised controlled trial. Lancet. 2006;368:1436.
28. Immunization against infectious disease. The stationery Office, London; 1998.
29. Simonsen O. Vaccination against tetanus and diphtheria: evaluations of immunity in the Danish population, guidelines for vaccination and methods for control of vaccination programmes. Dan Med J. 1989;36:24–47.
30. Liang JL, Tiwari T, Moro P, et al. Prevention of pertussis, tetanus, and diphtheria with vaccines in the United States: recommendations of the Advisory Committee on Immunization Practices (ACIP). MMWR Recomm Rep. 2018;67:1.
31. Cook TM, Protheroe RT, Handel JM, et al. Tetanus: a review of the literature. Br J Anaesthesia. 2001;87(3):477–87.
32. Sanford JP. Tetanus – forgotten but not gone. N Engl J Med. 1995;332:812–3.
33. Lisboa T. Guidelines for the management of accidental tetanus in adult patients. Rev Bras Ter Intensiva. 2011;23(4):394–409.

Tubercular Meningitis

7

M. Netravathi

Case Scenario

A 24-year-old woman presented with a 2-week history of ill health, decreased appetite and weight loss. There was a history of mild fever especially during the evenings for 10 days followed by diplopia and gait disturbances in the last 1 week. She had a significant history of contact with tuberculosis; her father had pulmonary Koch's 10 years previously for which he had taken treatment for 6 months. The rest of the past and family history was unremarkable. Her menstrual history was normal. On examination, she had tachypnoea (respiratory rate of 30/min) with occasional crepitations in the left infraclavicular region. No lymphadenopathy or hepatosplenomegaly was noted. Neurological examination revealed she was conscious and alert. She had bilateral abduction restriction (left side more than right side) of the eyes and mild papilledema bilaterally with normal visual acuity. Meningeal signs were present in the form of neck stiffness and Kernig's sign. The rest of the motor and sensory examinations were within normal limits.

Her investigations revealed the following: (i) normal hematological and biochemical parameters, (ii) CT brain plain and contrast revealed diffuse cerebral oedema with mild hydrocephalus, (iii) chest X-ray revealed infiltrates in the left axillary region with cavitatory changes, and (iv) CSF (cerebrospinal fluid) examination revealed xanthochromic fluid with pleocytosis, 126 cells (95% lymphocytes and the rest were neutrophils). Protein was 234 mg/dL and sugar 15 mg/dL. She was started on anti-oedema measures, four drug antitubercular agents and corticosteroids. Injectable steroids were given for 2 days followed by oral medications. She gradually showed improvement.

7.1 Introduction

Tubercular meningitis (TBM) is caused by Mycobacterium tuberculosis and is the most common form of central nervous system (CNS) tuberculosis (TB). TBM should be treated in the early stage, so as to avoid a high frequency of neurological sequelae and mortality. It is more common and has less favourable outcomes in vulnerable populations such as children below 4 years of age and HIV-infected individuals. TBM occurs due to dislodged and ruptured subependymal or subpial tubercles (Rich foci) from the bacillemia during primary infection (hematogenous spread) into the subarachnoid space. The various complications occur when the tubercle is released into the subarachnoid space causing impairment in the CSF flow to form hydrocephalus or tuberculomas or abscesses, or obliterative vasculitis causing infarction and

M. Netravathi (✉)
Department of Neurology, National Institute of Mental Health and Neurosciences (NIMHANS), Bangalore, India

© Springer Nature Singapore Pte Ltd. 2024
K. K. Oli et al. (eds.), *Case-based Approach to Common Neurological Disorders*,
https://doi.org/10.1007/978-981-99-8676-7_7

Table 7.1 Grades of tubercular meningitis (TBM)

Grade 1	GCS of 15 without any focal neurological deficits
Grade 2	GCS of 11–14 with focal neurological deficits
Grade 3	GCS of <10 with or without focal neurological deficits

Abbreviation: *GCS* Glasgow Coma Scale

stroke syndromes [1]. Risk factors for CNS TB include: age (children <4 years), malnutrition, recent measles in children, co-infection with HIV, alcoholism, malignancy and use of immunosuppressants [2].

TBM is classified into three grades of severity according to the British Medical Research Council TBM grade, which helps in stratification of patients and prediction of the patient's prognosis [3] (Table 7.1).

7.2 Epidemiology

TBM is rare in Western countries with only 100–150 cases occurring annually in the US. According to the estimation of the World Health Organization (WHO), one third of the world's population is infected with TB, among which Asia has the highest prevalence and India ranks the first among them [4]. The global prevalence of TB has been gradually declining with the advent of the Bacillus Calmette-Guerin (BCG) vaccination and the DOTS program for the treatment of TB. In India, the mortality rate is about 1.5 per 100,000 population with 20–50% mortality reported in various studies [4, 5].

7.3 Pathophysiology

Tubercular meningitis was first identified in 1832 with initial description of the disease in six children. It was first discovered by Robert Koch in 1882, who stained and cultured the bacterium, subsequently known as *Mycobacterium tuberculosis* [5]. It is an aerobic gram-positive rod with a thick cell wall that contains lipids, peptidogly-

cans and arabinomannans. The bacilli enter the host by droplet inhalation and later are engulfed by alveolar macrophages. Localized infection results with enlargement of the lymph nodes forming primary complex of Ghon's. Eventually mild bacteraemia develops during which it can be seeded on the CNS. The foci in the subpial and subependymal regions are called Rich foci (after Rich and McCordock) [6]. Rupture of this Rich foci into the subarachnoid space results in clinical manifestations of the disease. Usually this starts almost within 12 months from the onset of primary complex in 75% of cases (some reports within 3 months). The three pathological processes involved are: (i) Adhesion formation: especially in the basal region; exudates consist of activated macrophages, plasma cells, fibrin and lymphocytes that result in hydrocephalus; there is also cranial nerve palsy especially in the second, fourth and sixth nerves [1]. Other cranial nerves involved are: third, seventh and eighth cranial nerves. (ii) Obliterative vasculitis: especially the middle and small arteries of ICA, proximal MCA and the perforators supplying the basal ganglia which results in irreversible stroke and sequelae. (iii) Encephalopathy or myelitis due to oedema with raised intracranial pressure and white matter pallor [7]. The brain tissue adjacent to the basal exudates develops edema resulting in perivascular infiltration and microglial reaction and this is called "Border zone reaction". Cerebral infarction is usually common across the Sylvian fissure and basal ganglia. The infarcts involve the medial striate and thalamoperforating arteries.

7.4 Clinical Manifestations

Most patients develop vague prodromal symptoms of low-grade fever, headache, vomiting, malaise, anorexia, myalgia, dizziness and/or personality changes which may last for about 2–8 weeks. If left untreated, they progress to classic meningitis symptoms in the form of headache, fever, seizures, stiff neck, focal neurological deficits, altered sensorium and behavioural changes. Seizures are uncommon manifestations, usually seen in children. Children usually present with decreased food intake, irritability, bulging anterior fontanelle and incessant cry, in addition to mild fever and weakness. Tuberculous encephalopathy occurs when children present with profound decreased sensorium and seizures. Children and HIV-infected individuals with TBM develop acute symptoms with profound loss of consciousness and carry high mortality.

Cranial nerve palsy is seen in 20–30% of patients. The sixth cranial nerve is the most affected one. Visual dysfunction in patients occurs due to optochiasmatic arachnoiditis, compression of optic chiasma due to dilated third ventricle and optic nerve granuloma. Tuberculomas or tubercular abscess presents with focal neurological deficits such as seizures and weakness with or without features of raised intracranial tension. Movement disorders in the form of tremor, chorea, ballism or myoclonus may occur due to the presence of granuloma in the basal ganglia or as sequelae of the weakness following arteritis as neurological sequelae. The mortality rates in HIV-negative patients according to Medical Research Council grades are 15%, 30% and 50% respectively. This increases further in HIV-positive individuals to 25%, 50% and 80% respectively [8]. Hyponatremia is common in TBM due to hypothalamic dysfunction. The classification of CNS TB depends on the site of affection and the pathology as described in Table 7.2.

Table 7.2 Classification of CNS TB

Intracranial
Tuberculous meningitis (TBM)
Tuberculous encephalopathy
Tuberculous vasculopathy
CNS tuberculoma
Tuberculous brain abscess
Spinal
Pott's spine and Pott's paraplegia
Non-osseous spinal tuberculoma
Spinal meningitis

Adapted from [2]

7.5   Neurological Complications in TB Meningitis

(a) **Cranial nerve involvement:** Cranial nerve palsy can be seen in about 20–30% of patients. The commonly affected nerves are II, III, IV, VI and VIIth nerves. The VIth nerve is the most involved and can mimic as a false localizing sign. Sometimes isolated cranial nerve palsy can be a presenting complaint in tubercular infections [2]. The cranial nerve involvement occurs due to: (i) nerve trunk entrapment in thick basilar exudates, (ii) increased intracranial tension (ICT), (iii) adhesions of multiple nerve roots, and (iv) rarely, tuberculoma in the cerebellopontine (CP) angle or the brain stem that can compress the cranial nerves.

(b) **Hydrocephalus:** This is one of the most common complications [2, 3]. There are two types of hydrocephalus: the first is the communicating type, which is due to basal cistern blockage by the inflammatory exudates. The second is due to obstruction of these basal cisterns resulting from exudates; however, this is less commonly seen.

(c) **Visual dysfunction:** Visual dysfunction is one of the most serious complications as it leads to significant morbidity and dependence [1, 2]. The visual dysfunction occurs as a result of: (i) optochiasmatic arachnoiditis, (ii) compression of optic chiasma by the third ventricle in patients with a large hydrocephalus, (iii) optic nerve granuloma and (iv) ethambutol toxicity.

(d) **Focal neurological deficits:** Common focal neurological deficits include paraplegia, hemiplegia, monoplegia and aphasia. Paraplegia is commonly caused by tuberculous radiculomyelitis. Sometimes it may result due to intra-medullary/extra-medullary spinal cord tuberculoma, cavities due to spinal syringomyelia or rarely because of spinal cord infarcts. Ischemic infarcts in the brain are most commonly seen in basal ganglia and internal capsule. This is mainly due to vascular compression and occlusion of small perforator vessels due to inflammatory process. Middle cerebral and lenticulostriate arteries are commonly affected but sometimes it can even be multifactorial. Angiographic features (Fig. 7.2) in TBM show mainly the narrowing and/or occlusion of arteries at the base of the brain.

(e) **Tuberculoma:** These are due to enlarged Rich focus lesions [2, 4]. These granulomas are of two types: caseating and non-caseating. These tuberculomas may be either single or multiple in number and are often seen in frontal and parietal lobes.

(f) **Metabolic complications:** The most common metabolic complication is hyponatremia, seen in nearly 50% of cases. Previously it was believed to be due to inappropriate anti-diuretic hormone secretion; however, it has been found that many of these patients had low plasma volumes and persistent natriuresis even with normal anti-diuretic hormone (ADH) concentration. Currently it is hypothesized that hyponatremia occurs due to cerebral salt wasting syndrome. Other factors which may contribute are: excessive atrial natriuretic peptide and brain natriuretic peptide secretion, and direct neural influence on renal function. Hence sometimes it is also called "hyponatraemic natriuretic syndrome". Other metabolic complications are rare, but sometimes can have associated hypothalamic complications like hyperphagia and precocious puberty in adolescents.

7.6 Diagnosis

The diagnosis of TBM is challenging in view of atypical presentation, low sensitivity of CSF smear microscopy for acid fast bacilli (AFB), and the fact that it can take weeks to obtain the culture report due to slow growth of *M. tuberculosis*. Patients usually present with indolent symptoms of meningitis such as low-grade fever, headache,

neck stiffness, photophobia, vomiting, altered sensorium, seizures, limb weakness, cranial nerve palsies, stupor and coma. In the majority of cases, the diagnosis of TBM is empirical, based on the clinical, radiological and preliminary CSF results without definitive diagnosis. Classical CSF findings in TBM include increased white cell count with predominant lymphocytes, increased protein, and normal or low glucose levels. However, acid fast staining of CSF smear has low sensitivity. To increase the yield of sensitivity, few methods suggested are several daily large volumes (10–15 mL) CSF samples may increase the sensitivity to >85%. Sensitivity increases to >85% when four spinal taps are performed [4]. AFB staining can detect up to 80%, but the results largely depend on the high volume of CSF, timely transportation of the sample and prompt analysis and the expertise of the lab personnel for at least 30 min, centrifugation of the CSF sample and pre-treatment of CSF leukocytes with triton prior to ZN staining [9, 10]. The results of TB culture can take several weeks, and the culture also has low sensitivity of 40–80%. However, it has a role in determining the drug susceptibility pattern [4]. In patients with coexistent HIV, abnormal CSF features are normal cells with predominant polymorphonuclear leukocytes and normal glucose levels.

Other CSF tests include: (i) MODS (Microscopic Observation Drug Susceptibility Assay): This is an easy and rapid technique which uses the liquid culture method in the diagnosis of TBM and drug susceptibility testing. It is more sensitive than CSF smear, and more rapid than conventional TB culture. (ii) Becton Dickinson mycobacterial growth indicator tube (MGIT): Myocobacterial growth can be detected by a fluorescent growth indicator embedded in silicone at the bottom of an MGIT tube. (iii) Bactec MGIT 960 system for rapid mycobacterial detection. (iv) The Gene Xpert MTB/RIF: This is a fully automated PCR (polymerase chain reaction) which helps in diagnosis of tuberculosis as well as detection of rifampi-

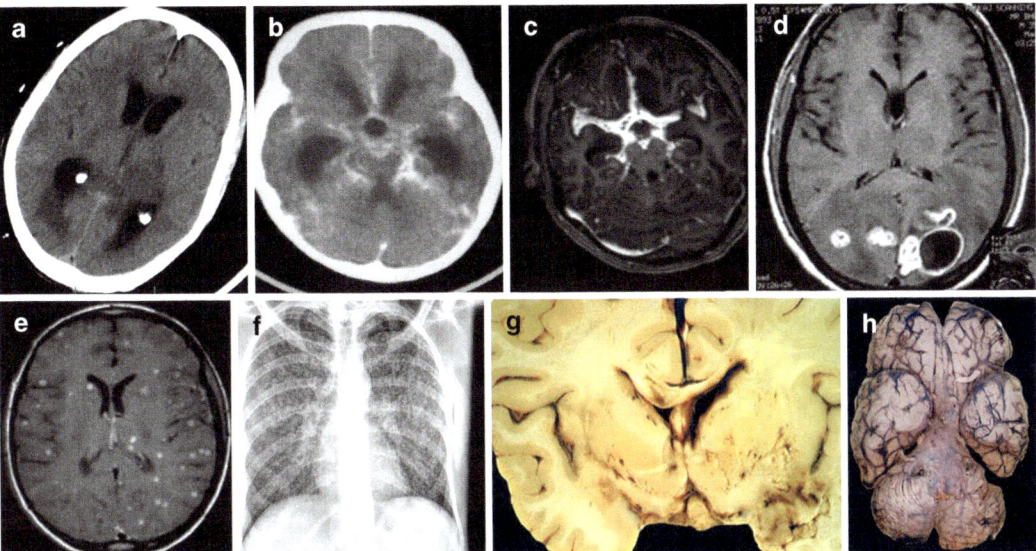

Fig. 7.1 Imaging and pathological features of various forms of tubercular meningitis: (**a**) CT of the brain plain shows hydrocephalus, hypodensity in left thalamus suggestive of infarct and diffuse cerebral oedema. (**b**) CT of the brain plain and contrast axial images show evidence of hydrocephalus with periventricular leukoariosis and basal exudates. (**c**) MRI brain T1 axial contrast images show the presence of basal exudates. (**d**) MRI brain T1 contrast axial images show multiple ring-enhancing tuberculomas in bilateral occipital regions. (**e**) MRI brain axial images of T1 contrast show multiple contrast-enhancing lesions suggestive of military form of CNS TB. (**f**) Chest X-ray showing military infiltrates in bilateral chest. (**g**) Gross specimen of a patient (post autopsy) showing ischemic infarct in left basal ganglia. Exudate is present along left Sylvian fissure entrapping MCA branches. (**h**) Gross specimen of a patient (post autopsy) showing basal exudates with obscuration of the basilar artery

cin drug resistance [11]. (v) Enzyme Linked Immuno Sorbent Assay (ELISA): This helps to detect antibodies against the mycobacterial antigens in CSF. (vii) Adenosine deaminase (ADA) levels of ≥10 U/L in CSF have >90% sensitivity and specificity in detecting mycobacterium. (viii) Tuberculin skin test: The diagnostic yield varies from 10 to 50%. The yield of the test varies according to age, HIV co-infection, BCG vaccination, nutritional status and administration technique [12].

Neuroimaging helps in the diagnosis of TBM (Figs. 7.1 and 7.2); MRI of the brain is more sensitive than CT in detecting the various pathologies. But CT may be helpful in the acute stage to rule out any complications and to decide about surgery for hydrocephalus. The imaging characteristics of TBM are basal meningeal enhancement, arteritis resulting in cerebral infarcts, cerebral edema, hydrocephalus, enhancing nodular lesions, tuberculoma, myelitis and arachnoiditis.

Fig. 7.2 (**a**) Flair images of the brain showing hyper intensity in anterior corpus callosum. (**b**) Diffusion restriction of the same areas. (**c**) T1 contrast showing ring-enhancing lesion–granuloma in the right temporal region. (**d**) T1 contrast showing evidence of exudates in anterior parasagittal region. (**e**) DSA: shows evidence of arteritis of MCA perforators. (**f**) DSA shows stenosis of distal MCA

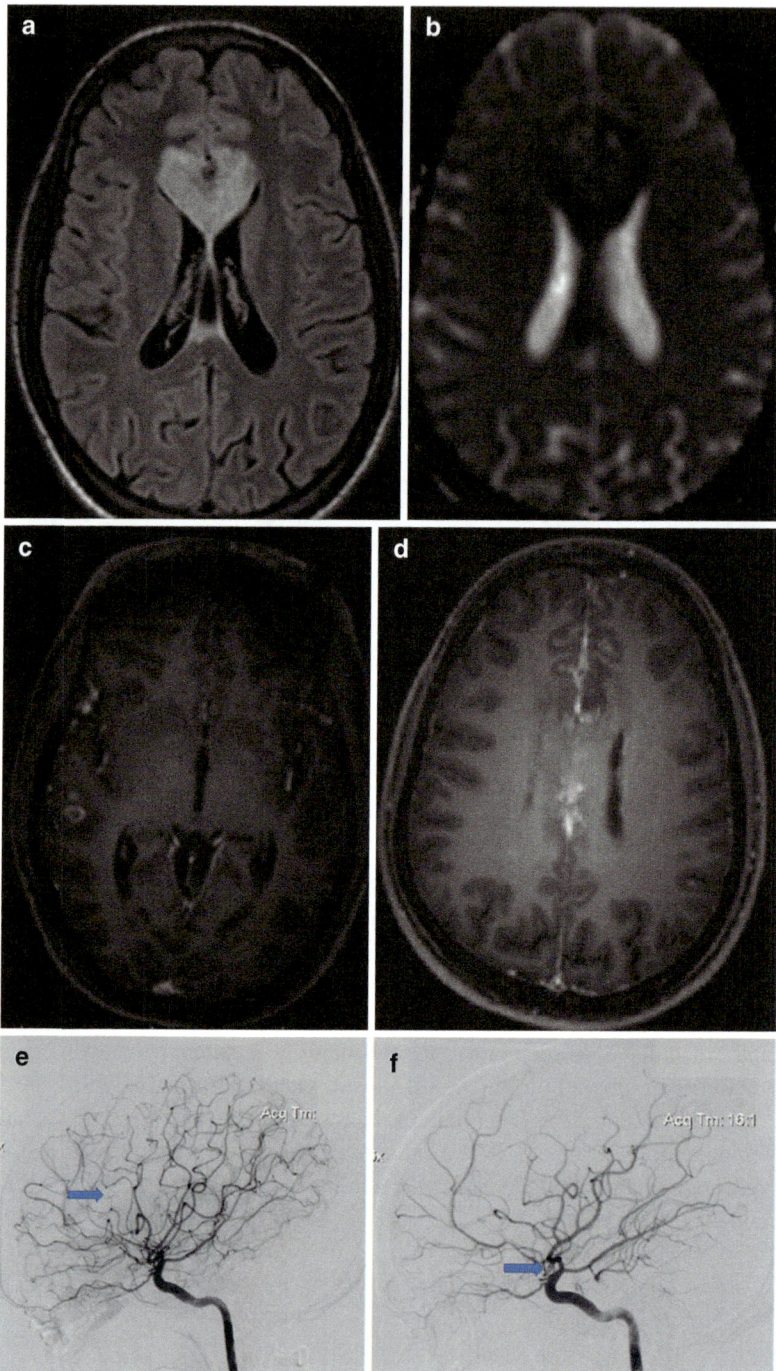

7.7 Treatment and Prognosis

Current treatment guidelines include an intensive phase in the first 2 months with a four-drug regimen (rifampicin, isoniazid, pyrazinamide and streptomycin) followed by a maintenance phase with an additional 10–16 months of two drugs (isoniazid and rifampicin). Recently, the Revised National Tuberculosis Control Programme has recommended adding ethambutol in the mainte-

Table 7.3 Recommended antituberculous treatment (ATT) regimen in the treatment of TBM

Drug	Dosage (children)	Dosage (adults)	Duration	Adverse events
Rifampicin	10 mg/kg	450 mg (<50 kg); 600 mg (>50 kg)	12–18 months	Hepatotoxicity, orange urine, drug interactions, rash, flu-like syndrome
Isoniazid	5 mg/kg	300 mg	12–18 months	Hepatotoxicity, peripheral neuropathy, lupus-like syndrome, confusion, seizures
Pyrazinamide	25 mg/kg	1500 mg	2 months	Hepatotoxicity, arthralgia, gout, gastrointestinal upset, anorexia, and photosensitization of the skin
Ethambutol	15 mg/kg	800 mg	2 months	Retrobulbar neuritis, peripheral neuritis, arthralgia and gastrointestinal upset
Streptomycin	15 mg/kg	0.75 mg	2 months	Nephrotoxicity, ototoxicity, vestibular toxicity
Moxifloxacin	10–20 mg/kg	400 mg	Throughout the course	Nausea, headache, tremor, confusion, tendon rupture (rare)

Corticosteroids
Adults: 0.4 mg/kg/day for 4 weeks followed by gradual taper over 6–8 weeks
Children: 0.6 mg/kg/day for 4 weeks followed by gradual taper over 6–8 weeks

nance phase [13]. There have been several studies which have shown better clinical outcomes with the following regimens: (i) intensified rifampicin (13 mg/kg of rifampicin intravenously) and standard therapy (10 mg/kg orally) for the first 14 days. The higher doses of rifampicin resulted in three-fold higher concentrations in plasma and CSF with an overall 50% reduction in the six-month mortality rate. (ii) Simultaneous treatment with moxifloxacin 800 mg instead of 400 mg, leading to higher concentrations in the CSF. Though there are wide variations in the treatment regimens in various countries with the duration of antituberculous treatment (ATT), the most important prognostic indicator is early diagnosis and treatment.

Corticosteroids decrease parenchymal and meningeal inflammation resulting in reduction of residual neurological deficits and mortality. Reduction in CSF inflammatory cytokines impairs the diapedesis of neutrophils and mononuclear cells, thus preventing death from vasculitis-induced stroke and obstructive hydrocephalus [3]. The corticosteroid regimen is shown in Table 7.3.

The co-infection of HIV with TBM results in a therapeutic challenge with higher morbidity and mortality. Introduction of antiretroviral therapy (ART) in the early course of ATT results in IRIS (immune reconstitution inflammatory syndrome) whereas morbidity and mortality can increase with late ART initiation. According to WHO guidelines, ART has to be started 8 weeks after starting ATT if CD4 count is more than 200 cells/μL. In case of severe disease and non-improvement, ART can be started 2 weeks after starting ATT, especially if CD4 count is <100 cells/μL [13–15]. Rifampicin induces the metabolism of protease inhibitors resulting in reduction of their drug levels. Hence, rifampicin has to be started with a non-nucleoside reverse transcriptase inhibitor, preferably efavirenz, at a higher dose of 800 mg. If the protease inhibitor has to be continued, then rifabutin has to be given instead of rifampicin.

References

1. Dastur DK, Manghani DK, Udani PM. Pathology and pathogenetic mechanisms in neurotuberculosis. Radiol Clin N Am. 1995;33:733–52.
2. Cherian A, Thomas SV. CNS TB. Afr Health Sci. 2011;11(1):116–27.
3. Thwaites GE, Nguyen DB, Nguyen HD, et al. Dexamethasone for the treatment of tuberculous

meningitis in adolescents and adults. N Engl J Med. 2004;351:1741–51.

4. Marx GE, Chan ED. Tuberculous meningitis: diagnosis and treatment review. Tuberculosis Res Treatment. 2011;2011:798764.

5. Lakshmi K, Santhanam R, Chithralekha S. Management of TBM: a review. Indian J Microbiol Res. 2017;4(1):1–6.

6. Koch R. Die aetiologie der tuberculosis. Berlin Klinische Wochenshrift. 1882;19:232–5.

7. Thwaites GE, Macmullen-Price J, Tran TH, et al. Serial MRI to determine the effect of dexamethasone on the cerebral pathology of tuberculous meningitis: an observational study. Lancet Neurol. 2007;6: 230–6.

8. Wilkinson RJ, Rohlwink U, Misra UK, van Crevel R, Mai NTH, Dooley KE, Caws M, Figaji A, Savic R, Solomons R, Thwaites GE. Tuberculous meningitis international research consortium. Nat Rev Neurol. 2017;13(10):581–98.

9. Thwaites GE, Chau TT, Farrar JJ. Improving the bacteriological diagnosis of tuberculous meningitis. J Clin Microbiol. 2004;42:378–9.

10. Chen P, Shi M, Feng GD, et al. A highly efficient Ziehl-Neelsen stain: identifying de novo intracellular Mycobacterium tuberculosis and improving detection of extracellular M. tuberculosis in cerebrospinal fluid. J Clin Microbiol. 2012;50:1166–70.

11. Pai M, Flores LL, Pai N, Hubbard A, Riley LW, Colford JM. Diagnostic accuracy of nucleic acid amplification tests for tuberculous meningitis: a systematic review and meta analysis. Lancet Infect Dis. 2003;3(10):633–43.

12. Joos TJ, Miller WC, Murdoch DM. Tuberculin reactivity in BCG vaccinated populations: a compilation of international dta. Int J Tuberc Lung Dis. 2006;10:883–91.

13. WHO. Treatment of tuberculosis: guidelines. 4th ed. The World Health Organization; 2010. p. 160.

14. Török ME, Yen NTB, Chau TTH, et al. Timing of initiation of antiretroviral therapy in human immunodeficiency virus (HIV)–associated tuberculous meningitis. Clin Infect Dis. 2011;52:1374–83.

15. Rich AR, Mc Cordock HA. The pathogenesis of tuberculous meningitis. Bull John Hopkins Hosp. 1933;52:5–37.

Subacute Sclerosing Panencephalitis

8

Madhu Nagappa and Sanjib Sinha

Case Scenario

A seven-year-old boy presented with inattentiveness in class for 6 months. His class teacher noted that his scholastic performance was gradually deteriorating. Over the next 2 months his grades dropped. Over the next 2 months, his parents noted that he became withdrawn, had reduced interaction, and did not show any interest in playing with his younger sister. Three months into the illness, he developed recurrent unprovoked falls. He had had an exanthematous fever at around 1 year of age. He was not immunized. At the time of evaluation, he was conscious with fluctuating alertness. Cranial nerve examination was normal. He had mild hypotonia of limbs. The striking feature was the presence of "slow" myoclonus resulting in extension of trunk and abduction of shoulders along with transient loss of "luster" in the eyes. His brain MRI was unremarkable. His EEG showed periodic complexes (Fig. 8.1). He was diagnosed as having subacute sclerosing panencephalitis.

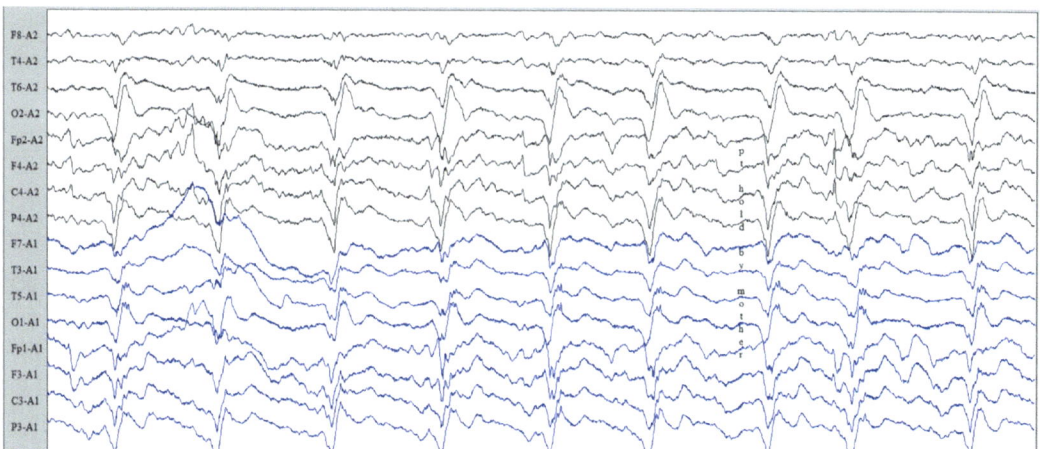

Fig. 8.1 Scalp EEG recording shows large amplitude complexes occurring every 2 s (recording parameters—time constant 0.30 s, high-frequency filter: 70 Hz, sweep speed: 1 s/div)

M. Nagappa · S. Sinha (✉)
Department of Neurology, National Institute of
Mental Health and Neurosciences (NIMHANS),
Bangalore, India

© Springer Nature Singapore Pte Ltd. 2024
K. K. Oli et al. (eds.), *Case-based Approach to Common Neurological Disorders*,
https://doi.org/10.1007/978-981-99-8676-7_8

8.1   Introduction

Subacute sclerosing panencephalitis (SSPE) is a progressive, neurodegenerative disorder of childhood caused by persistent infection of the central nervous system by a mutant measles virus. The name reflects the underlying clinical course and pathology, where "subacute" refers to progression over 9 months, "sclerosis" refers to the nature of pathological lesions, and "panencephalitis" refers to involvement of the entire brain. The disorder generally leads to death within 1–3 years of onset [1]. In this chapter, we provide a brief overview of the epidemiology of SSPE in relation to measles infection, its pathogenesis, clinical features, treatment, differential diagnosis, and preventive strategies.

8.2   History

Two consecutive papers in 1933 and 1934 from Dawson described two children from Tennessee who had rapidly progressive encephalitis, involuntary movements, cognitive decline, and intracellular eosinophilic inclusions in cortical neurons resembling viral inclusions. In 1939, Pette and Doring described a 17-year-old boy with progressive neurological deterioration, death, and nodular changes in gray and white matter resembling encephalomyelitis. Subsequently, van Bogaert (1945) described another patient, who had slower progression, demyelination, and glial proliferation in the brain. In 1949, Radermecher first described the abnormalities on electroencephalogram (EEG). In 1950, neuropathologist Greenfield coined the term subacute sclerosing panencephalitis. Boutellie et al. (1965) identified structures resembling nucleocapsids of paramyxovirus by electron microscopy. Connolly et al. (1967) reported very high titers of measles antibodies in blood and cerebrospinal fluid of all patients [2].

8.3   Epidemiology of SSPE Relative to Measles

There is a global decline in the prevalence of SSPE with the introduction of effective vaccination against measles [2]. Nevertheless due to gaps in immunization, it has not been eliminated. Outbreaks of measles occur and measles continues to be a public health problem in several geographic regions. The frequency of SSPE relative to that of measles varies with the age at acquisition of measles, being highest when measles is acquired during infancy (<1 year: 360/100,000, <5 years: 18/100,000, >5 years: 1.1/100,000). Overall, about 4–11 patients develop SSPE for every 100,000 subjects with measles. SSPE is more prevalent among Asians and Hispanics and the lower socio-economic classes. Higher birth order also predisposes to SSPE since there is a higher chance of coming in contact with a subject infected with measles before 5 years of age. Maternal measles or incomplete transfer of maternal antibodies to the newborn is associated with a higher risk for SSPE. Girls have reduced prevalence and longer latency from measles to onset of SSPE as compared to boys. Children born to mothers with acquired immunodeficiency syndrome (AIDS) and subjects with AIDS are also at an increased risk for SSPE and fulminant clinical course (Gutierrez et al., 2010) [1].

8.4   Pathogenesis

The underlying patho-mechanism in SSPE is persistent and chronic infection of the central nervous system by mutated measles virus; host immune factors also play a role. Mutations in the matrix (M), hemagglutinin (H), nucleocapsid (N), and fusion (F) genes of the measles virus confer on it the ability to maintain persistent infection in the brain, while negating the ability for transmission of viral particles. Mechanisms of entry of viral particles into the neurons are not clear. CD46 and signaling lymphocyte activation molecule may act as cellular receptors for the measles virus. Once neurons are infected, transneuronal spread occurs. Development of SSPE is dependent on genetically determined immune dysfunction in the host affecting cell-mediated immunity and inflammatory cytokines [3].

8.5   Pathology

Histologically, there is inflammation of meninges and brain parenchyma, demyelination, neuronal loss, and gliosis. Ultrastructural examination shows three types of inclusions: viral nucleocapsids in neurons and oligodendrocytes, and nuclear bodies and granulo-filamentous inclusions in astrocytic nuclei. These changes are noted initially in posterior regions of the brain, but eventually they spread and involve the entire brain including basal ganglia, brainstem, and spinal cord as well. In later stages, atrophy sets in [1, 3]. Immunohistochemistry for measles virus antigen is positive. Intranuclear viral inclusions are noted in the retina as well.

8.6   Clinical Manifestations

8.6.1   Classical SSPE

SSPE is a disorder of childhood. Onset is usually between 8 and 11years of age, i.e., the interval between SSPE and preceding measles infection is about 6 years. Classically, SSPE manifests first with scholastic decline and altered personality and behavior, followed by myoclonus and motor dysfunction and then rigidity, dysautonomia, vegetative or comatose state, and finally death. The initial manifestation of SSPE is myoclonus in 48.2%, seizures in 17.9%, intellectual decline in 16.3%, behavioral changes in 8.1%, visual disturbances in 2.6%, gait disturbances in 1.6%, extra-

pyramidal symptoms in 1.6%, speech disturbances in 1.3%, regression of milestones in 1.3%, and lateralizing motor weakness in 0.9% [4]. Based on the evolution of clinical features, the disease can be staged as follows [5]: Stage I: personality changes, decline in scholastic performance, abnormal behavior; Stage II: massive, repetitive, and frequent myoclonic jerks, seizures, and cognitive decline; Stage III: rigidity, extrapyramidal symptoms, and progressive unresponsiveness; and Stage IV: comatose or vegetative state, akineticmutism, and autonomic dysfunction.

Dyken proposed the definitions of acute, subacute, and chronic SSPE based on the speed of progression of clinical symptoms as follows [6]: (a) Acute or fulminant: development of severe neurological symptoms and disability within 3 months of onset of first symptom; (b) Subacute: development of neurologic disability within 9 months of onset of first symptom; and (c) Chronic: development of neurologic disability after 9 months of onset of first symptom.

8.7   Criteria for Diagnosis of SSPE

Garg RK in 2008 provided useful criteria: (i) a typical clinical picture of progressive subacute mental deterioration with stereotyped generalized myoclonus; (ii) characteristic electroencephalogram changes; (iii) elevated cerebrospinal fluid globulin levels greater than 20% of total cerebrospinal fluid protein; (iv) raised cerebrospinal fluid measles antibody titers, and (v) typical histopathologic findings in brain biopsy or autopsy. Visual disturbances occur due to involvement of retina, optic nerve, or occipital cortex. Ocular signs include necrotizing retinitis, which is the most characteristic, macular degeneration, optic atrophy, papilledema, and papillitis. Visual disturbances arising from cortical involvement include cortical blindness, visuo-spatial agnosias, hallucinations, Balint syndrome, and Anton syndrome [3].

8.8 Non-classical or Atypical SSPE

Atypical presentations are noted in about 10% of SSPE cases. Seizures may be the presenting feature of SSPE in 17.9% of subjects with SSPE [4]. The semiology may vary from generalized tonic clonic seizures, to complex partial seizures, partial motor seizures in clusters, epilepsia partialis continua, isolated facial twitching, and hemimyoclonus [7–10]. Recurrent febrile seizures may rarely be the initial manifestation [11]. Visual symptoms may be the initial and isolated manifestation for up to 2 years [1]. Other atypical presentations include abnormal gait, lateralizing motor deficit, and movement disorder [4]. Uncommon extrapyramidal features such as "Pisa" syndrome and severe rigidity and elevated creatine kinase as seen in neuroleptic malignant syndrome have been reported as the initial manifestation of SSPE [12, 13]. These atypical manifestations often mislead the clinician and delay the diagnosis unless there is a high index of suspicion. Brainstem involvement in SSPE can occur at any stage of the illness, more commonly in the third and fourth stages [14, 15]. This is independent of the supratentorial cortical involvement. Familial SSPE is rare, but reported [16].

8.9 Fulminant SSPE

This is defined as neurological deficit of 66% in the first 3 months or death within 6 months of disease onset. Risk factors include early age at infection with measles virus, viral virulence, immune-deficient state, and co-infection with other viruses [1]. Fulminant course occurs in 10% of cases of SSPE [17, 18].

8.10 Protracted Course in SSPE

SSPE has a progressive course resulting in vegetative state and death within a few months of diagnosis. In a proportion of patients, spontaneous stabilization/plateau period occurs for months to years [19, 20]. Remissions of varying degrees ranging from modest to substantial are also reported. They include subsidence of myoclonus and improvement from bed-bound or vegetative state to independence in ambulation or activities of daily living. Worsening or relapse after a variable period of stabilization or remission occurs. Later age at onset and onset in adulthood may correlate with slower progression [21, 22]. Visual symptoms and seizures are commoner among those with protracted clinical course [22]. Sustained remission for 8 to 10 years has been reported in 5%–10% of subjects [19].

8.11 SSPE in Adults

SSPE is a disorder of childhood. Uncommonly, adults are affected and they constitute about 1.75%–2.6% [23]. In a large study from India, adults constituted about 12.9% of all cases of SSPE [22]. Both genders are affected equally, but one study showed predominance of men with adult-onset SSPE [22]. Low virulence of the mutated virus and/or high immunological status of the host are the putative reasons for the unusually long interval between measles and onset of SSPE [22]. The clinical course is more fulminant in adult-onset SSPE compared to those with childhood onset [3, 24], but this is not a consistent observation [25]. SSPE with onset or worsening during pregnancy, as also reports of occurrence of conception in women following the diagnosis of SSPE [22, 24, 26]. Outcome of pregnancy was successful in most of the affected women [22].

8.12 HIV and Measles

Data on the effect of HIV on measles and risk of developing SSPE is not inadequate. Fulminant clinical course of SSPE in a patient with HIV has been reported. In cases of perinatally acquired HIV or a child born to an HIV-positive mother, there may be a shorter latency period for developing SSPE [27].

8.13   Investigations

Cerebrospinal fluid (CSF) analysis: Routine CSF analysis shows pleocytosis, normal or elevated protein, and normal glucose content. Elevated titers of measles antibodies (IgG) in CSF ranging from 1:40 to 1:1280 are diagnostic. CSF-serum ratio ranges from 5:1 to 40:1 reflecting intra-thecal synthesis of measles antibodies. Enzyme-linked immunosorbent assay (ELISA) has a sensitivity of 100%, a specificity of 93.3%, and a positive predictive value of 100%. Elevated soluble CD8 and reduced beta2-microglobulin in CSF correlates with clinical worsening [1].

Electroencephalogram (EEG): EEG plays a crucial role in the diagnosis of SSPE. The presence of periodic complexes is pathognomonic of SSPE. These are characterized by bilaterally symmetrical, periodic, generalized, high-amplitude (100–1000 microV) complexes that are stereotyped, last for 1–3 s, and recur every 2–20 s. They are present in 65%–83% of patients with SSPE [1]. These complexes precede or follow clinical myoclonus by about 200–800 ms [28]. The interval between complexes is varied and may be prolonged, particularly in the initial stages, when they may occur as infrequently as once in 5 min. These complexes may be present only during sleep, disappear with rise in body temperature, and may be elicited by extraneous stimuli [29]. These may be periodic, quasi-periodic, or aperiodic [30]. The morphology, frequency, and inter-burst intervals of these complexes are not altered by activation procedures like hyperventilation or photic or sensory stimulation. Periodic complexes disappear during advanced stages of the disease [3]. The following patterns of periodic complexes may aid in prognosis of SSPE [31]: Type I complexes (periodic giant delta waves, typical periodic complexes of SSPE) correlate with intermediate outcome; Type II complexes (periodic giant delta waves intermixed with rapid spikes or fast activity) correlate with best outcome; and Type III complexes (long spike wave discharges interrupted by giant delta waves) correlate with worst outcome.

A number of "atypical" EEG patterns have been recognized and reported. They include asymmetric, lateralized, focal, or regional complexes; this may be a reflection of asymmetry in cerebral hemispheric involvement [9]. Asynchronous discharges, commensurate with trans-callosal spread, are also recognized phenomena [32]. Other uncommon features are frontal rhythmic delta activity, frontal spikes, bisynchronous occipital spikes preceding periodic complexes, periodic generalized fast waves, and transient diffuse abnormal alpha in sleep. Prolonged discharges of sharp and slow waves for 4–7 s, followed by suppression for 1–4 s and periodic complexes comprising four or five sharp waves occurring every 2 s, have also been reported [33]. They seem to correlate with greater neurological disability, rapid progression, and longer duration of disease [33].

Brain MRI: MRI may be normal when done very early in the disease course. Initially, there is appearance of asymmetric T2/FLAIR hyperintensity of cerebral cortex and subcortical white matter, which initially affects the occipital region and then progresses to the frontal region. This is followed by atrophy and multifocal white matter hyperintensities. The basal ganglia, thalami, brainstem, cerebellum, and spinal cord may also be involved uncommonly [34–36]. Brainstem involvement in SSPE has been rarely mistaken for glioma [37]. The cerebral changes are replaced by symmetrical hyperintensities in periventricular white matter and atrophy [1]. Restricted diffusion and enhancement of involved areas may be seen. There are no characteristic patterns on MRI that are pathognomonic of SSPE. MRI changes do not correlate with the stage of SSPE and may continue to progress even when the patient is apparently stabilized or in remission [1, 30]. A high index of suspicion based on the clinical features is required. MRI aids in excluding other differential diagnosis.

8.14 Differential Diagnosis

When a child presents with acute/ rapidly progressive psychiatric disturbances, seizures, and movement disorder, autoimmune encephalitis, specifically that associated with N-methyl-D-aspartate receptor (NMDAR) antibodies, is a close differential diagnosis. Serological testing for NMDAR antibodies and EEG changes aid in distinguishing autoimmune encephalitis from SSPE. The presence of multifocal signal changes in brain MRI in a patient with poly-symptomatic presentation warrants consideration of acute disseminated encephalomyelitis (ADEM), pediatric multiple sclerosis (MS), neuromyelitis optica (NMO), and other causes of secondary demyelination. It is important to distinguish these disorders from SSPE in order to provide appropriate treatment and prognostication. Other differential diagnoses include progressive myoclonic epilepsy syndromes such as Lafora body disease, neuronal ceroid lipofuscinosis, and storage disorders [1].

8.15 Missed Diagnosis of SSPE

The initial diagnosis of SSPE may be missed in up to 78.8% [4]. SSPE is often mistaken for a variety of neuro-psychiatric disorders such as seizures, metachromatic leukodystrophy, Schilder's disease, cerebral palsy, hemiparkinsonism, Wilson's disease, vasculitis, spinocerebellar ataxia, motor neuron disease, nutritional amblyopia, tapetoretinal degeneration, catatonic schizophrenia, and malingering, among others. Misdiagnosis is commoner among those who present with atypical features, have onset in adulthood, or have an unusually fulminant or protracted clinical course. Besides these, the experience, knowledge, commitment, and confidence of the treating doctor may also contribute to missed diagnosis. Depending on the initial clinical manifestation, a patient may be seen by a pediatrician, physician, ophthalmologist, psychiatrist, or neurologist. Knowledge and awareness are necessary so that the disease is suspected at the bedside and focused evaluation is done. It is important to establish an early diagnosis for appropriate prognostication and to avoid unnecessary investigations and treatment.

8.16 Treatment

A number of drugs with anti-viral and immunomodulatory properties have been tried in SSPE. They slow the progression and prolong survival. At least one-third benefit and combination therapy are more effective than monotherapy [1]. However, none have any effect on the long-term outcome. Inosine pranobex (Isoprinosine), a complex of inosine and 2-hydroxypropyldimethyl ammonium-4-benzoate, was the first effective drug for SSPE. The recommended daily dose is 100 mg/kg. It acts by enhancing various components of the immune system including natural killer cells [38]. Clinical trials have shown that isoprinosine improves symptoms and increases life expectancy in patients with slowly progressive SSPE, but not in those with rapid disease [39, 40]. Interferon-alpha inhibits replication of measles virus as well as modulating the immune system so that there is enhanced expression and functions of natural killer cell, T cells, macrophages, and complement components. It is administered intrathecally or intra-ventricularly since interferon-alpha does not cross the blood–brain barrier. A combination of intra-ventricular interferon-alpha and oral isoprinosine stabilizes or brings about remission in 44%–50% of subjects [41, 42]. In a randomized trial of combined intraventricular interferon alpha2b and isoprinosine versus only isoprinosine by the International Consortium on SSPE, stabilization, improvement, and mortality were comparable between the two groups [43]. In a non-randomized retrospective study, a combination of subcutaneous interferon beta and isoprinosine was more beneficial than only interferon beta [44].

Anti-viral agents: Ribavirin and lamivudine are nucleoside analogs with anti-viral properties. Ribavirin inhibits viral mRNA synthesis, while lamivudine inhibits DNA polymerase and reverse transcriptase. Intraventricular ribavirin may be safe and effective [45]. Intravenous ribavirin in combination with intraventricular interferon and isoprinosine has been shown to have temporary benefit [46]. Lamivudine has better penetration into the cerebrospinal fluid. Subcutaneous administration of interferon-alpha2a along with oral isoprinosine and lamivudine resulted in remission in 36.8%, reduced mortality, and significantly longer survival [47]. Amantadine disrupts assembly of viral particles during replication. It does not have a beneficial role in SSPE [40].

Other agents: An isolated case report demonstrated the beneficial effect of intravenous immunoglobulin when co-administered with isoprinosine [48]. Propionibacterium granulosum, a bacterial immunomodulator, has been shown to be effective when combined with isoprinosine or intraventricular interferon [40]. Steroids, levamisole, cimetidine, plasmapheresis, thymus extracts, and rituximab do not have any beneficial role [40, 47, 49]. Retinoids upregulate interferon responses and effective elimination of the virus. Administration of vitamin A reduces mortality associated with measles [50]. Beta carotene levels are reduced in SSPE [51]. But the role of vitamin A in the treatment of SSPE remains to be explored. Anti-apoptotic agents like flupirtine when administered in combination with isoprinosine may slow disease progression. Trials exploring the role of novel therapeutic agents vizRNAi and antagonists of cyclophilin B and NK-1 are awaited [40].

Symptomatic treatment: Anticonvulsants are used for symptomatic treatment of myoclonus. Carbamazepine is relatively more effective in reducing myoclonus of SSPE and improves cognitive functions as well. This is surprising as carbamazepine is known to worsen multiple seizure types including myoclonic, absence, and atonic seizures in generalized epilepsies. However, the response to carbamazepine is not sustained as the disease eventually progresses. Carbamazepine does not have any significant effect on EEG changes [40, 52–54]. Levetiracetam has also been shown to improve myoclonus and cognition [55].

Immunization program: SSPE is a measure of the effectiveness and completeness of measles immunization in the community. The Government of India, through the Universal Immunization Programme (UIP), has been providing vaccination to all children less than 5 years of age. Measles is the commonest vaccine preventable disease and India has been providing measles vaccination under the UIP since 1985 in all states. Based on the recommendations of the National Technical Advisory Group on Immunization (NTAGI), a second dose of measles vaccine at 16–24 months was introduced in 2010. The rationale was that the first dose of measles vaccine administered at 9 months has an effectiveness of 85%, while the second dose administered after 12 months of age increases the effectiveness to 95%. Vaccination coverage in India is significantly short of the recommended global target of 95% at national and district level that is required to eliminate measles [56]. From 2014, the NTAGI recommended the introduction of measles-rubella vaccine and two doses are administered at 9 months and 16–24 months. The aim is to eliminate measles and rubella by 2020. There has been a recent increase in the number of cases of measles in developed countries like the USA, causing concerns among policy makers.

References

1. Gutierrez J, Issacson RS, Koppel BS. Subacute sclerosing panencephalitis: an update. Dev Med Child Neurol. 2010;52(10):901–7.
2. Gadoth N. Subacute sclerosing panencephalitis (SSPE) the story of a vanishing disease. Brain and Development. 2012;34:705–11.
3. Garg RK. Subacute sclerosing panencephalitis. J Neurol. 2008;255(12):1861–71.
4. Prashanth LK, Taly AB, Sinha S, Ravi V. Subacute sclerosing panencephalitis (SSPE): an insight into the diagnostic errors from a tertiary care university hospital. J Child Neurol. 2007;22(6):683–8.
5. Jabbour JT, Dueanas DA, Modlin J. SSPE: clinical staging, course and frequency. Arch Neurol. 1975;32:493.
6. Dyken PR. Neuroprogressive disease of postinfectious origin: a review of a resurging subacute sclerosing panencephalitis (SSPE). Ment Retard Dev Disabil Res Rev. 2001;7:217–25.
7. Kravljanac R, Jovic N, Djuric M, Nikolic L. Epilepsiapartialis continua in children with fulminant subacute sclerosing panencephalitis. Neurol Sci. 2011;32:1007–12.
8. Malhotra HS, Garg RK, Naphade P. Cluster of partial motor seizures heralding the onset of hemimyoclonic

subacute sclerosing panencephalitis. Mov Disord. 2012;27(8):958–9.

9. Shivji ZM, Al-Zahrani IS, Al-Said YA, Jan MM. Subacute sclerosing panencepahilits presenting with unilateral periodic myoclonic jerks. Can J NeurolSci. 2003;30(4):384–7.

10. Tuncel D, Ozbek AE, Demirpolat G, Karabiber H. Subacute sclerosing panencephalitis with generalized seizure as the first symptom: a case report. Jpn J Infect Dis. 2006;59:317–9.

11. Kartal A, Çıtak Kurt AN, Hirfanoğlu T, Aydın K, Serdaroğlu A. Subacute sclerosing panencephalitis in a child with recurrent febrile seizures. Case Rep Pediatr. 2015;2015:783936.

12. Garg D, Reddy V, Singh RK, Dash D, Bhatia R, Tripathi M. Neuroleptic malignant syndrome as a presenting feature of subacute sclerosing panencephalitis. J Neurovirol. 2018;24(1):128–31.

13. Pandey S, Tomar LR, Tater P. Pisa syndrome in a child with subacute sclerosing panencephalitis. JAMA Neurol. 2018;75(2):255–6.

14. Saini AG, Sankhyan N, Padmanabh H, Sahu JK, Vyas S, Singhi P. Subacute sclerosing panencephalitis presenting as acute cerebellar ataxia and brain stem hyperintensities. Eur J Paediatr Neurol. 2016;20(3):435–8.

15. Upadhyayula PS, Yang J, Yue JK, Ciacci JD. Subacute Sclerosing Panencephalitis of the brainstem as a clinical entity. Med Sci (Basel). 2017;5(4):pii: E26.

16. Sharma V, Gupta VB, Eisenhut M. Familial subacute sclerosing panencephalitis associated with short latency. Pediatr Neurol. 2008;38:215–7.

17. Anlar B, Yalaz K. Prognosis in subacute sclerosing panencephalitis. Dev Med Child Neurol. 2011;53(10):965.

18. Chung BH, Ip PP, Wong VC, Lo JY, Harding B. Acute fulminant subacute sclerosing panencephalitis with absent measles and PCR studies in cerebrospinal fluid. Pediatr Neurol. 2004;31(3):222–4.

19. Anlar B. Subacute sclerosing panencephalitis: diagnosis and drug treatment options. CNS Drugs. 1997;7:11–120.

20. Risk W, Haddad F. The variable natural history of subacute sclerosing panencephalitis: a study of 118 cases from the Middle East. Arch Neurol. 1979;36:610–4.

21. Srinivas K, Srinivasan AV, Kumaresan G, Sayeed ZA, Velumurugendran CU. Classical SSPE and its variants. An eight year prospective study. In: Pant B, Prabhakar S, editors. Proceedings of the third international symposium on SSPE. Vellore: Christian Medical College; 1989. p. 67–71.

22. Prashanth LK, Taly AB, Ravi V, Sinha S, Arunodaya GR. Adult onset subacute sclerosing panencephalitis: clinical profile of 39 patients from a tertiary care Centre. J Neurol Neurosurg Psychiatry. 2006;77(5):630–3.

23. Haddad FS, Risk WS, Jabbour JT. Subacute sclerosing panencephalitis in the Middle East: report of 99 cases. Ann Neurol. 1977;1:211–7.

24. Tan E, Namer IJ, Ciger A, et al. The prognosis of subacute sclerosing panencephalitis in adults. Report

of 8 cases and review of the literature. Clin Neurol Neurosurg. 1991;93:205–9.

25. Singer C, Lang AE, Suchowersky O. Adult onset subacute sclerosing panencephalitis: case reports and review of the literature. Mov Disord. 1997;12:342–53.

26. Chiu MH, Meatherall B, Nikolic A, Cannon K, Fonseca K, Joseph JT, MacDonald J, Pabbaraju K, Tellier R, Wong S, Koch MW. Subacute sclerosing panencephalitis in pregnancy. Lancet Infect Dis. 2016;16(3):366–75.

27. Sivadasan A, Alexander M, Patil AK, Balagopal K, Azad ZR. Fulminant subacute sclerosing panencephalitis in an individual with a perinatally acquired human immunodeficiency virus infection. Arch Neurol. 2012;69(12):1644–7.

28. Celesia GG. Pathophysiology of periodic EEG complexes in subacute sclerosing panencephalitis (SSPE). Electroencephalogr Clin Neurophysiol. 1973;35:293–300.

29. Farrel DF, Starr A, Freeman JM. The effect of body temperature on the periodic complexes of subacute sclerosing panencephalitis (SSPE). Electroencephalogr Clin Neurophysiol. 1971;30:415–21.

30. Praveen-kumar S, Sinha S, Taly AB, Jayasree S, Ravi V, Vijayan J, Ravishankar S. Electroencephalographic and imaging profile in a subacute sclerosing panencephalitis (SSPE) cohort: a correlative study. Clin Neurophysiol. 2007;118(9):1947–54.

31. Yakub BA. Subacute sclerosing panencephalitis (SSPE) early diagnosis, prognostic factors and natural history. J Neurol Sci. 1996;39:227–34.

32. Gurses C, Ozturk A, Baykan B, Gokyigit A, Eraksoy M, Barlas M, Caliskan A, Ozcan H. Correlation between clinical stages and EEG findings of subacute sclerosing panencephalitis. Clin Electroencephalogr. 2000;31:201–6.

33. Ekmekci O, Karasoy H, Gökçay A, Ulkü A. Atypical EEG findings in subacute sclerosing panencephalitis. Clin Neurophysiol. 2005;116(8):1762–7.

34. Tatli B, Ekici B, Ozmen M. Current therapies and future perspectives in subacute sclerosing panencephalitis. Expert Rev Neurother. 2012;12(4):485–92.

35. Anlar B, Saatçi I, Köse G, Yalaz K. MRI findings in subacute sclerosing panencephalitis. Neurology. 1996;47:1278–83.

36. Tuncay R, Akman-Demir G, Gökyigit A, Eraksoy M, Barlas M, Tolun R, et al. MRI in subacute sclerosing panencephalitis. Neuroradiology. 1996;38:636–40.

37. Ozturk A, Gurses C, Baykan B, Gokyigit A, Eraksoy M. Subacute sclerosing panencephalitis: clinical and magnetic resonance imaging evaluation of 36 patients. J Child Neurol. 2002;17:25–9.

38. Kalane U, Kulkarni S. Atypical neuroimaging findings with involvement of brainstem and cerebellum as well as basal ganglia in a case of SSPE misinterpreted as glioma. J Pediatr Neurol. 2009;4:397–400.

39. Huttenlocher PR, Mattson RH. Isoprinosine in subacute sclerosing panencephalitis. Neurology. 1979;29:763–71.

40. Jones CE, Dyken PR, Huttenlocher PR, Jabbour JT, Maxwell KW. Inosiplex therapy in subacute sclerosing panencephalitis. A multicentre, non-randomised study in 98 patients. Lancet. 1982;1(8280):1034–7.

41. Yalaz K, Anlar B, Oktem F, Aysun S, Ustacelebi S, Gurcay O, Gucuyener K, Renda Y. Intraventricular interferon and oral inosiplex in the treatment of subacute sclerosing panencephalitis. Neurology. 1992;42(3 Pt 1):488–91.

42. Gascon G, Yamani S, Crowell J, Stigsby B, Nester M, Kanaan I, Jallu A. Combined oral isoprinosine-intraventricular alpha-interferon therapy for subacute sclerosing panencephalitis. Brain and Development. 1993;15(5):346–55.

43. Gascon GG, International Consortium on Subacute Sclerosing Panencephalitis. Randomized treatment study of inosiplex versus combined inosiplex and intraventricular interferon-alpha in subacute sclerosing panencephalitis (SSPE): international multicenter study. J Child Neurol. 2003;18(12):819–27.

44. Anlar B, Aydin OF, Guven A, Sonmez FM, Kose G, Herguner O. Retrospective evaluation of interferon-beta treatment in subacute sclerosing panencephalitis. Clin Ther. 2004;26(11):1890–4.

45. Tomoda A, Nomura K, Shiraishi S, Hamada A, Ohmura T, Hosoya M, et al. Trial of intraventricular ribavirin therapy for subacute sclerosing panencephalitis in Japan. Brain and Development. 2003;25:514–7.

46. Solomon T, Hart CA, Vinjamuri S, Beeching NJ, Malucci C, Humphrey P. Treatment of subacute sclerosing panencephalitis with interferon-alpha, ribavirin, and inosiplex. J Child Neurol. 2002;17(9):703–5.

47. Aydin OF, Senbil N, Kuyucu N, Gürer YK. Combined treatment with subcutaneous interferon-alpha, oral isoprinosine, and lamivudine for subacute sclerosing panencephalitis. J Child Neurol. 2003;18(2):104–8.

48. Gürer YK, Kükner S, Sarica B. Intravenous gamma-globulin treatment in a patient with subacute sclerosing panencephalitis. Pediatr Neurol. 1996;14(1):72–4.

49. Titomanlio L, Soyah N, Guerin V, Delanoe C, Sterkers G, Evrard P, Husson I. Rituximab in subacute sclerosing panencephalitis. Eur J Paediatr Neurol. 2007;11(1):43–5.

50. Huiming Y, Chaomin W, Meng M. Vitamin A for treating measles in children. Cochrane Database Syst Rev. 2005;(4):CD001479.

51. Gungor S, Olmez A, Firat PA, Haliloğlu G, Anlar B. Serum retinol and beta-carotene levels in subacute sclerosing panencephalitis. J Child Neurol. 2007;22(3):341–3.

52. Yiğit A, Sarikaya S. Myoclonus relieved by carbamazepine in subacute sclerosing panencephalitis. Epileptic Disord. 2006;8(1):77–80.

53. Schimmel M, Penzien J. Improvement of SSPE after carbamazepine: natural course or therapeutic effect? Neuropediatrics. 2010;41:1380.

54. Ravikumar S, Crawford JR. Role of carbamazepine in the symptomatic treatment of subacute sclerosing panencephalitis: a case report and review of the literature. Case Rep Neurol Med. 2013;2013:327647.

55. Becker D, Patel A, Abou-Khalil BW, Pina-Garza JE. Successful treatment ofencephalopathy and myoclonus with levetiracetam in a case of subacute sclerosing panencephalitis. J Child Neurol. 2009;24(6):763–7.

56. Centers for Disease Control and Prevention (CDC). Progress in implementing measles mortality reduction strategies—India, 2010–2011. MMWR Morb Mortal Wkly Rep. 2011;60(38):1315–9.

Brain Abscess

9

A. Shobhana

Case Scenario

A 35-year-old male was admitted with complaints of intermittent headache of 1 year duration. He had suffered two episodes of generalized tonic-clonic convulsion twice, few days prior to admission. He had no known medical co-morbidities at the time of admission. He was conscious but somewhat confused with a left hemiparesis (upper limb 0/5; lower limb 3/5). He was afebrile with blood pressure of 110/74 mmHg and pulse of 88/min. Initial CT scan of the brain was suggestive of a right frontal space-occupying lesion (SOL) with surrounding edema. Routine blood parameters including TC WBC, renal, liver function tests, and C-reactive protein (CRP) were normal. Contrast MRI of the brain (Fig. 9.1a–e) revealed a large ring-enhancing lesion in the right frontal lobe with central necrosis, surrounding edema, and mass effect suggestive of a brain abscess. A trans-thoracic echocardiography revealed a mobile mass on the tricuspid valve. Transesophageal echocardiography facility was not available. Empirical antibiotics, i.v. ceftriaxone, vancomycin, and metronidazole were started. The patient's family members denied any addictions. Since there was a lot of mass effect a right frontal craniotomy and excision of the abscess were done. Histopathology of the biopsy specimen revealed a necrotic brain abscess (Fig. 9.2a, b). Blood cultures were negative. Microbiological tests from the biopsy specimen revealed gram-positive cocci on gram stain; however, culture was negative. Unfortunately, the patient died as a result of a sudden cardiac event on the second postoperative day before any cardiac intervention could be done.

A. Shobhana (✉)
Institute of Neurosciences Kolkata, Kolkata, India

© Springer Nature Singapore Pte Ltd. 2024
K. K. Oli et al. (eds.), *Case-based Approach to Common Neurological Disorders*,
https://doi.org/10.1007/978-981-99-8676-7_9

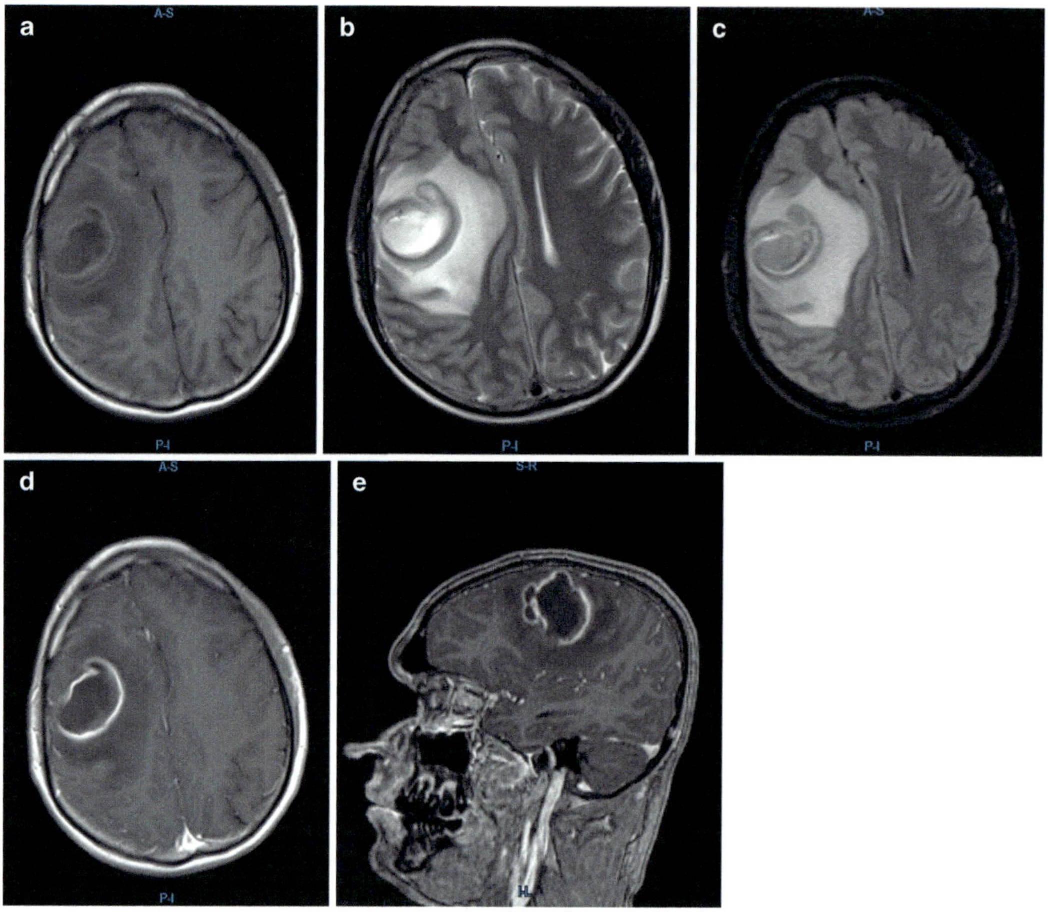

Fig. 9.1 (**a**) T1-weighted MRI image showing right frontal central hypointense lesion with surrounding hyperintense rim and perilesional hypointense area; (**b**) T2 MRI showing central hyperintense lesion with surrounding hypointense rim and outer hyperintense area; (**c**) FLAIR sequence showing central isointense mixed with hypointense lesion with surrounding hyperintense rim with outer hyperintense area; (**d**) T1 contrast sequence showing central hypointense lesion with surrounding enhanced hyperintense rim and perilesional hypointense area; (**e**) sagittal T1 contrast sequence showing additional conglomerate-enhanced lesions

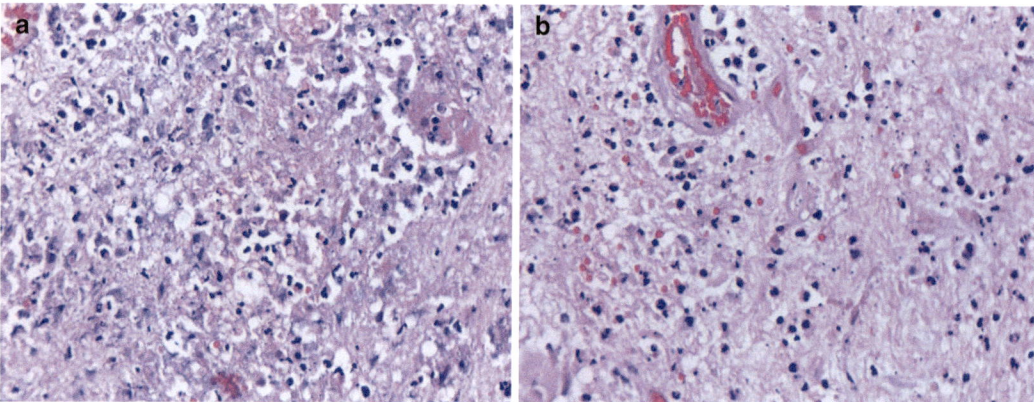

Fig. 9.2 (**a**) Biopsy specimen showing necrosis and neutrophilic infiltrates (lower resolution); (**b**) Biopsy specimen showing thick neutrophilic infiltrates along with blood vessel invasion (higher resolution)

9.1 Introduction

Central nervous system (CNS) infections may be caused by bacteria, viruses, fungi, protozoa, or helminths and are important as they should be recognized early for immediate and effective treatment to decrease the mortality and morbidity of the illness [1–3]. Focal CNS infections include brain abscess, subdural empyema, and infectious thrombophlebitis [1, 3]. The clinical features depend on the route of spread of infection, CNS location, and severity of raised intracranial pressure (ICP) [1].

A brain abscess is a focal suppurative collection within the brain parenchyma beginning as cerebritis and later surrounded by a well-defined vascularized capsule. The incidence of bacterial brain abscess is about 0.3–1.3/100,000 persons per year with a male predominance [2, 3]. Bacteria enter the brain through contiguous spread in about half of cases, through hematogenous dissemination in about one third of cases, and unknown mechanisms accounting for the remaining cases [4].

9.2 Etiology

Predisposing conditions and microbiology of brain abscesses are as given in Table 9.1 [2, 4]. In Latin America and Asia brain abscesses due to *Taenia solium*, that is, neurocysticercosis (NCC) and Mycobacteria, are quite common.

A brain abscess may develop (1) directly by spreading from a contiguous focus of infection like paranasal sinusitis, otitis media, or dental infections; (2) following a head trauma or a neurosurgical procedure; or (3) as a result of hematogenous spread from a remote site of infection. In a few cases no primary source is identified.

Table 9.1 Predisposing conditions and microbiology of brain abscesses

Predisposing condition	Common microbial isolates
Immunocompromised	
• HIV infection	• *Toxoplasma gondii*, *Nocardia* and *Mycobacterium* species, *Listeria monocytogenes*, *Cryptococcus neoformans*
• Neutropenia	• Aerobic gram-negative bacilli, A*spergillus*, *Mucorales*, *Candida*, and *Scedosporium* species
• Transplantation	• *Aspergillus*, *Candida*, *Mucorales*, *Scedosporium* Enterobacteriaceae, and *Nocardia* species, *Toxoplasma gondii*, *Mycobacterium tuberculosis*
Contiguous spread of bacteria	
• Penetrating trauma or neurosurgery	• *Staphylococcus aureus*, *Staphylococcus epidermidis*, *Streptococcus* species (anaerobic and aerobic), *Enterobacteriaceae*, *Clostridium* species
• Otitis media or mastoiditis	• *Streptococcus* species (anaerobic and aerobic), *Bacteroides*, *Prevotella*, and *Enterobacteriaceae* species
• Paranasal sinusitis	• *Streptococcus* species (anaerobic and aerobic), *Bacteroides*, *Enterobacteriaceae*, *Staphylococcus aureus*, and *Haemophilus* species
Hematogenous spread of bacteria	
• Lung abscess, empyema, bronchiectasis	• *Fusobacterium*, *Actinomyces*, *Bacteroides*, *Prevotella*, *Nocardia*, and *Streptococcus species*
• Bacterial endocarditis	• *Staphylococcus aureus*, *Streptococcus species*
• Congenital heart disease	• *Streptococcus and Haemophilus species*
• Dental infection	• *Mixed infection with Fusobacterium*, *Prevotella*, *Actinomyces*, *Bacteroides*, and *Streptococcus species (anaerobic and aerobic)*

9.3 Bacterial Brain Abscess

Streptococci (aerobic, anaerobic, microaerophilic) are grown in almost 70% of bacterial brain abscesses [2]. They are found in oropharyngeal, infective endocarditis as well as post-neurosurgery brain abscesses. *Staphylococcus aureus* (often **Methicillin-resistant Staphylococcus aureus**) is found in 10–20% cases, mainly post-trauma or infective endocarditis cases. Anaerobes like bacteroides may be isolated with better culture techniques. Enteric gram-negative organisms are often causative agents where otitis media is the source, post neurosurgery and in immunocompromised hosts. Listeria may cause abscesses along with meningitis in immunocompromised patients or those with hematological malignancies. Nocardia (most often asteroids) cause isolated brain abscess or occur along with lung and skin involvement. Although it is common in those with defective cell-mediated immunity, those on steroids, and those who have received organ transplants, many cases of normal host infection have also been reported [2]. Burkholderia are known to cause abscesses when infecting the nervous system. In the Asian population focal CNS lesions caused by Mycobacteria, both tuberculous and non-tuberculous, are quite common.

9.4 Fungal Brain Abscess

Fungal brain abscesses are more often seen now than earlier due to wider use of immunosuppressants, broad spectrum antibiotics, and corticosteroids. Candida species are more common these days with diabetic, immunosuppressed patients in hospitals as well as those on hyperalimentation and central venous catheters. Apergillosis and mucormycosis are other fungi seen in paranasal sinus infections spreading to the brain as well as in other low-immunity states. Scedosporium may cause disease even in normal hosts. Cladophialophora is another cause being increasingly reported. Cryptococcus, histoplasma, and coccidiodes are other organisms that can cause brain abscess.

9.5 Protozoal and Helminthic Brain Abscess

NCC is the most common parasitic disease of the CNS especially in developing countries. It usually manifests as a new-onset partial seizure with or without secondary generalization [2, 3]. The disease is caused by ingestion of food contaminated with eggs of the parasite *Taenia solium*. Toxoplasma gondii is the most common protozoa causing brain abscess due to ingestion of undercooked meat or handling of cat feces [3]. Primary infection is often asymptomatic; however, parasites may spread to the CNS in a latent phase. Reactivation of this phase occurs in immunocompromised hosts, for example in HIV infections, immunosuppressive therapy, or cytotoxic therapy or due to reticuloendothelial malignances [2, 3] manifesting as intracranial mass lesion or encephalitis. *Trypanosoma cruzi, Entamoeba histolytica*, Schistosoma spp., and Paragonimus spp. have all been reported to cause brain abscesses [2].

9.6 Mycobacterial Abscesses

Abscesses may form following tuberculous meningitis and tuberculoma formation when there is central cavitation with chronic inflammatory infiltrate and fibrosis in the wall but lacking granulation tissue in the wall [5]. Treatment of extrapulmonary tuberculosis has to be patient-centered, and where accessible a tissue-based diagnosis is recommended [6].

9.7 Pathogenesis and Pathophysiology

About 30–40% of brain abscesses are spread from otitis media and mastoiditis [2, 3] and localize most often to the temporal lobe or cerebellum. The frontal lobe is often affected in paranasal sinusitis. Hematogenously spread abscesses are often located in the territory of the middle cerebral artery in the posterior frontal or parietal lobe at the junction of the gray and white matter. Brain abscess also occurs secondary to open cranial fractures due to trauma with dural breach. CSF leak is the third common cause. Nosocomial brain abscesses after neurosurgery are also encountered. It is cryptogenic in 10–15% cases.

Once the organism invades the otherwise resistant brain parenchyma the infection passes through the stages of development depending upon the infecting organism and the host immune status [1, 3]. The different stages of abscess formation are as follows:

1. **Early cerebritis stage** (days 1–4)
   Perivascular infiltration of inflammatory cells with a core of necrosis and marked edema.
2. **Late cerebritis stage** (days 4–9)
   Pus formation; enlargement of necrotic center surrounded by a border of macrophages and fibroblasts.
3. **Early capsule formation** (day 10–13)
   The capsule is formed better in the cortical side than the ventricular side, making rupture into the ventricular system more common than into the subarachnoid space.
4. **Late capsule formation** (>14 days)
   There is a dense necrotic center surrounded by a dense collagenous capsule which is again surrounded by edema that later decreases, but marked gliosis develops.

features of raised intracranial pressure. Management is seen only when the abscess ruptures into the ventricles or the infection has spread to the subarachnoid space. The clinical features in an immunosuppressed patient may be masked due to diminished inflammatory response [2].

Frontal lobe lesions present with headache, drowsiness, inattention, hemiparesis, and motor speech defects, while temporal lobe lesions present with ipsilateral headache and aphasia if in the dominant hemisphere or upper homonymous quadrantanopia. Cerebellar lesions present with ataxia, nystagmus, dysmetria, and vomiting. Brian stem lesions may have cranial nerve involvement like facial weakness. These lesions often spread longitudinally along the tracts rather than transversely.

Some organisms have peculiar manifestations like Nocardial disease suspected in the presence of pulmonary, skin, or muscle involvement. Aspergillosis may present as a stroke syndrome. Tuberculosis may have multisystem involvement. Rhinocerebral mucormycosis may initially present with complaints referable to the eyes or sinuses, necrotic nasal turbinates, or involvement of hard palate [2]. CNS toxoplasmosis in immunosuppressed patients may have variable features like focal seizures, altered behavior, confused state, or symptoms localizing to the basal ganglia or brain stem regions.

9.8 Clinical Presentation

A brain abscess may present in an indolent or fulminant manner. Most of them clinically present like an intracranial space-occupying lesion depending on the location rather than as an infection [2, 3]. The classical triad of headache, fever, and focal neurological deficit is found in less than half of these patients [2]. Headache is the most common symptom in >75% cases. Focal or generalized defects which are new in onset are seen in 15–20% patients. Focal neurological defects like hemiparesis, aphasias, or visual field deficits are seen in >60% cases. Papilledema, nausea, vomiting, drowsiness, and altered sensorium are

9.9 Diagnosis

Diagnosis may be difficult and a multidisciplinary approach involving neurosurgeons, microbiologists, and infectious disease experts is usually required. Histopathological and microbiological examinations including studies for bacteria, Mycobacteria, and fungi often become mandatory in evolving intracerebral mass lesions. Although a contrast-enhanced CT scan is an excellent initial examination showing a hypodense center with peripheral uniform ring enhancement (early cerebritis phase shows hypodensity with no contrast enhancement), MRI is better in the early stages, in posterior fossa lesions and to pick up satellite lesions. In the cerebritis stage, MRI T1 sequences show low signal intensity with irregular post-gadolinium enhancement with increased signal intensity on T2. A mature abscess reveals a contrast-enhanced capsule surrounding a hypodense center itself surrounded by a hypodense area of edema on post-contrast T1 images. The T2 image shows a hyperintense central area of pus surrounded by a well-defined hypointense capsule and hyperintense area of surrounding edema. The features of the capsule may be altered with glucocorticoid therapy. Diffusion-weighted imaging sequence is done to differentiate abscess from other lesions as abscesses show restricted diffusion. Magnetic resonance spectroscopy has limited scope in small, peripheral, or skull base lesions. Sometimes MRI findings may help to pinpoint the etiology as well. Presence of infarcts may indicate aspergillosis while immunosuppressed patients may not show contrast enhancement in aspergillosis. Presence of sinus opacification, bone erosion, obliteration of facial planes, or cavernous sinus involvement in CT/MRI may indicate rhinocerebral mucormycosis. Toxoplasmosis typically is present in the corticomedullary junction and basal ganglia and shows marked edema as well as mass effect. Neurocysticercosis has variable findings on brain imaging [3]. Viable cysts will show an acystic area with scolex with contrast enhancement and surrounding edema. Nonviable cysts are calcified. CT guided aspiration or biopsy of abscesses is often possible.

Microbiological diagnosis of the etiology is most accurately determined by gram stain and culture (both aerobic and anaerobic) of the abscess material. Blood cultures should be sent. Lumbar puncture for CSF study should not be done in suspected focal intracranial SOL. For mycobacterial organisms, ZN stain of pus, culture, and Mycobacterium tuberculosis PCR are important. Modified AFB stain and culture may isolate Nocardia. Toxoplasmosis is diagnosed by CSF PCR for toxoplasma antigen; serum toxoplasma IgG if positive is more suggestive [2, 3]. Multiple 16S ribosomal DNA sequencing has increased the yield of infecting agents [2]. Other special stains used are methenamine silver and mucicarmine. Aspergillus has septated hyphae which branch at acute angles while mucormycosis has irregular hyphae branching at right angles with lack of septation [2]. For CNS toxoplasmosis special stains as well as monoclonal antibodies in brain tissue preparations are available [2].

Other ancillary tests like total white cell count, erythrocyte sedimentation rate, and CRP provide more information. For abscesses more than 2.5 cm in diameter, excision or stereotactic aspiration should be done.

9.10 Differential Diagnosis

1. Cerebral hematoma
2. Primary and metastatic brain tumors
3. Cerebral venous (superior sagittal sinus) thrombosis
4. Subdural empyema
5. Meningitis and meningoencephalitis
6. Acute disseminated encephalomyelitis

9.11 Treatment

Apart from the general supportive care, empirical antimicrobials should be started as soon as possible based on the patient's predisposing conditions pending microbiology reports. The choice of antibiotics as well as dosage are illustrated in Tables 9.2 and 9.3.

In case of significant edema or mass effect corticosteroids are administered. Antiepileptics are added for at least 3 months and can be stopped if a follow-up EEG is normal. A minimum of 6–8 weeks of parenteral antibiotics are given. Continuation of oral antibiotics is debatable [3].

Table 9.2 Selection of antibiotics

Indication	Antibiotic
Preterm infants to infants <1 month	Ampicillin + cefotaxime
Infants 1–3 months	Ampicillin + cefotaxime or ceftriaxone
Immunocompetent children >3 months and adults <55	Cefotaxime, ceftriaxone, or cefepime + vancomycin
Adults >55 and adults of any age with alcoholism or other debilitating illnesses	Ampicillin + cefotaxime, ceftriaxone or cefepime + vancomycin
Hospital-acquired meningitis, posttraumatic or postneurosurgery meningitis, neutropenic patients, or patients with impaired cell-mediated immunity	Ampicillin + ceftazidime or meropenem + vancomycin

Table 9.3 Total daily dose and dosing interval

Antimicrobial agent	Child	Adult
Ampicillin	300 (mg/kg)/d, q6h	12 g/d, q4h
Cefepime	150 (mg/kg)/d, q8h	6 g/d, q8h
Cefotaxime	225–300 (mg/kg)/d, q6h	12 g/d, q4h
Ceftriaxone	100 (mg/kg)/d, q12h	4 g/d, q12h
Ceftazidime	150 (mg/kg)/d, q8h	6 g/d, q8h
Gentamicin	7.5 (mg/kg)/d, q8hb	7.5 (mg/kg)/d, q8h
Meropenem	120 (mg/kg)/d, q8h	6 g/d, q8h
Metronidazole	30 (mg/kg)/d, q6h	1500–2000 mg/d, q6h
Nafcillin	100–200 (mg/kg)/d, q6h	9–12 g/d, q4h
Penicillin G	400,000 (U/kg)/d, q4h	20–24 million U/d, q4h
Vancomycin	45–60 (mg/kg)/d, q6h	45–60 (mg/kg)d, q6–12hb

Some abscesses, especially multiple ones, may require surgical drainage. Serial MRI/CT are needed every 1 or 2 months to document resolution of disease. A small amount of enhancement may remain even after successful treatment [3].

Prognosis depends upon the rapidity of progression of disease and low GCS on admission, and the fact that immunosuppressed individuals have an uncertain outcome must be taken into account. Mortality has decreased substantially due to better diagnostics procedures and availability of newer antibiotics [2, 3]. Twenty to seventy percent of patients may have one or more sequel-like seizures, or cognitive defects underscoring the importance of early as well as accurate diagnosis and appropriate management.

References

1. Tunkel AR. Approach to the patient with central nervous system infection. In: Mandell GL, Bennett JE, Dolin R, editors. Mandell, Douglas, and Bennet's principles and practice of infectious diseases, vol. 1. Philadelphia: Churchill Livingstone (Elsevier); 2010. p. 1183–8.
2. Tunkel AR. Brain abscess. In: Mandell GL, Bennett JE, Dolin R, editors. Mandell, Douglas, and Bennet's principles and practice of infectious diseases, vol. 1. Philadelphia: Churchill Livingstone (Elsevier); 2010. p. 1265–78.
3. Roos KL, Tyler KL. Meningitis, encephalitis, brain abscess, and empyema. In: Kasper DL, Fauci AS, Hauser SL, Longo DL, Jameson JL, Loscalzo J, editors. Harrison's principles of internal medicine, vol. 2. McGraw Hill; 2015. p. 883–905.
4. Brouwer CM, Tunkel AR, McKhann GM II, van de Beek D. Brain abscess. N Engl J Med. 2014;371:447–56.
5. Modi M, Prabhakar S, Gupta K, Vasishta RK, Ahuja C, Khandelwal N, Kajsekhar V. CNS tuberculomas. In: Chopra JS, Sawhney IMS, editors. Neurology in tropics. Elsevier; 2016. p. 206–21.
6. Index-TB Guidelines—Guidelines on extrapulmonary tuberculosis for India. From Central TB Division, Ministry of Health and Family Welfare, Govt Of India.

Part II

Cardiovascular Disorders

Acute Ischemic Stroke

10

Deependra Raj Khanal

Case Discussion

A 62-year-old right-handed male with a history of hypertension (on lisinopril) presented with acute left-sided weakness. He was seen in his usual state of health at 8 am. His wife heard a noise at 10 am. He was unable to stand up and could not move his left side. Family brought him to the local emergency department 3 h after symptom onset. During assessment, he had left hemiparesis, left facial droop, dysarthria, left hemi-neglect, and right gaze preference. He did not have any evidence of aphasia. His National Institute of Health Stroke Scale (NIHSS) was 12. Computerized tomography (CT) scan of head showed no hemorrhage. Computerized tomography angiography (CTA) of head showed an abrupt cutoff at the onset of anterior division of right middle cerebral artery (commonly referred as right anterior M2 branch). CTA neck showed about 80% stenosis of right internal carotid artery (ICA).

After completion of neurological examination (including NIHSS), we went through exclusion criteria for tissue plasminogen activator (t-PA). He had no contraindications. t-PA treatment was started 4 h 15 min after symptom onset. He was then taken from emergency department to interventional radiology suite for catheter-directed endovascular therapy. Clot was identified, and retrieval was attempted but was unsuccessful. The patient was then admitted to the neurological intensive care unit for post-thrombolysis monitoring. Follow-up CT of the head showed mild hypodensity in the right anterior middle cerebral artery territory (Fig. 10.1). No hemorrhage was seen. His workup revealed mild left ventricular

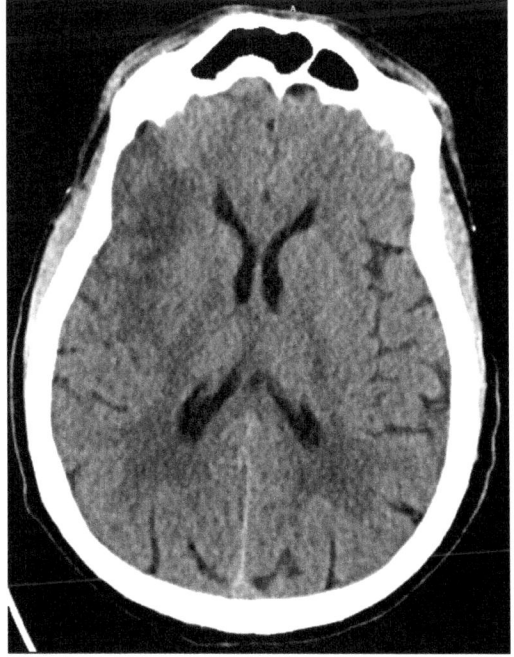

Fig. 10.1 Non-contrast CT head. Subtle hypodensity seen in the anterior division of right middle cerebral artery territory

D. R. Khanal (✉)
Neurology Critical Care, Regional Hospital, Health Partners, St. Paul, MN, USA
e-mail: Deependra.R.Khanal@HealthPartners.Com

© Springer Nature Singapore Pte Ltd. 2024
K. K. Oli et al. (eds.), *Case-based Approach to Common Neurological Disorders*,
https://doi.org/10.1007/978-981-99-8676-7_10

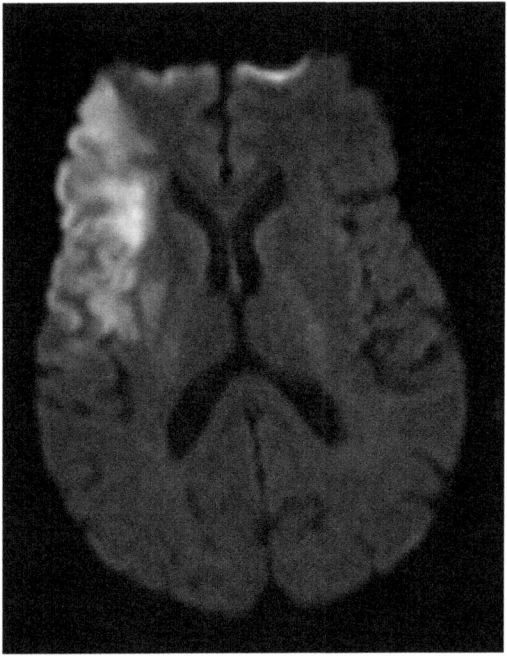

Fig. 10.2 Diffusion weight imaging (DWI) MRI sequence. Axial image. Brightness seen in the anterior division of right middle cerebral artery territory

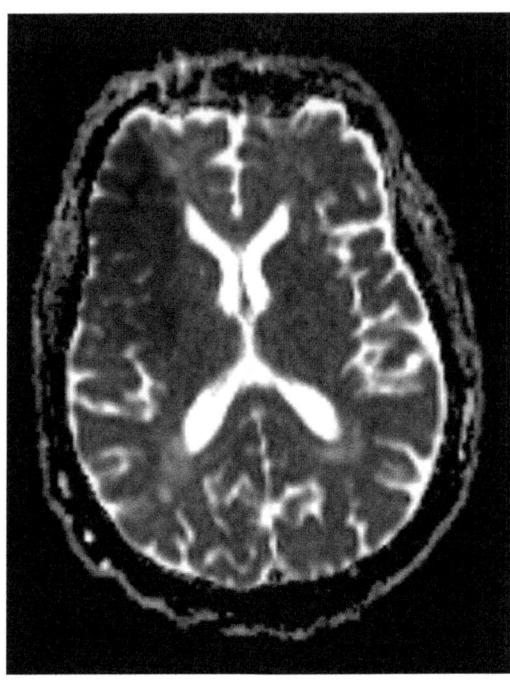

Fig. 10.3 Apparent diffusion coefficient (ADC) MRI sequence. Axial image. Darkness seen in the anterior division of right middle cerebral artery territory

hypertrophy on echocardiogram. No wall motion abnormality was found. Agitated saline contrast did not reveal intra-cardiac shunt. The 48-h telemetry did not show any evidence of atrial fibrillation. Conventional cerebral angiogram showed 80% stenosis of right internal carotid artery. This correlated with earlier CTA study. His LDL cholesterol was 121. He was started on high-dose statin (atorvastatin 80 mg daily) along with aspirin 325 mg daily. Magnetic resonance imaging (MRI) was done to look at the extent of stroke. Figure 10.2 shows a diffusion-weighted image (DWI). It is seen bright in acute stroke. Figure 10.3 shows apparent diffusion coefficient (ADC) image. It is seen dark in cytotoxic stroke (seen in ischemic stroke—as seen in our case) and bright in vasogenic stroke (usually seen in edema around brain tumor). Additional MRI image was thought to help evaluate the extent of infarct and therefore the timing of carotid revascularization. He clinically improved during the hospital stay and was discharged home with minimal weakness on his left hand. He was successfully treated with right carotid endarterectomy 10 days after the event.

10.1 Introduction

Stroke is defined as an acute neurological dysfunction due to disturbances in the blood supply to the brain. It is broadly categorized into ischemic and hemorrhagic strokes. Ischemic stroke is caused by the occlusion of a blood vessel, leading to distal ischemia. Closely related to ischemic stroke is transient ischemic stroke (TIA), which is mechanistic but resolves clinically on its own. TIA is a major risk factor for a stroke. Symptoms of stroke are immediate and involve weakness, numbness, and speech disturbance (slurred speech and difficulty in comprehension and/or expression). Symptoms correspond to the area of the brain supplied by the occluded blood vessel. Knowledge that a stroke causes acute neurological symptoms and information about vascular territory and corresponding symptoms help to suspect a diagnosis of stroke. This leads to timely workup and treatment.

Stroke is broadly categorized into ischemic and hemorrhagic strokes. Ischemic stroke is caused by an obstruction of blood flow, while hemorrhagic stroke is caused by bleeding and subsequent compression of the surrounding brain structures. Ischemic stroke accounts for about 87% of all strokes in developed countries, while it is slightly less at 68% in developing countries [1*, 2].

10.2 Epidemiology

Stroke is the second leading cause of death and third leading cause of disability worldwide [3]. This statistic is slightly different in developing and developed countries. In the United States, stroke became the fifth leading cause of death from fourth leading cause in 2013. Burden of stroke is estimated to be 34 billion USD in the United States. Stroke incidence is different among different ethnic groups. Incidence among blacks is twice compared to whites. Stroke is still a major cause of serious disability for adults [1, 4, 5*]. Disability related to stroke is not only limited to paralysis and speech difficulty. It is also an important cause of dementia, seizure, and depression [6]. Stroke incidence is decreasing in developed countries due to proper management of risk factors. It is, however, increasing in developing countries [7]. The lifetime risk of stroke for adult men and women (25 years of age and older) is approximately 25%. The highest risk of stroke is found in East Asia, Central Europe, and Eastern Europe [3]. On average, stroke occurs 15 years earlier and causes more deaths in low- and middle-income countries when compared to those in high-income countries [6*].

10.3 Risk Factors

Stroke risk factors are similar to other risk factors for vascular events, including ischemic heart disease and peripheral vascular disease. They include modifiable and non-modifiable risk factors. Modifiable risk factors include hypertension, dyslipidemia, diabetes mellitus, cigarette smoking, alcohol consumption, physical inactivity, diet, and obesity.

About 90% of the stroke risk could be attributed to modifiable risk factors (such as high blood pressure, obesity, hyperglycemia, hyperlipidemia, and renal dysfunction), and 74% could be attributed to behavioral risk factors, such as smoking, sedentary lifestyle, and an unhealthy diet. Globally, 29% of the risk of stroke is attributable to air pollution. Although global age-adjusted mortality rates for ischemic and hemorrhagic strokes decreased between 1990 and 2015, the absolute number of people who have strokes annually, as well as related deaths and disability-adjusted life-years lost, increased. The majority of global stroke burden is in low- and middle-income countries, as stated above in Sect. 10.2 [8*].

Hypertension is the single most important modifiable risk factor for ischemic as well as hemorrhagic strokes. Studies have consistently shown a linear relationship between blood pressure and stroke risk. In some studies, 10 mm reduction in blood pressure is associated with a 33% reduction in stroke risk [9]. In Secondary Prevention of Small Subcortical Strokes (SPS3) trial, systolic BP of less than 130 is likely associated with decrease in recurrent stroke {hazard ratio 0.81, 95% CI 0.64–1.03, $p = 0.08$} [10]. Hypertension is also responsible for silent cerebrovascular events, which in turn lead to diseases like vascular dementia [11].

Dyslipidemia is another risk factor for stroke. While the association between high cholesterol and coronary artery disease and peripheral vascular disease is well established, the relationship between high cholesterol and stroke is less clear [11]. In a prospective study that compared cases of ischemic stroke and hemorrhagic stroke with controls, elevated total cholesterol and lower high-density lipoprotein (HDL) levels were associated with an increased risk of ischemic stroke, especially for large-artery atherosclerotic and lacunar stroke subtypes [12].

In a randomized trial named SPARCL (Stroke Prevention by Aggressive Reduction of Cholesterol Levels), high-dose statin (e.g., atorvastatin 80 mg) was associated with 16% relative risk reduction in stroke incidence. Those achieving 50% reduction in low-density lipoprotein (LDL) cholesterol level had 38% relative risk reduction [13].

Atrial fibrillation is the most common cause of cardioembolic stroke [14]. Identification of atrial fibrillation (either permanent or paroxysmal) is important, as it is amenable to treatment with anticoagulation [15]. Other cardiac risk factors include myocardial infarction, left ventricular dysfunction, valvular disease, left ventricular thrombus, atrial septal defects, and complex atheroma in the ascending aorta or proximal arch.

Other medical conditions that lead to hypercoagulability also increase the risk of stroke. These include the following:

- Antiphospholipid antibody syndrome
- Protein C deficiency
- Protein S deficiency
- Antithrombin deficiency
- Activated protein C resistance
- Factor V Leiden as a cause of activated protein C resistance
- Prothrombin G20210A mutation
- Methylenetetrahydrofolate reductase (MTHFR) mutations associated with hyperhomocysteinemia [16]

10.4   Clinical Features

A hallmark of stroke is the sudden onset of neurological deficits. Ischemic stroke causes symptoms almost immediately. Hemorrhagic stroke symptoms are also sudden onset but may progress over time if bleeding is slow. Some intracranial hemorrhages like epidural hematoma produces initial symptom followed by a lucid interval and a progressive neurological deficit related to hematoma expansion. Clinical symptoms associated with stroke correspond to the area of the brain affected. Most common symptoms include weakness, numbness, facial droop, and speech difficulty. FAST (facial droop, arm weakness, speech difficulties, and time to call emergency services) acronym is commonly used to educate the general public about the symptoms

of stroke. Hemiplegia is usually the most common sign of cerebrovascular disease, whether in the cerebral hemisphere or the brainstem. Other stroke symptoms include numbness, aphasia, dysarthria, dizziness, diplopia, and symptoms related to particular cranial nerve if that is affected by stroke. These symptoms could present either in isolation or in combination. Sometimes, stroke in a particular brain area produces well-recognized clinical syndromes.

Some of the well-known clinical syndromes caused by ischemic stroke include the following:

Name of syndrome	Symptoms	Area of brain affected
Weber syndrome	Oculomotor palsy with crossed hemiplegia	Base of midbrain
Claude syndrome	Ipsilateral oculomotor nerve palsy, contralateral hemiparesis, contralateral ataxia	Oculomotor nerve, red nucleus, and brachium conjunctivum
Miller-Gubler syndrome	Ipsilateral palsy of CN VI and VII with contralateral hemiplegia	Ventral pons
Locked-in syndrome	Limb paralysis and loss of speech with retained consciousness, alertness, and cognition	Ventral pons affecting corticospinal, corticopontine, and corticobulbar tracts
Perinaud's syndrome	Upward gaze palsy	Compression of the vertical gaze center at the rostral interstitial nucleus of medial longitudinal fasciculus
Wallenberg syndrome	Sensory deficits contralateral to lesion in trunk and extremities and ipsilateral to the lesion in face and cranial nerves	Lateral medulla in the brainstem
Alexia without agraphia	Can write, but not read	Left occipital lobe and extend to the splenium of the corpus callosum

10.5   Diagnosis

Suspicion that the presenting symptom is related to stroke is the first step in diverting the diagnostic pathway in an accurate direction. Sudden onset of neurological deficit is the core feature of acute ischemic stroke. During the evaluation of stroke, it is important to keep in mind other differential diagnoses that could potentially produce similar symptoms.

Differential diagnosis of acute ischemic stroke includes the following:

- Other stroke types including intracranial hemorrhage and cerebral venous sinus thrombosis
- Seizure
- Encephalitis
- CNS infection including brain abscess
- Brain tumor
- Transient global amnesia
- Wernicke's encephalopathy

Immediate non-contrast head CT is the most important diagnostic test in patients who present with focal neurological deficit. It rules out intracranial hemorrhage and is an adequate radiological test before starting intravenous reperfusion therapy with t-PA. Additional diagnostic tests could be considered. They include CT angiograms of the head and neck. This will help to show vascular occlusion, critical stenosis, or vessel dissection. This is needed before considering interventional procedures for the treatment of stroke. CT perfusion or magnetic resonance (MR) perfusion could be done to find out the ratio of infarcted core to penumbra. This is mostly useful in patients who present as a wake-up stroke or when the last known normal time is unknown. Some of the acute stroke treatment recommendations are based on the perfusion results [17, 18]. Other diagnostic consideration is MRI. MRI is very sensitive for the identification of an acute stroke. However, it is expensive, takes time, and is not widely available in all hospitals. A conventional cerebral angiogram rarely has diagnostic value in acute ischemic stroke. However, it is considered when therapeutic intervention is contemplated. Other essential tests include fingerstick glucose and oxygen saturation, which are usually performed during the initial evaluation. International normalized ratio (INR) and electrocardiogram (EKG) are recommended but are not essential before treatment is initiated. Platelet count and INR should always be drawn before starting t-PA. However, it is not recommended that we wait for results in patients not suspected to have coagulopathy. It is a common practice to stop t-PA infusion after it is started if the results of INR and platelet count come unexpected.

Ecarin clotting time, thrombin time, or appropriate direct factor Xa activity assay are not usually done but could be considered in special circumstances. They could be useful if it is known or suspected that the patient is taking a direct thrombin inhibitor or a direct factor Xa inhibitor and is a candidate for thrombolytic therapy with t-PA. However, it is not essential before thrombolytic therapy is started unless the patient is on an anticoagulant or there is a suspicion of bleeding disorders or thrombocytopenia.

10.6   Treatment

Treatment of acute ischemic stroke with reperfusion therapy started after a landmark trial in 1995 [19]. This was the first study to show benefit if t-PA is given within 3 h of symptom onset. Many stroke trials have failed before this. This study did not show any change in mortality but did show improvement in functional outcome at 3 months. In 2008, another trial showed benefit of t-PA within 4.5 h of symptom onset [20]. Currently, treatment with intravenous t-PA is recommended in patients >18 years of age with symptom onset within 4.5 h. Treatment with t-PA involves significant risks. The most feared complication of this treatment is intracranial hemorrhage, some of which could be fatal. In the initial trial, risk of intracranial hemorrhage was 6.4 in treatment arm vs. 0.6 in placebo group [19]. Therefore, all patients should be stringently evaluated for any risk factors that increase the chance of intracranial hemorrhage or other complications.

10.7 Exclusion Criteria for Treatment with t-PA [21*]

Onset	>3 h from symptom onset OR >4.5 h from symptoms onset (with an additional exclusion criteria[a])
CT	Evidence of hemorrhage on CT
History	1. Intracranial hemorrhage 2. Stroke or traumatic brain injury (TBI) in the last 3 months 3. Brain or spinal surgery in the last 3 months
Bleeding	Gastrointestinal or genitourinary bleeding in the last 3 months
Coagulopathy	Platelets <100,000/mm³ INR >1.7 OR or prothrombin time (PT) >15 s Activated partial thromboplastin time (aPTT) >40 s
Antithrombotic use	Treatment dose Low-molecular-weight heparin use within 24 h (prophylactic dose is not a contraindication) Factor Xa inhibitors/direct thrombin inhibitors use within 48 h OR abnormal aPTT, INR, platelet count, Ecarin clotting time, thrombin time, Xa assay

[a] Additional exclusion criteria for treatment between 3 and 4.5 h

- Age >80 years
- Oral anticoagulant use regardless of INR
- Severe stroke (NIHSS score >25)
- Combination of both previous ischemic stroke and diabetes mellitus

10.8 Special Considerations in a Select Group of Patients [21]

Stroke mimics	It is reasonable to treat with t-PA in the case of uncertainly. Risk of intracranial hemorrhage is quite low
Rapidly improving symptoms	Recommend treatment unless improved symptoms cause no disability
Seizure at the onset of stroke	Treatment is reasonable if residual symptom is likely caused by a stroke and not a seizure
Abnormal blood glucose	Treatment is reasonable if symptoms persist despite controlling glucose to 50–400 mg/dL range

Preexisting disability	Treatment is reasonable, but decisions should take into account relevant factors, including quality of life, social support, and goals of care
Menstruation	It is reasonable to treat unless the bleeding is heavy. Utero-vaginal packing could be considered to stop bleeding if necessary
Recent dural puncture	It could be considered
Brain tumor	It is "probably recommended" if tumor is extra-axial (e.g., meningioma) [21]
Unruptured brain aneurysm	If aneurysm is small or moderate-sized (<10 mm), IV t-PA is reasonable and probably recommended
Dissection	It is considered reasonably safe, and treatment is recommended
Myocardial infarction	It is probably reasonable to treat and consider additional treatment for myocardial infarction (MI). Need for heparin use after MI treatment could be an issue

10.9 Secondary Prevention of Acute Ischemic Stroke

All patients with acute ischemic stork should adapt strategies to reduce overall cardiovascular risk. They include management of the following:

- Hypertension
- Diabetes
- Obesity
- Sedentary lifestyle
- Sleep apnea

The mainstay of acute ischemic treatments includes the use of antithrombotic therapy (antiplatelets and anticoagulants) along with cholesterol-lowering drugs.

Antiplatelet Therapy All antiplatelet therapy irreversibly inhibits platelet function. After exposure to an antiplatelet medication, platelet aggregation is reduced for the remainder of platelet's lifespan (~7–10 days). Multiple researches have proven the efficacy of antiplatelet therapy in the prevention of acute ischemic stroke. Aspirin

75–325 mg has been used in most of the research studies [22]. The International Stroke Trial and Chinese Acute Stroke Trial are two of the largest trials to study the effect of aspirin in the prevention of ischemic stroke [23, 24].

Clopidogrel 75 mg daily and a combination of dipyridamole 200 mg + aspirin 25 mg are other alternatives. Multiple studies have compared different antiplatelet agents. Although some studies revealed the superiority of clopidogrel or dipyridamole 200 mg + aspirin 25 mg over aspirin, the majority of studies showed similar efficacy [25].

Reasonable alternative therapies to aspirin include:

1. Clopidogrel 75 mg daily
2. Dipyridamole 200 mg + aspirin 25 mg
3. Dual antiplatelet therapy (short-term dual antiplatelet therapy is reasonable in high-risk TIA or stroke patients who were on monotherapy at the time of stroke onset)

Anticoagulants Use of warfarin or other similar medication is recommended in patients with atrial fibrillation. This is proven in multiple clinical trials and their meta-analyses [26]. Reasonable alternatives to warfarin are:

1. Heparin (unfractionated or low molecular weight)—intravenous or subcutaneous
2. Direct thrombin inhibitors (e.g., dabigatran)—oral
3. Factor Xa inhibitors (e.g., apixaban, rivaroxaban)—oral

Surgical Treatments for Secondary Prevention of Stroke Patients with carotid stenosis benefit from revascularization with either carotid endarterectomy (CEA) or carotid stent placement. It was demonstrated by North American Symptomatic Carotid Endarterectomy Trial (NASCET) in 1991 [27*]. It was initially studied in patients with >70% stenosis. Another trial called European Carotid Surgery Trial (ECST) again showed the benefit of surgery in patients with high-grade stenosis [28]. Veterans Affairs trial also proved efficacy of surgery. In a pooled

analysis of above three trials, it was found that patients with lesser degree of stenosis also benefited from surgery. Number needed to treat (NNT) to prevent one stroke over 5 years for patients with >70% stenosis was 6.3, while NNT for patients with 50–70% stenosis was 22 [29]. Currently it is widely accepted to treat patients with >50% carotid stenosis on symptomatic side. Treatment of asymptomatic carotid stenosis is less clear. Carotid artery stenting is another reasonable alternative to CEA. In 2010, endarterectomy compared to stenting in the treatment of carotid artery stenosis (CREST) trial was published. It showed that among patients with carotid stenosis, stenting and CEA were associated with similar rates of stroke, MI, and death, although stenting was associated with fewer peri-procedural MIs and endarterectomy with fewer peri-procedural strokes [30].

In patients >50 years with cryptogenic non-lacunar stroke and patent foramen ovale (PFO), closure of PFO could be considered. Thorough evaluation should be undertaken to rule out cariogenic causes, including long-term (unto 30 days) cardiac rhythm evaluation [31].

Left atrial appendage occlusion with a device (e.g., WATCHAMN) could be considered in certain patients with atrial fibrillation who cannot tolerate anticoagulation [32].

References

1. Benjamin EJ, Blaha MJ, Chiuve SE, et al. Heart disease and stroke statistics-2017 update: a report from the American Heart Association. Circulation. 2017;135:e146.
2. Krishnamurthi RV, Feigin VL, Forouzanfar MH, et al. Global and regional burden of first-ever ischaemic and haemorrhagic stroke during 1990–2010: findings from the Global Burden of Disease Study 2010. Lancet Glob Health. 2013;1:e259.
3. Lozano R, Naghavi M, Foreman K, et al. Global and regional mortality from 235 causes of death for 20 age groups in 1990 and 2010: a systematic analysis for the Global Burden of Disease Study 2010. Lancet. 2012;380(9859):2095–128.
4. Kochanek KD, Xu JQ, Murphy SL, Arias E. Mortality in the United States, 2013. NCHS Data Brief, No. 178. National Center for Health Statistics, Centers

for Disease Control and Prevention, Department of Health and Human Services: Hyattsville, MD; 2014.

5. Mozzafarian D, Benjamin EJ, Go AS, Arnett DK, Blaha MJ, Cushman M, et al., on behalf of the American Heart Association Statistics Committee and Stroke Statistics Subcommittee. Heart disease and stroke statistics—2016 update: a report from the American Heart Association. Circulation. 2016;133(4):e38–360.

6. Owolabi MO, Akarolo-anthony S, Akinyemi R, et al. The burden of stroke in Africa: a glance at the present and a glimpse into the future. Cardiovasc J Afr. 2015;26(2 Suppl 1):S27–38.

7. Feigin VL, Forouzanfar MH, Krishnamurthi R, et al. Global and regional burden of stroke during 1990–2010: findings from the Global Burden of Disease Study 2010. Lancet. 2014;383(9913):245–54.

8. Benjamin EJ, Muntner P, Alonso A, et al. Heart disease and stroke statistics-2019 update: a report from the American Heart Association. Circulation. 2019;139(10):e56–66.

9. Lawes CM, Bennett DA, Feigin VL, Rodgers A. Blood pressure and stroke: an overview of published reviews. Stroke. 2004;35(3):776–85.

10. Benavente OR, Coffey CS, Conwit R, et al. Blood-pressure targets in patients with recent lacunar stroke: the SPS3 randomised trial. Lancet. 2013;382(9891):507–15.

11. Prabhakaran S, Wright CB, Yoshita M, et al. Prevalence and determinants of subclinical brain infarction: the Northern Manhattan Study. Neurology. 2008;70(6):425–30.

12. Tirschwell DL, Smith NL, Heckbert SR, Lemaitre RN, Longstreth WT, Psaty BM. Association of cholesterol with stroke risk varies in stroke subtypes and patient subgroups. Neurology. 2004;63(10):1868–75.

13. Castilla-guerra L, Fernandez-moreno MDC, Leon-jimenez D, Rico-corral MA. Statins in ischemic stroke prevention: what have we learned in the post-SPARCL (the stroke prevention by aggressive reduction in cholesterol levels) decade? Curr Treat Options Neurol. 2019;21(5):22.

14. Hart RG, Pearce LA, Miller VT, et al. Cardioembolic vs. noncardioembolic strokes in atrial fibrillation: frequency and effect of antithrombotic agents in the stroke prevention in atrial fibrillation studies. Cerebrovasc Dis. 2000;10(1):39–43.

15. Stroke Prevention in Atrial Fibrillation Study. Final results. Circulation. 1991;84(2):527–39.

16. Levine SR. Hypercoagulable states and stroke: a selective review. CNS Spectr. 2005;10(7):567–78.

17. Nogueira RG, Jadhav AP, Haussen DC, et al. Thrombectomy 6 to 24 hours after stroke with a mismatch between deficit and infarct. N Engl J Med. 2018;378(1):11–21.

18. Albers GW, Lansberg MG, Kemp S, et al. A multicenter randomized controlled trial of endovascular therapy following imaging evaluation for ischemic stroke (DEFUSE 3). Int J Stroke. 2017;12(8):896–905.

19. Tissue plasminogen activator for acute ischemic stroke. N Engl J Med. 1995;333(24):1581–7.

20. Hacke W, Kaste M, Bluhmki E, et al. Thrombolysis with alteplase 3 to 4.5 hours after acute ischemic stroke. N Engl J Med. 2008;359(13):1317–29.

21. Powers WJ, Rabinstein AA. Response by Powers and Rabinstein to letter regarding article, "2018 guidelines for the early management of patients with acute ischemic stroke: a guideline for healthcare professionals from the American Heart Association/American Stroke Association". Stroke. 2019;50(9):e277–8.

22. Guyatt GH, Akl EA, Crowther M, Gutterman DD, Schünemann HJ. Executive summary: Antithrombotic therapy and prevention of thrombosis, 9th ed: American College of Chest Physicians Evidence-Based Clinical Practice Guidelines. Chest. 2012;141(2 Suppl):7S–47S.

23. International Stroke Trial Collaborative Group. The International Stroke Trial (IST): a randomised trial of aspirin, subcutaneous heparin, both, or neither among 19435 patients with acute ischaemic stroke. Lancet. 1997;349(9065):1569–81.

24. CAST (Chinese Acute Stroke Trial) Collaborative Group. CAST: randomised placebo-controlled trial of early aspirin use in 20,000 patients with acute ischaemic stroke. Lancet. 1997;349(9066):1641–9.

25. CAPRIE Steering Committee. A randomised, blinded, trial of clopidogrel versus aspirin in patients at risk of ischaemic events (CAPRIE). Lancet. 1996;348(9038):1329–39.

26. Hart RG, Pearce LA, Aguilar MI. Meta-analysis: antithrombotic therapy to prevent stroke in patients who have nonvalvular atrial fibrillation. Ann Intern Med. 2007;146(12):857–67.

27. North American Symptomatic Carotid Endarterectomy Trial. Methods, patient characteristics, and progress. Stroke. 1991;22(6):711–20.

28. European Carotid Surgery Trialists' Collaborative Group. MRC European Carotid Surgery Trial: interim results for symptomatic patients with severe (70–99%) or with mild (0–29%) carotid stenosis. Lancet. 1991;337(8752):1235–43.

29. Rothwell PM, Eliasziw M, Gutnikov SA, et al. Analysis of pooled data from the randomised controlled trials of endarterectomy for symptomatic carotid stenosis. Lancet. 2003;361(9352):107–16.

30. Brott TG, Hobson RW, Howard G, et al. Stenting versus endarterectomy for treatment of carotid-artery stenosis. N Engl J Med. 2010;363(1):11–23.

31. Shah R, Nayyar M, Jovin IS, et al. Device closure versus medical therapy alone for patent foramen ovale in patients with cryptogenic stroke: a systematic review and meta-analysis. Ann Intern Med. 2018;168(5):335–42.

32. Whang W, Holmes DR, Miller MA, et al. Does left atrial appendage closure reduce mortality? A vital status analysis of the randomized PROTECT AF and PREVAIL clinical trials. J Atr Fibrillation. 2018;11(4):2119.

Subarachnoid Hemorrhage

11

Prakash Kafle, S. Vignesh, Sabin Bhandari, and Gentle Sunder Shrestha

Case Scenario

A 48-year-old right-handed male presented to the emergency department (ED) with chief complaint of headache of 8 h duration, which was sudden in onset, severe from the onset, and progressively increasing in intensity, diffuse, non-radiating, without any aggravating or relieving factors, associated with multiple episodes of projectile non-bilious vomiting. The patient doesn't give a history of loss of consciousness and abnormal body movements. There was no history of head trauma or similar attacks in the past. There was no history of fever, burning micturition, palpitation, chest pain, or heaviness. He is a known case of hypertension for 12 years under regular medication of losartan 50 mg once a day. He is also a known case of type 2 diabetes mellitus for the last 10 years for which he is taking metformin. He occasionally consumes homemade alcohol and smokes cigarettes, around 10 packs per year for the last 20 years. On examination in ED, he was well oriented to time, place, and person with the Glasgow Coma Scale (GCS) of 15. His vital parameters were stable. His neurological examination was within normal limits, and other systemic examinations did not reveal any abnormalities. He underwent a plain CT head, which showed diffuse subarachnoid hemorrhage (SAH) more on the left sylvian fissure. He subsequently underwent cerebral CT angiography (CTA), which showed a bilateral middle cerebral artery (MCA) aneurysm. The provisional diagnosis of spontaneous SAH due to bilateral MCA aneurysm rupture with the World Federation of Neurological Surgeons (WFNS) grade-1 was made, and he was posted for the surgery as a semi-emergency case. He underwent left pterional craniotomy and microsurgical clipping of the aneurysm. The immediate post-operative period was uneventful. On the second post-operative day, he became drowsy and developed hemiparesis of right half of the body. Transcranial Doppler study showed features of vasospasm. He was then managed with blood pressure (BP) augmentation therapy, maintaining the normal central venous pressure (CVP). Over the next 6 h of treatment, there was a gradual improvement in his level of consciousness and hemiparesis. He was shifted to the ward on the fourth post-operative day and was discharged from hospital on the seventh post-operative day with the GCS of 15 and no focal neurological deficits with advice for endovascular coiling of the right-sided aneurysm at a later date.

P. Kafle (✉) · S. Vignesh
Department of Neurosurgery, Nobel Medical College Teaching Hospital, Biratnagar, Nepal

S. Bhandari · G. S. Shrestha
Tribhuvan University Institute of Medicine, Maharajgunj Medical Campus, Kathmandu, Nepal

© Springer Nature Singapore Pte Ltd. 2024
K. K. Oli et al. (eds.), *Case-based Approach to Common Neurological Disorders*,
https://doi.org/10.1007/978-981-99-8676-7_11

11.1 Introduction

Headache is one of the most common clinical symptoms for which a patient visits ED [1]. Subarachnoid hemorrhage (SAH), characterized by bleeding in the subarachnoid space between the arachnoid mater and pia mater, is a rare but extremely lethal cause of headaches seen in the emergency department. It has an incidence of 1% and a median case-fatality rate of 27–44% [2, 3]. While trauma is the most frequent cause of subarachnoid hemorrhage (SAH), approximately 85% of cases of non-traumatic spontaneous SAH are attributed to a ruptured aneurysm, leading to the sudden onset of a severe headache; therefore, it is crucial to promptly recognize and differentiate SAH as the underlying cause of the headache to greatly reduce the patient's risk of mortality [4, 5].

11.2 Epidemiology

The incidence of SAH is about 9.1 cases per 100,000 people per year in population-based studies including out-of-hospital deaths. The incidence of aneurysmal subarachnoid hemorrhage (aSAH) varies across regions, with higher rates observed in Japan (22.7 cases per 100,000 people per year, 21.9–23.5), Finland (19.7 cases per 100,000 people per year), and China, while lower rates are seen in South and Central America [6, 7].

The average age at which aneurysm rupture tends to happen is higher as individuals get older, typically occurring between the ages of 50 and 60; however, it is important to note that young children and older adults can also experience this condition [8–10]. aSAH is 1.6 times more common in female population after the age of 50 [11]. The factors associated with the increased prevalence of unruptured intracranial aneurysm include female sex; age more than 30 years; descendants of Japanese, Chinese, Korean, and Finnish; presence of hypertension; increased wall stress due to arteriovenous malformation (AVM); hypoplasia of cerebral arteries; vascular disease; high cholesterol level; genetic conditions like collagen vascular disease (polycystic kidney, Marfan's disease, and Ehlers-Danlos syndrome); smoking; diabe-

Table 11.1 Annual rupture risk of unruptured aneurysm as described in the International Study of Unruptured Intracranial Aneurysms (ISUIA)

Aneurysm size (mm)	Aneurysm location	
	Anterior[a] (%)	Posterior[b] (%)
<7	0	2.5
7–12	2.6	14.5
13–24	14.5	18.4
≥25	40	50

[a] Anterior: Includes aneurysms in internal carotid artery, anterior communicating artery, anterior cerebral artery, and middle cerebral artery
[b] Posterior: Includes aneurysm located in posterior circulation and posterior communicating artery

tes; and alcohol consumption [11, 12]. Unruptured intracranial aneurysm has its natural course with a risk of rupture depending upon the location and size of the aneurysm, as shown in Table 11.1 [13].

The overall risk of rupture of untreated aneurysms is 1.2–1.3% [12]. Multiple factors interplay for the unruptured aneurysm to rupture. Risk factors for aneurysm rupture are higher age, female gender, Japanese or Finnish descent, and smoking. Aneurysm characteristics that include aneurysm larger than 10 mm, presence of wall stress, posterior circulation aneurysm, multiple aneurysms, irregularity with the daughter sac aspect ratio, height-to-width ratio, bottleneck factor, growing aneurysm, and presence of inflammation were significantly and positively correlated with rupture risk, while aneurysms located at the internal carotid artery (ICA) and neck width (N) correlated negatively with rupture risk [9, 13, 14–18].

11.3 Pathophysiology

Most of the aneurysms develop spontaneously, and only few develop following trauma, tumor, or infection (1–2%) [19–21]. The precise mechanisms involved in the development, enlargement, and rupture of spontaneous cerebral aneurysms remain unclear, but several interrelated factors such as abnormalities and degradation of the extracellular matrix, hemodynamic stress, and inflammatory reactions have been identified as potentially contributing to this process [22].

The dysregulation between matrix metalloproteinases (MMPs) and tissue inhibitors of metalloproteinases, which are generated by smooth muscle cells and inflammatory cells, plays a role in the degradation and restructuring of the extracellular matrix. This process is believed to be involved in the onset and advancement of cerebral aneurysms. Similarly, elevated wall shear stress caused by turbulent blood flow at arterial junctions, wider bifurcation angles, or sharp changes in vascular angles leads to endothelial cell injury, degeneration of smooth muscle cells, and thinning of the media layer, which ultimately may lead to the formation of aneurysm. Multiple immune-related elements, such as monocyte chemoattractant protein 1, NF-κB, angiotensin II, prostaglandin E2, Interleukin (IL) 1β, IL6, tumor necrosis factor-α, TLR4, Fas, nitric oxide, and complements, synergistically contribute to the weakening of the vessel wall, leading to the formation of aneurysmal dilatation and eventual rupture [18, 22, 23]. The final common pathway for aneurysm formation thus involves endothelial dysfunction/injury triggered by high shear stress, a mounting inflammatory response, vascular smooth muscle cell (VSMC) phenotypic modulation, extracellular matrix remodeling, and subsequent cell death and vessel wall degeneration [18].

Recent studies utilizing computational fluid dynamics models have revealed that although high wall shear stress contributes to the development of aneurysms, low stress levels have been related to the rupture of aneurysm. Surprisingly, the wall shear stress is notably lower at the site of rupture, and pooled analyses have shown that reduced wall shear stress may serve as a predictive factor for aneurysm rupture [24–26].

On the basis of pathogenesis, the shape of aneurysm can be saccular aneurysm (berry aneurysm), which are outpouching on blood vessels; fusiform aneurysm, which are blood vessel dilatations resulted from dissection of the blood vessels; and infective aneurysm, which arises from focal necrosis of the arterial wall following either bacterial or fungal infection.

11.4 Etiology of SAH

The etiology of SAH can be divided into:

11.4.1 Traumatic SAH

1. The commonest cause of SAH [4]

11.4.2 Spontaneous SAH

It can be further subclassified into:

1. Vascular
   Ruptured intracranial aneurysms: Accounts for 75–80% of spontaneous SAHs
   Cerebral arteriovenous malformation (AVM): Accounts for 4–5% of cases
   Hypertensive bleed, amyloid, vasculitis due to polyarteritis nodosa, eclampsia, hypercoagulable states, etc.
   Spinal AVMs
2. Infection
   Bacterial, tuberculous and fungal meningitis, syphilis, malaria, dengue, viral encephalitis, herpes simplex, etc.
3. Tumor
   Gliomas, meningiomas, hemangiomas, pituitary adenoma, choroid plexus papilloma and others.
4. Toxins
   Amphetamines, cocaine, nicotine, alcohol, lead, insulin, snake venom
5. Hematological
   Coagulopathy, leukemia, sickle cell anemia, lymphomas, melanoma
6. Pretruncal nonaneurysmal SAH
7. Idiopathic—14–22%

11.5 Clinical Manifestation

Patient with spontaneous SAH typically presents as sudden onset of severe thunderclap headache, described as "the worst headache of my life" [27]. The typical description of the headache is characterized by its sudden and intense nature, reaching its peak intensity at the onset or within a few minutes, although some studies have expanded the timeframe to include headaches that become severe in intensity within 1 h. This type of headache has been likened to a sudden loud sound, which is why it is referred to as a "thunderclap headache" [5, 28]. The headache typically lasts a few days, and it is atypical to be resolved in less than 2 h [29]. In two-thirds of patients, the headache is accompanied by loss of consciousness or focal deficits, and in up to one-third of patients with aSAH, symptoms or signs consist of headache alone [30]. Other associated symptoms include seizures (6–9%), delirium (16%), stroke, visual disturbances, nausea, vomiting, dizziness, neck stiffness, and photophobia [5].

In 10–40% of patients, the headache is preceded by a warning leak or "sentinel headache," which consists of severe headache of sudden onset associated with nausea, vomiting, and dizziness that reaches maximum intensity within minutes. However, unlike SAH, patients with sentinel headaches generally do not have meningismus, altered consciousness, or focal neurological symptoms and signs [5, 31]. Minor leak has been widely accepted as the principal cause of these warning leaks; however, vascular and parenchymal ischemic origins have also been suggested as the possible cause [31].

The signs and symptoms produced by SAH are also dependent on the site and size of aneurysm. Anterior cerebral artery aneurysm may present with transient bilateral lower limb paresis. Middle cerebral artery aneurysm may present with contralateral hemiparesis, paresthesia, hemianopsia, and dysphasia. Posterior cerebral artery aneurysm may present with symptoms of brainstem dysfunction. Internal carotid and posterior communicating artery aneurysm may present with third cranial nerve palsy and retro-orbital pain. Visual field defect or vision loss may be the presenting feature in carotid-ophthalmic artery aneurysm [32].

Apart from neurological manifestations, SAH may also present with cardiac arrhythmias, pulmonary edema, and intraocular hemorrhage (Terson syndrome) [33, 34].

11.6 Grading of SAH

Numerous grading systems have been developed to grade patients with SAH to assess the clinical severity of the initial injury, guide the treatment decision, know the prognosis regarding outcome, and standardize patient evaluation for the purpose of scientific study. Currently, the common SAH grading scales are the Hunt and Hess scale, Fisher scale, Glasgow Coma Scale (GCS), and the World Federation of Neurological Surgeons (WFNS) scale. The GCS, the WFNS (Table 11.2), and Hunt and Hess grading scale (Table 11.3) are used to predict the patient clinical outcome, and the Fisher grade (Table 11.4) helps to predict the event of vasospasm [35]. Vasograde scale (Table 11.5) is used for the prediction of delayed cerebral ischemia (DCI) after SAH [36]. Although multiple scoring systems have been developed to

Table 11.2 World Federation of Neurological Surgeons (WFNS) grading [38*]

WFNS[a] grade	GCS score[b]	Major focal deficits[c]
0[d]	–	–
1	15	–
2	13–14	–
3	13–14	+
4	7–12	±
5	3–6	±

[a] *WFNS* World Federation of Neurological Surgeons
[b] *GCS* Glasgow Coma Scale
[c] Hemiparesis or hemiplegia/aphasia
[d] Intact aneurysm

Table 11.3 Hunt and Hess grading [39*]

Grade	Clinical status	Survival (%)
1	Asymptomatic/minimal headache and slight nuchal rigidity	70
2	Moderate-to-severe headache, nuchal rigidity, no neurological deficits or CN palsy	60
3	Drowsy, confusion, or mild focal deficits	50
4	Stupor, moderate-to-severe hemiparesis, nearly decerebrate rigidity and vegetative disturbance	20
5	Deep coma, decerebrate rigidity, moribund appearance	10

Table 11.4 Modified Fisher's CT grading [40*]

Grade	Blood in CT	Symptomatic vasospasm (%)
0	**No SAH or IVH**	
1	Minimal or thin SAH, no IVH in B/L lateral ventricles	24
2	Minimal or thin SAH, with IVH in B/L lateral ventricles	33
3	Thick SAH, no IVH in B/L lateral ventricles	33
4	Thick SAH, with IVH in B/L lateral ventricles	40

B/L Bilateral

Table 11.5 Vasograde scale [36*]

Vasograde	WFNS	Modified Fisher scale
Green	1–2	1–2
Yellow	1–2	3–4
Red	4–5	Any

predict different patient-centered outcomes and prognosis, none of these specific scores demonstrated superior performance compared to the Glasgow Coma Scale (GCS) [35, 37].

11.7 Diagnosis

11.7.1 Diagnostic Tools

11.7.1.1 Computed Tomography

When there is a clinical suspicion for SAH, non-contrast computed tomography (CT) is the first diagnostic tool. The probability of detecting SAH in non-contrast CT head is proportional to the amount of blood in the subarachnoid space, the time after the event, and the quality of the CT scan. Non-contrast CT (Fig. 11.1) if done within 6 h of ictus has a sensitivity of 98.7% with confidence intervals of 97.1–99.4%, the sensitivity declines to 86% after 1 day, 76% after 2 days, 58% after 5 days, and 50% at 1 week for detecting SAH [27, 41].

Various scoring system requires non-contrast CT to prognosticate patients regarding outcome, angiographic vasospasm, and delayed cerebral ischemia based on the location and volume of

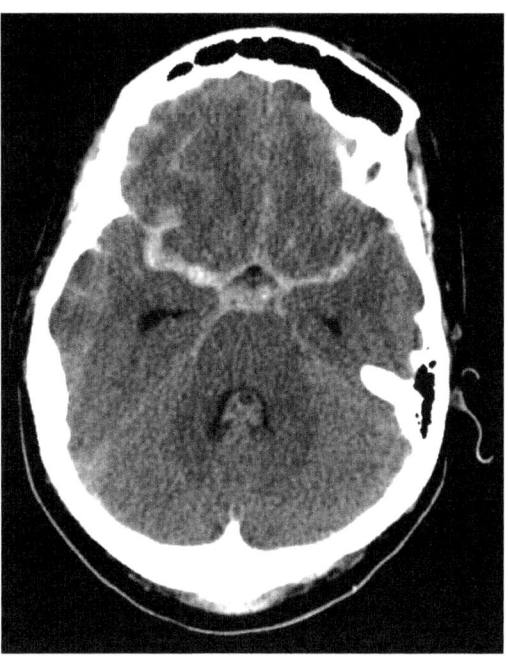

Fig. 11.1 Plain computed tomography of a 48-year-old male with diffuse subarachnoid hemorrhage

blood in SAH. In addition to showing SAH, a non-contrast CT head also helps to show the presence of hydrocephalus, mass effect, and cerebral edema, which might be important in deciding management strategies [28].

Some authors have claimed that the negative CT scan after 6 h rules out SAH, but this is controversial because severely anemic patients may have a normal CT head even after SAH if CT is done very late following ictus [41].

11.7.1.2 Lumbar Puncture

Lumbar puncture (LP) is an indispensable tool for the diagnosis of SAH with a convincing clinical history and negative brain CT [42]. The presence of erythrocytes and xanthochromia in CSF raises the suspicion of SAH. The presence of erythrocytes can also be seen in "traumatic tap" in 30% of LP and can confound the result [28]. Typically, the identification of red blood cells (RBCs) in the fourth tube of cerebrospinal fluid (CSF) is considered indicative of subarachnoid hemorrhage (SAH), while a decrease in the number of erythrocytes in subsequent tubes is an indication of a traumatic tap [43]. Nevertheless,

Table 11.6 CSF features in subarachnoid hemorrhage and in traumatic tap

SN	Features	Subarachnoid hemorrhage	Traumatic tap
1	RBCs	RBC count usually >100,000 RBCs/mm³. Compare RBC count in first to last tube	Decreasing numbers of RBC count on serial tubes
2	Clotting	Non-clotting bloody fluid that does not clear with sequential tubes	Clots with the time
3	Xanthochromia	Present when centrifuged after 12th hours of ictus	Absent
4	Free Hb	>0.04 AU	<0.04 AU
5	Bilirubin	>350 nm/L	<350 nm/L
6	RBC-to-WBC ratio	Decreased	Same as in peripheral blood sample
7	CSF glucose	Normal or reduced	Normal
8	CSF opening pressure	High/elevated	Normal

several authors have demonstrated the unreliability of the method that involves comparing the first and fourth tubes [44, 45].

Xanthochromia or yellowish discoloration of CSF is considered by many authors to be pathognomonic of SAH. Xanthochromia can be identified either through visual examination of the CSF tube compared to a tube of water or by using spectrophotometry. It takes approximately 12 h for xanthochromia to develop [27, 28]. Visual inspection of the CSF is however unreliable and had a sensitivity of less than 50% [46]. Hence, spectrophotometry is the recommended test to detect xanthochromia [28]. The CSF characteristic to differentiate SAH from traumatic tap is as shown in Table 11.6.

11.7.2 Angiographic Studies

Angiographic studies are the investigation of choice to locate and visualize the aneurysm [47].

11.7.2.1 CT Cerebral Angiography

CT angiography (Fig. 11.2) is an alternative diagnostic method that exhibits high sensitivity (98%) and specificity (100%) in detecting cerebral aneurysms in patients with confirmed SAH [28, 48]. This imaging technique can be performed rapidly and without invasive procedures. In situa-

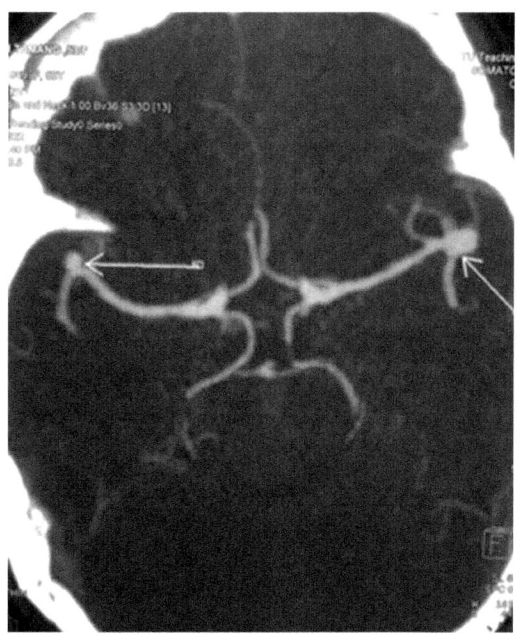

Fig. 11.2 Cerebral CT angiogram of the same patient showing saccular aneurysms at bilateral MCA

tions where LP is not feasible due to factors like coagulopathy, CTA can be utilized to guide treatment, with awareness of its limitations taken into account [28]. The sensitivity of CTA for aneurysms <4 mm is 92.3%; thus, small aneurysms and those adjacent to the skull base may be missed [49, 50].

11.7.2.2 Digital Subtraction Angiography

Digital subtraction angiography (DSA) with three-dimensional reconstruction remains the "gold standard" in the investigation of spontaneous SAH, which also defines relevant anatomy for treatment [51]. CTA has a maximum spatial resolution between 0.35 and 0.5 mm, whereas 3D rotational angiography can resolve vessels between 0.2 and 0.3 mm, and conventional DSA can resolve vessels as small as 0.1 mm [52]. DSA is thus indicated in a diffuse aneurysmal pattern of SAH with a negative CTA and for confirmation of vasculitis if blood is peripherally located [51].

11.7.2.3 Magnetic Resonance Imaging and MR Angiography

The feasibility of doing MR angiography is only 51%, and the sensitivity of MRA is only 95%, which is inferior to CTA [53]. Likewise, in cases of SAH, the blood mixes with CSF containing high levels of oxygen, which slows down the process of blood products transitioning into a deoxy-hemoglobin state and can be visualized more effectively using magnetic resonance imaging (MRI) [54]. MRI with fluid-attenuated inversion recovery (FLAIR), proton density, and gradient-echo sequences, when performed more than 24 h after the onset of headache, exhibits a sensitivity of 100% in detecting SAH [55]. MRI is not suggested as a primary imaging method in SAH but can be beneficial in specific uncommon situations, particularly for patients who experience a significant time lapse between the occurrence of symptoms and their presentation [28].

11.7.3 Differential Diagnosis

1. Reversible cerebral vasoconstriction syndrome
2. Meningitis
3. Cluster headache
4. Encephalitis
5. Hypertensive emergency
6. Intracranial hemorrhage
7. Migraine headache

11.8 Management

The rupture of an intracranial aneurysm sets off a sequence of events that unfolds over a period of days to weeks, often necessitating an extended stay in the intensive care unit (ICU) [56, 57]. The initial stage is the acute phase, lasting for the first 24 h, during which the abrupt release of blood into the subarachnoid space leads to a rapid increase in intracranial pressure (ICP). In cases of severe and prolonged elevation of ICP, cerebral perfusion may be compromised, resulting in overall cerebral ischemia. Subsequently, the subacute phase takes place within the first 72 h, characterized by imbalances in oxygen supply and demand that trigger the activation of pathways leading to cell death and early brain injury (EBI). The final phase, referred to as the delayed or chronic phase, occurs more than a week after the rupture and is characterized by vasospasm and delayed cerebral ischemia (DCI) [58]. The management of aneurysmal SAH patients focuses on the anticipation, prevention, and management of these phases and different complications arising in it.

11.8.1 Acute Phase

11.8.1.1 Initial Stabilization

Upon recognizing the presence of an SAH, timely referring the patient to a specialized medical facility with a high volume of cases (>35 cases per year) with access to neurocritical care, neurosurgery, and endovascular specialists has been linked to reduced mortality, enhanced outcomes, and an increased proportion of patients being discharged to their homes [59–61]. The primary objectives that require prompt attention involve ensuring a stable airway, stabilizing cardiovascular function, and addressing seizures [57].

11.8.1.2 Prevention of Rebleeding

The immediate focus should be on lowering systolic blood pressure (BP) and reversing anticoagulation in order to minimize the possibility of aneurysm re-rupture [28]. According to the American Heart Association/American Stroke Association (AHA/ASA) [62], it is recommended to maintain systolic blood pressure below 160 mmHg, while the Neurocritical Care [63] guidelines advise to keep the mean arterial blood pressure below 110 mmHg. On the other hand, the European guidelines suggest to maintain the systolic blood pressure below 180 mmHg [64] for ruptured unsecured aneurysm. The target BP however varies after the aneurysm has been secured. Similarly, the guidelines have also suggested to prevent wide fluctuations in BP and hypotension, which may result in a drop in cerebral perfusion pressure (CPP) [62–64].

The reversal of anticoagulation should be initiated without delay. Phytonadione (vitamin K), prothrombin complex concentrate (PCC), or fresh frozen plasma can be used to reverse the effects of vitamin K antagonists. PCC is the preferred option due to its quick action, elimination of the need for thawing or blood type matching, and the ability to be administered rapidly with lower volume and reduced risk of fluid overload [65]. While it is advisable to keep the platelet count above 100,000/mm³ in SAH patients eligible for neurosurgical treatment, administering platelet infusions to patients on antiplatelet therapy has been associated with higher mortality rates [66]. Research has shown that direct thrombin inhibitors like dabigatran can be reversed using idarucizumab, and factor Xa inhibitors such as apixaban, edoxaban, and rivaroxaban can be reversed using andexanet alfa.

Another potential treatment to reduce rebleeding is antifibrinolytic agents, such as tranexamic acid, which may stabilize the initial thrombus at the bleeding site. In a randomized, controlled clinical trial, tranexamic acid, given for a short course (1 g every 6 h), until the aneurysm was repaired (maximum up to 72 h), reduced the risk of rebleeding, albeit without a significant improvement in outcome [67]. They were also associated with an increased risk of deep venous thrombosis and delayed cerebral ischemia [68]. Currently European [64] and recently published Italian guidelines [69] have neither supported nor refuted the use of antifibrinolytics; however, AHA/ASA and the Neurocritical Care Society have suggested short-term (<72 h) therapy with tranexamic acid or aminocaproic acid to reduce the risk of early aneurysm rebleeding for patients

with an unavoidable delay in obliteration of aneurysm, a significant risk of rebleeding, and no compelling medical contraindications [62, 63].

Once a bleeding aneurysm is identified, the ultimate therapeutic goal is to secure it by coiling or clipping. Two randomized trials have compared endovascular coiling with neurosurgical clipping for ruptured intracranial aneurysms: the International Subarachnoid Aneurysm Trial (ISAT) and the Barrow Ruptured Aneurysm Trial (BRAT). Despite a significantly higher rate of obliteration and greater durability with open-surgical treatment than with endovascular treatment, both trials showed better functional outcomes at 1 year with endovascular treatment than with open-surgical treatment [70–73]. However, the ISAT study faced the problem of selection bias as the majority of patients who underwent coiling had aneurysms smaller than 1 cm, were classified as WFNS grades 1–3 (mostly 1–2), and only 3% of aneurysms in posterior circulation were included. Similarly, BRAT study revealed a significant proportion of patients initially assigned to the coiling group switched to the surgical clipping group (38%). This raises doubts about the benefits of coiling in a small subset of posterior circulation aneurysms [32].

The selection of endovascular coiling or neurosurgical clipping for repairing an aneurysm is influenced by several factors. These factors include the age and overall health of the patient, the presence of large intracranial hematomas, comorbidity, characteristics of the ruptured aneurysm (size, shape, and location), the presence of other aneurysms, and the certainty regarding the aneurysm with bleeding. Additionally, the estimated risks associated with both clipping and coiling procedures, as well as the availability of appropriate equipment and the expertise of the medical professionals involved, are important considerations [74]. As a rough guidance, aneurysms with a wide neck, branching vessels out of the aneurysm sack, middle cerebral artery aneurysms, or patients with intracerebral hematoma should preferably be treated by clipping, while aneurysms of the basilar artery, elderly patients (patients >70 years, small aneurysm neck, posterior circulation), and those presenting with poor grade (World Federation of Neurological

Surgeons classification IV/V) should be coiled [62, 64]. For aneurysms treatable by either endo-vascular coiling or neurosurgical clipping, endovascular repair is recommended [62, 75].

The timing of aneurysm repair is another area where evidences are limited. Early repair of aneurysm rupture, within 72 h after the onset of first symptoms, has been recommended by the American Heart Association/American Stroke Association, which has also been corroborated by their European counterparts and Neurocritical Care Society [62–64]. The superiority of ultra-early treatment (within 24 h) compared to early aneurysm repair (within 72 h) and the potential for improved outcomes with early treatment (within 3 days) compared to intermediate (days 4–7) or late (after day 7) treatment in patients with poor-grade subarachnoid hemorrhage remain uncertain [76, 77].

11.8.1.3 Management of Intracranial Hypertension

Intracranial hypertension, which is characterized by elevated pressure within the skull (at least 20 mmHg), is a frequently observed complication in cases of subarachnoid hemorrhage (SAH). It occurs in over 50% of patients with SAH. Various factors, including cerebral swelling, bleeding within the brain tissue, rapid accumulation of fluid in the brain cavities (acute hydrocephalus), bleeding into the ventricles (intraventricular hemorrhage), re-rupture of the aneurysm, complications arising from aneurysm treatment, early brain injury (EBI), and delayed cerebral ischemia (DCI), have been identified as contributors to the development of intracranial hypertension [78].

To effectively manage raised intracranial pressure (ICP), the following interventions are recommended: elevating the head of the bed by 30°–45° to optimize cerebral venous drainage, maintaining normoventilation with arterial partial pressure of carbon dioxide ($PaCO_2$) between 35 and 40 mmHg, utilizing short periods of hyperventilation as a temporary measure, administering sedation and analgesia to achieve a state of calmness (targeting a Richmond Agitation Sedation Scale score of −5 or Sedation-Agitation Scale score of 1), maintaining ICP below 20 mmHg and cerebral perfusion pressure between 50 and 70 mmHg, considering surgical intervention for mass-occupying lesions and cerebrospinal fluid drainage, and employing barbiturate sedation, decompressive craniectomy, or hypothermia in refractory cases [79, 80].

Hyperosmolar agents, such as mannitol (20%) and hypertonic saline, are usually considered in SAH with features of raised ICP. But their role in clinical outcome is unclear owing to the lack of well-designed RCTs; however, a meta-analysis and systemic review from TBI reported better control of elevated ICP with the use of hypertonic saline compared with mannitol, though with a different patient population, it remains uncertain whether to extrapolate this result to SAH [81].

The use of therapeutic hypothermia has demonstrated effectiveness in managing ICP in SAH. However, it has not been linked to enhanced functional recovery or decreased mortality rates in patients with SAH of poor grade. As a result, further evidence is needed before promoting its widespread utilization [82].

Decompressive craniectomy is a potential approach to address high ICP in patients with SAH who do not respond to other treatments. While decompressive craniectomy has been linked to lower mortality rates, notable decreases in ICP, improved oxygenation, and metabolism in the brain, it often leads to unfavorable outcomes, such as severe disability or death, for most patients. Experts suggest that the greatest benefit from decompressive craniectomy can be achieved when the procedure is performed early (within 48 h of the bleeding) and when there are no signs of cerebral infarction in radiological images [80, 83, 84].

11.8.1.4 Management of Hydrocephalus

Hydrocephalus, defined as a bicaudate index on the CT scan exceeding the 95th percentile for age, occurs in approximately 20% of patients during the acute phase and in about 10% during the chronic phase after SAH [85]. An external ventricular drain (EVD) should be inserted to allow CSF drainage and ICP monitoring when the hydrocephalus is associated with a decreased level of consciousness. The placement of an EVD prior to treating an aneurysm has been proven to be secure and does not result in a higher likelihood of the aneurysm re-rupturing [86, 87]. Roughly 30% of patients experiencing severe SAH show neurological improvement following the insertion of an EVD and drainage of CSF. Nevertheless, it is important to exercise caution when draining CSF prior to repairing the aneurysm, as excessive and rapid drainage can raise the transmural pressure, thereby elevating the risk of aneurysm re-rupture [87, 88]. A randomized trial investigated the impact of lumbar drainage and found that it decreased the occurrence of delayed cerebral ischemia. However, there was no observable influence on the overall outcome after 6 months [89].

11.8.1.5 Management of Seizure

Seizure is an early complication that can occur in up to 26% of patients when an aneurysm ruptures. Most seizures happen within the first 24 h, with only about 2–8% occurring later [58]. Risk factors for seizures after SAH include surgical repair of the aneurysm in patients over 65 years of age, a thick clot in the subarachnoid space, and possibly the presence of intraparenchymal hematoma or infarction [90, 91]. Various studies have shown that using antiepileptic drugs can lead to poor cognitive outcomes and increase complications during hospitalization [58]. If seizure prevention is deemed necessary, alternative anticonvulsants other than phenytoin can be used, but only for a short duration of 3–7 days, as this has been shown to be as effective as longer treatment [92]. Patients with severe bleeding or unexplained neurological symptoms should undergo continuous electroencephalogram monitoring to detect non-convulsive seizures, although the impact of successfully treating these non-convulsive seizures has not been studied [63].

11.8.1.6 Management of Cardiopulmonary Dysfunction

Cardiopulmonary dysfunction is common after aSAH, especially in poor-grade SAH, and is related to high catecholamine release and sympathetic overstimulation [93]. The cardiac

issues that occur after SAH can vary from minor alterations in the electrocardiogram to severe cardiogenic shock, which may necessitate the use of an intra-aortic balloon pump and apical ballooning of the left ventricle [94, 95]. Supportive care is the primary approach to treatment, and the majority of cases will naturally improve within a period of 2 weeks. Around one-third of patients may experience pulmonary complications following a subarachnoid hemorrhage, including hospital-acquired pneumonia, cardiogenic or neurogenic pulmonary edema, aspiration pneumonitis, pulmonary embolism, and potentially acute respiratory distress syndrome [96–98].

11.8.2 Subacute Phase

The primary goal during this stage is to avoid further harm to the brain by ensuring sufficient oxygen supply and meeting the brain's metabolic requirements. Achieving this objective involves optimizing cerebral perfusion pressure (CPP), as recent evidence indicates that maintaining a CPP level above 70 mmHg in the early stages can enhance brain tissue oxygenation and overall brain blood flow. This, in turn, reduces metabolic strain and enhances outcomes [99].

For the treatment of anemia, recent guideline from Italian society of anesthesia and intensive care has recommended to maintain an Hb level > 8 g/dL in poor-grade SAH patients without DCI-related vasospasm and an Hb level > 9 g/dL in case of DCI associated with cerebral vasospasm [69]. It is strongly recommended to monitor for fever and any infection to reduce metabolic demand on the brain [62, 63, 100].

11.8.3 Chronic/Delayed Phase

The delayed stage is characterized by the emergence of vasospasm and delayed cerebral ischemia (DCI), which typically occur between 3 and 14 days following aSAH [101]. The management is focused on the prevention and treatment of vasospasm and DCI in this phase.

11.8.3.1 Prevention of Vasospasm and DCI

Nimodipine

Nimodipine is a calcium channel antagonist which has been proven to be the only medication that enhances results following SAH. Studies [62–64] have demonstrated that nimodipine reduces the entry of calcium after cerebral ischemia caused by DCI. Additionally, it decreases the occurrence of microthrombi by promoting the body's natural fibrinolysis process and may counteract cortical spreading ischemia [80]. A randomized, double-blind, placebo-controlled trial involving multiple centers and 188 patients with severe-grade SAH (Hunt and Hess grade 3–5) revealed an improvement in functional outcomes after 3 months (29.2% in the nimodipine group compared with 9.8% in the placebo group), despite similar rates of moderate and severe angiographic vasospasm observed during follow-up angiography [102].

Magnesium

Magnesium is a calcium antagonist that operates in a non-competitive manner and is neuroprotective as well [103]. According to the Magnesium in Aneurysmal Subarachnoid Hemorrhage (MASH) trial, which was a phase II randomized controlled trial (RCT), intravenous (IV) magnesium demonstrated an improvement in neurological outcomes [104]. Nevertheless, these results were not successfully reproduced in subsequent trials, namely the Magnesium in Aneurysmal Subarachnoid Hemorrhage (MASH-2) trial, a phase III trial, and the Intravenous Magnesium for Subarachnoid Hemorrhage (IMASH) trial, a phase III multicenter RCT [105, 106].

Statins

Statins maintain the endothelial function by enhancing the production of nitric oxide and reducing the endothelin-1. They also possess properties that reduce inflammation, oxidative stress, and blood clot formation, which were believed to be advantageous in cases of SAH [80]. However, a phase III clinical trial called STASH (SimvaSTatin in Aneurysmal Subarachnoid Hemorrhage), which was conducted across multiple centers and involving randomization and a placebo control group, did not find any positive effects of simvastatin in patients with SAH after a period of 6 months [107].

Clazosentan

Clazosentan is an endothelin-I antagonist that was initially thought to be helpful in reducing vasospasm and DCI in SAH patients. Though CONSCIOUS-1, a phase II multicenter RCT, found it to be effective in the reducing the angiographic vasospasm, subsequent phase III trials—CONSCIOUS-2 and CONSCIOUS-3—failed to show significant effect on outcome [107–109].

11.9 Other Treatments

Meta-analyses of fasudil, intrathecal fibrinolytics, and cilostazol hint at efficacy, but these findings require further study [110–112]. Similarly, trials involving the use of antiplatelet agents and low-molecular-weight heparin for the prevention and management of microthrombi in DCI have not yielded positive results in the management of DCI [113, 114]. The combination of induced hypertension, hypervolemia, and hemodilution (triple-H therapy) carries significant medical morbidity, including pulmonary edema, myocardial infarction, hyponatremia, renal medullary washout, indwelling catheter-related complications, cerebral hemorrhage, and cerebral edema [115].

11.9.1 Treatment for Vasospasm and Delayed Cerebral Ischemia

If a person experiences a newly developed impairment in a specific area of their brain or a decrease in their level of alertness, and there are no other known reasons for these symptoms, such as hydrocephalus or rebleeding, it is important to consider the possibility of symptomatic vasospasm and DCI. In such cases, it is crucial to begin aggressive treatment promptly [116]. If patients do not recover from the new deficit even after attempting to reverse it with a fluid challenge, they can be subjected to a gradual trial of hypertension using a vasopressor [62, 63]. The goal of hemodynamic optimization should focus on alleviating clinical symptoms and/or radiological findings. This should be done until the mean arterial pressure (MAP) reaches 120 mmHg and the systolic blood pressure reaches 220 mmHg. The patient's cardiovascular condition should be considered to minimize the risks associated with increasing MAP. In cases where vasospasm does not respond to MAP augmentation, more invasive intra-arterial procedures such as angioplasty and the use of vasodilators like milrinone, verapamil, and nicardipine, along with advanced hemodynamic monitoring, may be employed [117, 118].

11.10 Recent Advances in the Management of Ruptured Aneurysm

11.10.1 Endovascular Flow Diversion

This is a relatively recent endovascular approach, where a specialized device made of a tightly woven, porous mesh with a high metal content is placed across the neck of an aneurysm. Its purpose is to redirect the blood flow away from the aneurysm and toward the main blood vessel. This redirection leads to the reconstruction and reshaping of the main artery while blocking the connection between the aneurysm and the main vessel. However, this technique is associated with a high occurrence of complications, such as the aneurysm tearing or bursting during the procedure, cerebral ischemia, cerebral edema surrounding the aneurysm, intraparenchymal bleeding, occlusion of side branches, delayed rupture of the aneurysm, and narrowing or blockage of the parent artery due to neointimal overgrowth [119–121].

11.11 Prognosis

Spontaneous aSAH carries a high risk of early mortality and long-term disability in survivors. A meta-analysis study revealed that the mortality rate among patients with SAH ranged from 8.3% to 66.7%. In their study, about 55% of patients achieved independent functioning, 19% continued to rely on assistance, and 26% succumbed to the disease [122]. Long-term mortality, as reported in 2014, is 17.9% at 10 years, 29.5% at 15 years, and 43.6% at 20 years after SAH [123]. Though little information is available regarding functional outcome, Taufique et al. found that 35% of patients had poor overall quality of life after SAH, and poor prognosis (modified Rankin Scale [mRS] score 3–6) was observed in 42.4% of patients with SAH by Hammer et al. [124, 125].

References

1. Edlow JA, Panagos PD, Godwin SA, Thomas TL, Decker WW, American College of Emergency Physicians. Clinical policy: critical issues in the evaluation and management of adult patients presenting to the emergency department with acute headache. Ann Emerg Med. 2008;52(4):407–36.
2. Ramirez-Lassepas M, Espinosa CE, Cicero JJ, Johnston KL, Cipolle RJ, Barber DL. Predictors of intracranial pathologic findings in patients who seek emergency care because of headache. Arch Neurol. 1997;54(12):1506–9.
3. Nieuwkamp DJ, Setz LE, Algra A, Linn FH, de Rooij NK, Rinkel GJ. Changes in case fatality of aneurysmal subarachnoid haemorrhage over time, according to age, sex, and region: a meta-analysis. Lancet Neurol. 2009;8(7):635–42.
4. Ziu E, Mesfin FB. Subarachnoid hemorrhage. StatPearls Publishing; 2019. https://www.ncbi.nlm.nih.gov/books/NBK441958/. Accessed 7 Aug 2022.
5. Schwedt TJ, Matharu MS, Dodick DW. Thunderclap headache. Lancet Neurol. 2006;5(7):621–31.
6. de Rooij NK, Linn FH, van der Plas JA, Algra A, Rinkel GJ. Incidence of subarachnoid haemorrhage: a systematic review with emphasis on region, age, gender and time trends. J Neurol Neurosurg Psychiatry. 2007;78(12):1365–72.
7. Bederson JB, Awad IA, Wiebers DO, Piepgras D, Haley EC Jr, Brott T, et al. Recommendations for the management of patients with unruptured intracranial aneurysms: a statement for healthcare professionals from the Stroke Council of the American Heart Association. Circulation. 2000;102(18):2300–8.

8. Zacharia BE, Hickman ZL, Grobelny BT, DeRosa P, Kotchetkov I, Ducruet AF, Connolly ES. Epidemiology of aneurysmal subarachnoid hemorrhage. Neurosurg Clin. 2010;21(2):221–33.

9. Rinkel GJ, Djibuti M, Algra A, Van Gijn J. Prevalence and risk of rupture of intracranial aneurysms: a systematic review. Stroke. 1998;29(1):251–6.

10. Jordan LC, Johnston SC, Wu YW, Sidney S, Fullerton HJ. The importance of cerebral aneurysms in childhood hemorrhagic stroke: a population-based study. Stroke. 2009;40(2):400–5.

11. Vlak MH, Algra A, Brandenburg R, Rinkel GJ. Prevalence of unruptured intracranial aneurysms, with emphasis on sex, age, comorbidity, country, and time period: a systematic review and meta-analysis. Lancet Neurol. 2011;10(7):626–36.

12. Zacks DJ, Russell DB, Miller JD. Fortuitously discovered intracranial aneurysms. Arch Neurol. 1980;37:39–41.

13. Wang GX, Zhang D, Wang ZP, Yang LQ, Yang H, Li W. Risk factors for ruptured intracranial aneurysms. Indian J Med Res. 2018;147(1):51–7. https://doi.org/10.4103/ijmr.IJMR_1665_15. PubMed PMID: 29749361; PubMed Central PMCID: PMC5967217

14. Wiebers DO, International Study of Unruptured Intracranial Aneurysms Investigators. Unruptured intracranial aneurysms: natural history, clinical outcome, and risks of surgical and endovascular treatment. Lancet. 2003;362(9378):103–10.

15. Juvela S, Porras M, Heiskanen O. Natural history of unruptured intracranial aneurysms: a long-term follow-up study. J Neurosurg. 1993;79:174–82.

16. Can A, Mouminah A, Ho AL, et al. Effect of vascular anatomy on the formation of basilar tip aneurysms. Neurosurgery. 2015;76:62–66, discussion 6.

17. Mount LA, Brisman R. Treatment of multiple aneurysms—symptomatic and asymptomatic. Clin Neurosurg. 1974;21:166–70.

18. Chalouhi N, Ali MS, Jabbour PM, et al. Biology of intracranial aneurysms: role of inflammation. J Cereb Blood Flow Metab. 2012;32:1659–76.

19. Benoit BG, Wortzman G. Traumatic cerebral aneurysms. Clinical features and natural history. J Neurol Neurosurg Psychiatry. 1973;36:127.

20. Clare CE, Barrow DL. Infectious intracranial aneurysms. Neurosurg Clin N Am. 1992;3:551.

21. Damasio H, Seabra-Gomes R, da Silva JP, et al. Multiple cerebral aneurysms and cardiac myxoma. Arch Neurol. 1975;32:269.

22. Jung KH. New pathophysiological considerations on cerebral aneurysms. Neurointervention. 2018;13(2):73–83.

23. Fennell VS, Kalani MY, Atwal G, Martirosyan NL, Spetzler RF. Biology of saccular cerebral aneurysms: a review of current understanding and future directions. Front Surg. 2016;3:43.

24. Can A, Du R. Association of hemodynamic factors with intracranial aneurysm formation and rupture: systematic review and meta-analysis. Neurosurgery. 2016;78(4):510–20.

25. Li M, Wang J, Liu J, Zhao C, Yang X. Hemodynamics in ruptured intracranial aneurysms with known rupture points. World Neurosurg. 2018;118:e721–6.

26. Zhou G, Zhu Y, Yin Y, Su M, Li M. Association of wall shear stress with intracranial aneurysm rupture: systematic review and meta-analysis. Sci Rep. 2017;7:5331.

27. Edlow JA, Caplan LR. Avoiding pitfalls in the diagnosis of subarachnoid hemorrhage. N Engl J Med. 2000;342(1):29–36.

28. Marcolini E, Hine J. Approach to the diagnosis and management of subarachnoid hemorrhage. Western J Emerg Med. 2019;20(2):203.

29. Warlow CP, Van Gijn J, Dennis MS, Wardlaw JM, Bamford JM, Hankey GJ, Sandercock PA, Rinkel G, Langhorne P, Sudlow C, Rothwell P. Stroke: practical management. Wiley; 2011.

30. Linn FH, Rinkel GJ, Algra A, Van Gijn J. Headache characteristics in subarachnoid haemorrhage and benign thunderclap headache. J Neurol Neurosurg Psychiatry. 1998;65(5):791–3.

31. Bassi P, Bandera R, Loiero M, Tognoni G, Mangoni A. Warning signs in subarachnoid hemorrhage: a cooperative study. Acta Neurol Scand. 1991;84(4):277–81.

32. D'Souza S. Aneurysmal subarachnoid hemorrhage. J Neurosurg Anesthesiol. 2015;27(3):222–40.

33. Czorlich P, Skevas C, Knospe V, Vettorazzi E, Richard G, Wagenfeld L, Westphal M, Regelsberger J. Terson syndrome in subarachnoid hemorrhage, intracerebral hemorrhage, and traumatic brain injury. Neurosurg Rev. 2015;38(1):129–36.

34. Weir B. Headaches from aneurysms. Cephalalgia. 1994;14(2):79–87.

35. Rosen DS, Macdonald RL. Subarachnoid hemorrhage grading scales. Neurocrit Care. 2005;2(2):110–8.

36. de Oliveira Manoel AL, Jaja BN, Germans MR, Yan H, Qian W, Kouzmina E, Marotta TR, Turkel-Parrella D, Schweizer TA, Macdonald RL, SAHIT collaborators. The VASOGRADE: a simple grading scale for prediction of delayed cerebral ischemia after subarachnoid hemorrhage. Stroke. 2015;46(7):1826–31.

37. Kapapa T, Tjahjadi M, König R, Wirtz CR, Woischneck D. Which clinical variable influences health-related quality of life the most after spontaneous subarachnoid hemorrhage? Hunt and Hess scale, Fisher score, World Federation of Neurosurgeons score, Brussels coma score, and Glasgow coma score compared. World Neurosurg. 2013;80(6):853–8.

38. Drake CG. Report of World Federation of Neurological Surgeons Committee on a universal subarachnoid hemorrhage grading scale. J Neurosurg. 1988;68:985–6.

39. Hunt WE, Hess RM. Surgical risk as related to time of intervention in the repair of intracranial aneurysms. J Neurosurg. 1968;28(1):14–20.

40. Frontera JA, Claassen J, Schmidt JM, Wartenberg KE, Temes R, Connolly ES, Macdonald RL, Mayer SA. Prediction of symptomatic vasospasm after sub-

arachnoid hemorrhage: the modified Fisher scale. Neurosurgery. 2006;59(1):21–7.

41. Dubosh NM, Bellolio MF, Rabinstein AA, et al. Sensitivity of early brain computed tomography to exclude aneurysmal subarachnoid hemorrhage: a systematic review and meta-analysis. Stroke. 2016;47(3):750–5.

42. Backes D, Rinkel GJ, Kemperman H, Linn FH, Vergouwen MD. Time-dependent test characteristics of head computed tomography in patients suspected of nontraumatic subarachnoid hemorrhage. Stroke. 2012;43(8):2115–9.

43. Long B, Koyfman A. Controversies in the diagnosis of subarachnoid hemorrhage. J Emerg Med. 2016;50(6):839–47.

44. Perry JJ, Alyahya B, Sivilotti ML, Bullard MJ, Émond M, Sutherland J, Worster A, Hohl C, Lee JS, Eisenhauer MA, Pauls M. Differentiation between traumatic tap and aneurysmal subarachnoid hemorrhage: prospective cohort study. BMJ. 2015;350:h568.

45. Heasley DC, Mohamed MA, Yousem DM. Clearing of red blood cells in lumbar puncture does not rule out ruptured aneurysm in patients with suspected subarachnoid hemorrhage but negative head CT findings. Am J Neuroradiol. 2005;26(4):820–4.

46. Arora S, Swadron SP, Dissanayake V. Evaluating the sensitivity of visual xanthochromia in patients with subarachnoid hemorrhage. J Emerg Med. 2010;39:13–6.

47. Sailer AM, Wagemans BA, Nelemans PJ, et al. Diagnosing intracranial aneurysms with MR angiography: systematic review and meta-analysis. Stroke. 2014;45:119–26.

48. Menke J, Larsen J, Kallenberg K. Diagnosing cerebral aneurysms by computed tomographic angiography: meta-analysis. Ann Neurol. 2011;69:646–54.

49. Mckinney AM, Palmer CS, Truwit CL, Karagulle A, Teksam M. Detection of aneurysms by 64-section multidetector CT angiography in patients acutely suspected of having an intracranial aneurysm and comparison with digital subtraction and 3D rotational angiography. Am J Neuroradiol. 2008;29(3):594–602.

50. Westerlaan HE, Van Dijk JM, Jansen-van der Weide MC, de Groot JC, Groen RJ, Mooij JJ, Oudkerk M. Intracranial aneurysms in patients with subarachnoid hemorrhage: CT angiography as a primary examination tool for diagnosis—systematic review and meta-analysis. Radiology. 2011;258(1):134–45.

51. Agid R, Andersson T, Almqvist H, Willinsky RA, Lee SK, Farb RI, Söderman M. Negative CT angiography findings in patients with spontaneous subarachnoid hemorrhage: when is digital subtraction angiography still needed? Am J Neuroradiol. 2010;31(4):696–705.

52. Kallmes DF, Layton K, Marx WF, Tong F. Death by nondiagnosis: why emergent CT angiography should not be done for patients with subarachnoid hemorrhage. Am J Neuroradiol. 2007;28(10):1837–8.

53. Pierot L, Portefaix C, Rodriguez-Régent C, Gallas S, Meder JF, Oppenheim C. Role of MRA in the detection of intracranial aneurysm in the acute phase of subarachnoid hemorrhage. J Neuroradiol. 2013;40(3):204–10.

54. Kidwell CS, Wintermark M. Imaging of intracranial haemorrhage. Lancet Neurol. 2008;7(3):256–67.

55. Verma RK, Kottke R, Andereggen L, Weisstanner C, Zubler C, Gralla J, Kiefer C, Slotboom J, Wiest R, Schroth G, Ozdoba C. Detecting subarachnoid hemorrhage: comparison of combined FLAIR/SWI versus CT. Eur J Radiol. 2013;82(9):1539–45.

56. Macdonald RL, Schweizer TA. Spontaneous subarachnoid haemorrhage. Lancet. 2017;389(10069):655–66.

57. Lawton MT, Vates GE. Subarachnoid hemorrhage. N Engl J Med. 2017;377(3):257–66.

58. Osgood ML. Aneurysmal subarachnoid hemorrhage: review of the pathophysiology and management strategies. Curr Neurol Neurosci Rep. 2021;21(9):1.

59. Mirski MA, Chang CW, Cowan R. Impact of a neuroscience intensive care unit on neurosurgical patient outcomes and cost of care: evidence-based support for an intensivist-directed specialty ICU model of care. J Neurosurg Anesthesiol. 2001;13(2):83–92.

60. Rush B, Romano K, Ashkanani M, McDermid RC, Celi LA. Impact of hospital case-volume on subarachnoid hemorrhage outcomes: a nationwide analysis adjusting for hemorrhage severity. J Crit Care. 2017;37:240–3.

61. Varelas PN, Schultz L, Conti M, Spanaki M, Genarrelli T, Hacein-Bey L. The impact of a neurointensivist on patients with stroke admitted to a neurosciences intensive care unit. Neurocrit Care. 2008;9(3):293–9.

62. Connolly ES Jr, Rabinstein AA, Carhuapoma JR, Derdeyn CP, Dion J, Higashida RT, Hoh BL, Kirkness CJ, Naidech AM, Ogilvy CS, Patel AB. Guidelines for the management of aneurysmal subarachnoid hemorrhage: a guideline for healthcare professionals from the American Heart Association/American Stroke Association. Stroke. 2012;43(6):1711–37.

63. Diringer MN, Bleck TP, Claude Hemphill JI, Menon D, Shutter L, Vespa P, Bruder N, Connolly ES, Citerio G, Gress D, Hänggi D. Critical care management of patients following aneurysmal subarachnoid hemorrhage: recommendations from the Neurocritical Care Society's Multidisciplinary Consensus Conference. Neurocrit Care. 2011;15(2):211–40.

64. Steiner T, Juvela S, Unterberg A, Jung C, Forsting M, Rinkel G. European Stroke Organization guidelines for the management of intracranial aneurysms and subarachnoid haemorrhage. Cerebrovasc Dis. 2013;35(2):93–112.

65. Christos S, Naples R. Anticoagulation reversal and treatment strategies in major bleeding: update 2016. Western J Emerg Med. 2016;17(3):264.

66. Baharoglu MI, Cordonnier C, Salman RA, De Gans K, Koopman MM, Brand A, Majoie CB, Beenen LF, Marquering HA, Vermeulen M, Nederkoorn

PJ. Platelet transfusion versus standard care after acute stroke due to spontaneous cerebral haemorrhage associated with antiplatelet therapy (PATCH): a randomised, open-label, phase 3 trial. Lancet. 2016;387(10038):2605–13.

67. Hillman J, Fridriksson S, Nilsson O, Yu Z, Säveland H, Jakobsson KE. Immediate administration of tranexamic acid and reduced incidence of early rebleeding after aneurysmal subarachnoid hemorrhage: a prospective randomized study. J Neurosurg. 2002;97(4):771–8.

68. Starke RM, Kim GH, Fernandez A, Komotar RJ, Hickman ZL, Otten ML, Ducruet AF, Kellner CP, Hahn DK, Chwajol M, Mayer SA. Impact of a protocol for acute antifibrinolytic therapy on aneurysm rebleeding after subarachnoid hemorrhage. Stroke. 2008;39(9):2617–21.

69. Picetti E, Berardino M, Bertuccio A, Bertuetti R, Boccardi EP, Caricato A, Castioni CA, Cenzato M, Chieregato A, Citerio G, Gritti P. Early management of patients with aneurysmal subarachnoid hemorrhage in a hospital without neurosurgical/neuroendovascular facilities: a consensus and clinical recommendations of the Italian Society of Anesthesia and Intensive Care (SIAARTI). J Anesth Analg Crit Care. 2021;1(1):1–7.

70. Molyneux A, Kerr R, International Subarachnoid Aneurysm Trial (ISAT) Collaborative Group. International Subarachnoid Aneurysm Trial (ISAT) of neurosurgical clipping versus endovascular coiling in 2143 patients with ruptured intracranial aneurysms: a randomized trial. J Stroke Cerebrovasc Dis. 2002;11(6):304–14.

71. Molyneux AJ, Birks J, Clarke A, Sneade M, Kerr RS. The durability of endovascular coiling versus neurosurgical clipping of ruptured cerebral aneurysms: 18 year follow-up of the UK cohort of the International Subarachnoid Aneurysm Trial (ISAT). Lancet. 2015;385(9969):691–7.

72. Spetzler RF, McDougall CG, Albuquerque FC, Zabramski JM, Hills NK, Partovi S, Nakaji P, Wallace RC. The barrow ruptured aneurysm trial: 3-year results. J Neurosurg. 2013;119(1):146–57.

73. Spetzler RF, McDougall CG, Zabramski JM, Albuquerque FC, Hills NK, Russin JJ, Partovi S, Nakaji P, Wallace RC. The barrow ruptured aneurysm trial: 6-year results. J Neurosurg. 2015;123(3):609–17.

74. Darsaut TE, Kotowski M, Raymond J. How to choose clipping versus coiling in treating intracranial aneurysms. Neurochirurgie. 2012;58(2–3):61–7.

75. Frazer D, Ahuja A, Watkins L, Cipolotti L. Coiling versus clipping for the treatment of aneurysmal subarachnoid hemorrhage: a longitudinal investigation into cognitive outcome. Neurosurgery. 2007;60(3):434–42.

76. Oudshoorn SC, Rinkel GJ, Molyneux AJ, Kerr RS, Dorhout Mees SM, Backes D, Algra A, Vergouwen MD. Aneurysm treatment <24 versus 24–72 h after subarachnoid hemorrhage. Neurocrit Care. 2014;21(1):4–13.

77. Zhang Q, Ma L, Liu Y, He M, Sun H, Wang X, Fang Y, Hui XH, You C. Timing of operation for poor-grade aneurysmal subarachnoid hemorrhage: study protocol for a randomized controlled trial. BMC Neurol. 2013;13(1):1–6.

78. Heuer GG, Smith MJ, Elliott JP, Winn HR, Leroux PD. Relationship between intracranial pressure and other clinical variables in patients with aneurysmal subarachnoid hemorrhage. J Neurosurg. 2004;101(3):408–16.

79. de Oliveira Manoel AL, Turkel-Parrella D, Duggal A, Murphy A, McCredie V, Marotta TR. Managing aneurysmal subarachnoid hemorrhage: it takes a team. Cleve Clin J Med. 2015;82(3):177–92.

80. de Oliveira Manoel AL, Goffi A, Marotta TR, Schweizer TA, Abrahamson S, Macdonald RL. The critical care management of poor-grade subarachnoid haemorrhage. Crit Care. 2016;20(1):1–9.

81. Mortazavi MM, Romeo AK, Deep A, Griessenauer CJ, Shoja MM, Tubbs RS, Fisher W. Hypertonic saline for treating raised intracranial pressure: literature review with meta-analysis: a review. J Neurosurg. 2012;116(1):210–21.

82. Inamasu J, Ichikizaki K. Mild hypothermia in neurologic emergency: an update. Ann Emerg Med. 2002;40(2):220–30.

83. Schirmer CM, Hoit DA, Malek AM. Decompressive hemicraniectomy for the treatment of intractable intracranial hypertension after aneurysmal subarachnoid hemorrhage. Stroke. 2007;38(3):987–92.

84. Buschmann U, Yonekawa Y, Fortunati M, Cesnulis E, Keller E. Decompressive hemicraniectomy in patients with subarachnoid hemorrhage and intractable intracranial hypertension. Acta Neurochir. 2007;149(1):59–65.

85. Heros RC. Acute hydrocephalus after subarachnoid hemorrhage. Stroke. 1989;20(6):715–7.

86. Hellingman CA, van den Bergh WM, Beijer IS, van Dijk GW, Algra A, van Gijn J, Rinkel GJ. Risk of rebleeding after treatment of acute hydrocephalus in patients with aneurysmal subarachnoid hemorrhage. Stroke. 2007;38(1):96–9.

87. McIver JI, Friedman JA, Wijdicks EF, Piepgras DG, Pichelmann MA, Toussaint LG, McClelland RL, Nichols DA, Atkinson JL. Preoperative ventriculostomy and rebleeding after aneurysmal subarachnoid hemorrhage. J Neurosurg. 2002;97(5):1042–4.

88. Nornes H. The role of intracranial pressure in the arrest of hemorrhage in patients with ruptured intracranial aneurysm. J Neurosurg. 1973;39(2):226–34.

89. Al-Tamimi YZ, Bhargava D, Feltbower RG, Hall G, Goddard AJ, Quinn AC, Ross SA. Lumbar drainage of cerebrospinal fluid after aneurysmal subarachnoid hemorrhage: a prospective, randomized, controlled trial (LUMAS). Stroke. 2012;43(3):677–82.

90. Choi KS, Chun HJ, Yi HJ, Ko Y, Kim YS, Kim JM. Seizures and epilepsy following aneurysmal

subarachnoid hemorrhage: incidence and risk factors. J Kor Neurosurg Soc. 2009;46(2):93.

91. Rhoney DH, Tipps LB, Murry KR, Basham MC, Michael DB, Coplin WM. Anticonvulsant prophylaxis and timing of seizures after aneurysmal subarachnoid hemorrhage. Neurology. 2000;55(2):258–65.

92. Chumnanvej S, Dunn IF, Kim DH. Three-day phenytoin prophylaxis is adequate after subarachnoid hemorrhage. Neurosurgery. 2007;60(1):99–103.

93. Yoneda H, Nakamura T, Shirao S, Tanaka N, Ishihara H, Suehiro E, Koizumi H, Isotani E, Suzuki M. Multicenter prospective cohort study on volume management after subarachnoid hemorrhage: hemodynamic changes according to severity of subarachnoid hemorrhage and cerebral vasospasm. Stroke. 2013;44(8):2155–61.

94. Mayer SA, Limandri G, Sherman D, Lennihan L, Fink ME, Solomon RA, Ditullio M, Klebanoff LM, Beckford AR, Homma S. Electrocardiographic markers of abnormal left ventricular wall motion in acute subarachnoid hemorrhage. J Neurosurg. 1995;83(5):889–96.

95. Taccone FS, Lubicz B, Piagnerelli M, Van Nuffelen M, Vincent JL, De Backer D. Cardiogenic shock with stunned myocardium during triple-H therapy treated with intra-aortic balloon pump counterpulsation. Neurocrit Care. 2009;10(1):76–82.

96. Banki N, Kopelnik A, Tung P, Lawton MT, Gress D, Drew B, Dae M, Foster E, Parmley W, Zaroff J. Prospective analysis of prevalence, distribution, and rate of recovery of left ventricular systolic dysfunction in patients with subarachnoid hemorrhage. J Neurosurg. 2006;105(1):15–20.

97. Friedman JA, Pichelmann MA, Piepgras DG, McIver JI, Toussaint LG III, McClelland RL, Nichols DA, Meyer FB, Atkinson JL, Wijdicks EF. Pulmonary complications of aneurysmal subarachnoid hemorrhage. Neurosurgery. 2003;52(5):1025–32.

98. Kahn JM, Caldwell EC, Deem S, Newell DW, Heckbert SR, Rubenfeld GD. Acute lung injury in patients with subarachnoid hemorrhage: incidence, risk factors, and outcome. Crit Care Med. 2006;34(1):196–202.

99. Cahill WJ, Calvert JH, Zhang JH. Mechanisms of early brain injury after subarachnoid hemorrhage. J Cereb Blood Flow Metab. 2006;26(11):1341–53.

100. Commichau C, Scarmeas N, Mayer SA. Risk factors for fever in the neurologic intensive care unit. Neurology. 2003;60(5):837–41.

101. Vergouwen MD, Vermeulen M, van Gijn J, Rinkel GJ, Wijdicks EF, Muizelaar JP, Mendelow AD, Juvela S, Yonas H, Terbrugge KG, Macdonald RL. Definition of delayed cerebral ischemia after aneurysmal subarachnoid hemorrhage as an outcome event in clinical trials and observational studies: proposal of a multidisciplinary research group. Stroke. 2010;41(10):2391–5.

102. Petruk KC, West M, Mohr G, Weir BK, Benoit BG, Gentili F, Disney LB, Khan MI, Grace M, Holness RO, Karwon MS. Nimodipine treatment in poor-grade aneurysm patients: results of a multicenter double-blind placebo-controlled trial. J Neurosurg. 1988;68(4):505–17.

103. Chang JJ, Mack WJ, Saver JL, Sanossian N. Magnesium: potential roles in neurovascular disease. Front Neurol. 2014;5:52.

104. van den Bergh WM. Magnesium sulfate in aneurysmal subarachnoid hemorrhage: a randomized controlled trial. Stroke. 2005;36(5):1011–5.

105. Mees SM, Algra A, Vandertop WP, van Kooten F, Kuijsten HA, Boiten J, van Oostenbrugge RJ, Salman RA, Lavados PM, Rinkel GJ, van den Bergh WM. Magnesium for aneurysmal subarachnoid haemorrhage (MASH-2): a randomised placebo-controlled trial. Lancet. 2012;380(9836):44–9.

106. Wong GK, Poon WS, Chan MT, Boet R, Gin T, Ng SC, Zee BC, IMASH Investigators. Intravenous magnesium sulphate for aneurysmal subarachnoid hemorrhage (IMASH). Stroke. 2010;41(5):921–6.

107. Macdonald RL, Kassell NF, Mayer S, Ruefenacht D, Schmiedek P, Weidauer S, Frey A, Roux S, Pasqualin A. Clazosentan to overcome neurological ischemia and infarction occurring after subarachnoid hemorrhage (CONSCIOUS-1) randomized, double-blind, placebo-controlled phase 2 dose-finding trial. Stroke. 2008;39(11):3015–21.

108. Macdonald RL, Higashida RT, Keller E, Mayer SA, Molyneux A, Raabe A, Vajkoczy P, Wanke I, Bach D, Frey A, Marr A, Roux S, Kassell N. Clazosentan, an endothelin receptor antagonist, in patients with aneurysmal subarachnoid haemorrhage undergoing surgical clipping: a randomised, double-blind, placebo-controlled phase 3 trial (CONSCIOUS-2). Lancet Neurol. 2011;10(7):618–25.

109. Clazosentan in Aneurysmal Subarachnoid Hemorrhage (CONSCIOUS-3). ClinicalTrials.gov [Internet]. Bethesda (MD): National Library of Medicine (US). 2009–2012. http://clinicaltrials.gov/showclinicalTrails.govidentifierNCT00940095.

110. Liu GJ, Wang ZJ, Wang YF, Xu LL, Wang XL, Liu Y, Luo GJ, He GH, Zeng YJ. Systematic assessment and meta-analysis of the efficacy and safety of fasudil in the treatment of cerebral vasospasm in patients with subarachnoid hemorrhage. Eur J Clin Pharmacol. 2012;68(2):131–9.

111. Amin-Hanjani S, Ogilvy CS, Barker FG. Does intracisternal thrombolysis prevent vasospasm after aneurysmal subarachnoid hemorrhage? A meta-analysis. Neurosurgery. 2004;54(2):326–35.

112. Niu PP, Yang G, Xing YQ, Guo ZN, Yang Y. Effect of cilostazol in patients with aneurysmal subarachnoid hemorrhage: a systematic review and meta-analysis. J Neurol Sci. 2014;336(1–2):146–51.

113. Mees SD, van den Bergh WM, Algra A, Rinkel GJ. Antiplatelet therapy for aneurysmal subarachnoid haemorrhage. Cochrane Database Syst Rev. 2007;(4):CD006184.

114. Wurm G, Tomancok B, Nussbaumer K, Adelwöhrer C, Holl K. Reduction of ischemic sequelae fol-

lowing spontaneous subarachnoid hemorrhage: a double-blind, randomized comparison of enoxaparin versus placebo. Clin Neurol Neurosurg. 2004;106(2):97–103.

115. Lee KH, Lukovits T, Friedman JA. "Triple-H" therapy for cerebral vasospasm following subarachnoid hemorrhage. Neurocrit Care. 2006;4(1):68–76.

116. Washington CW, Zipfel GJ, Participants in the International Multi-disciplinary Consensus Conference on the Critical Care Management of Subarachnoid Hemorrhage. Detection and monitoring of vasospasm and delayed cerebral ischemia: a review and assessment of the literature. Neurocrit Care. 2011;15(2):312–7.

117. Kimball MM, Velat GJ, Hoh BL. Critical care guidelines on the endovascular management of cerebral vasospasm. Neurocrit Care. 2011;15(2):336–41.

118. Picetti E, Barbanera A, Bernucci C, Bertuccio A, Bilotta F, Boccardi EP, Cafiero T, Caricato A, Castioni CA, Cenzato M, Chieregato A. Early management of patients with aneurysmal subarachnoid hemorrhage in a hospital with neurosurgical/neuroendovascular facilities: a consensus and clinical recommendations of the Italian Society of Anesthesia and Intensive Care (SIAARTI)—Part 2. J Anesth Analg Crit Care. 2022;2(1):1–1.

119. D'Urso PI, Lanzino G, Cloft HJ, Kallmes DF. Flow diversion for intracranial aneurysms: a review. Stroke. 2011;42(8):2363–8.

120. Lanzino G. Flow diversion for intracranial aneurysms. J Neurosurg. 2013;118(2):405–7.

121. Brinjikji W, Murad MH, Lanzino G, Cloft HJ, Kallmes DF. Endovascular treatment of intracranial aneurysms with flow diverters: a meta-analysis. Stroke. 2013;44(2):442–7.

122. Bor AS, Rinkel GJ, van Norden J, Wermer MJ. Long-term, serial screening for intracranial aneurysms in individuals with a family history of aneurysmal subarachnoid haemorrhage: a cohort study. Lancet Neurol. 2014;13(4):385–92.

123. Nieuwkamp DJ, de Wilde A, Wermer MJ, Algra A, Rinkel GJ. Long-term outcome after aneurysmal subarachnoid hemorrhage—risks of vascular events, death from cancer and all-cause death. J Neurol. 2014;261(2):309–15.

124. Taufique Z, May T, Meyers E, Falo C, Mayer SA, Agarwal S, Park S, Connolly ES, Claassen J, Schmidt JM. Predictors of poor quality of life 1 year after subarachnoid hemorrhage. Neurosurgery. 2016;78(2):256–64.

125. Hammer A, Steiner A, Ranaie G, Yakubov E, Erbguth F, Hammer CM, Killer-Oberpfalzer M, Steiner H, Janssen H. Impact of comorbidities and smoking on the outcome in aneurysmal subarachnoid hemorrhage. Sci Rep. 2018;8(1):1–7.

Intracerebral Hemorrhage

Gopal Sedain, Sachit Sharma,
and Gentle Sunder Shrestha

Case Scenario

A 60-year-old female presented to the emergency department in a state of unconsciousness. She was found unconscious on the floor of her bedroom by her daughter in the morning. She had gone to bed at 9 pm the day before and was in a state of good health. She had hypertension for the previous 20 years and was on irregular medications. In the emergency department, she had a Glasgow Coma Scale (GCS) of E3V aphasia and M5 (GCS 8/10) and had weakness of the right half of the body. She had blood pressure of 220/100 mmHg, pulse of 60/min and regular breathing. Bilateral pupils were round, regular and reactive to light. She was started on injection labetalol and after her blood pressure stabilised was sent for computed tomography (CT) of the head with suspicion of stroke. CT of the head revealed a large intracerebral hematoma in the left putamen with an approximate volume of 24 mL with effacement of the sulci and lateral ventricle (Fig. 12.1). She was then managed in the ICU with regular BP monitoring with invasive arterial blood pressure monitoring and hourly monitoring of GCS. She was not on any anticoagulants and her coagulation profile was normal. She had an uneventful recovery, but with residual weakness of the right half of the body.

G. Sedain (✉)
Department of Neurosurgery, Tribhuvan University
Teaching Hospital, Kathmandu, Nepal

S. Sharma · G. S. Shrestha
Department of Critical Care Medicine, Tribhuvan
University Teaching Hospital, Kathmandu, Nepal

© Springer Nature Singapore Pte Ltd. 2024
K. K. Oli et al. (eds.), *Case-based Approach to Common Neurological Disorders*,
https://doi.org/10.1007/978-981-99-8676-7_12

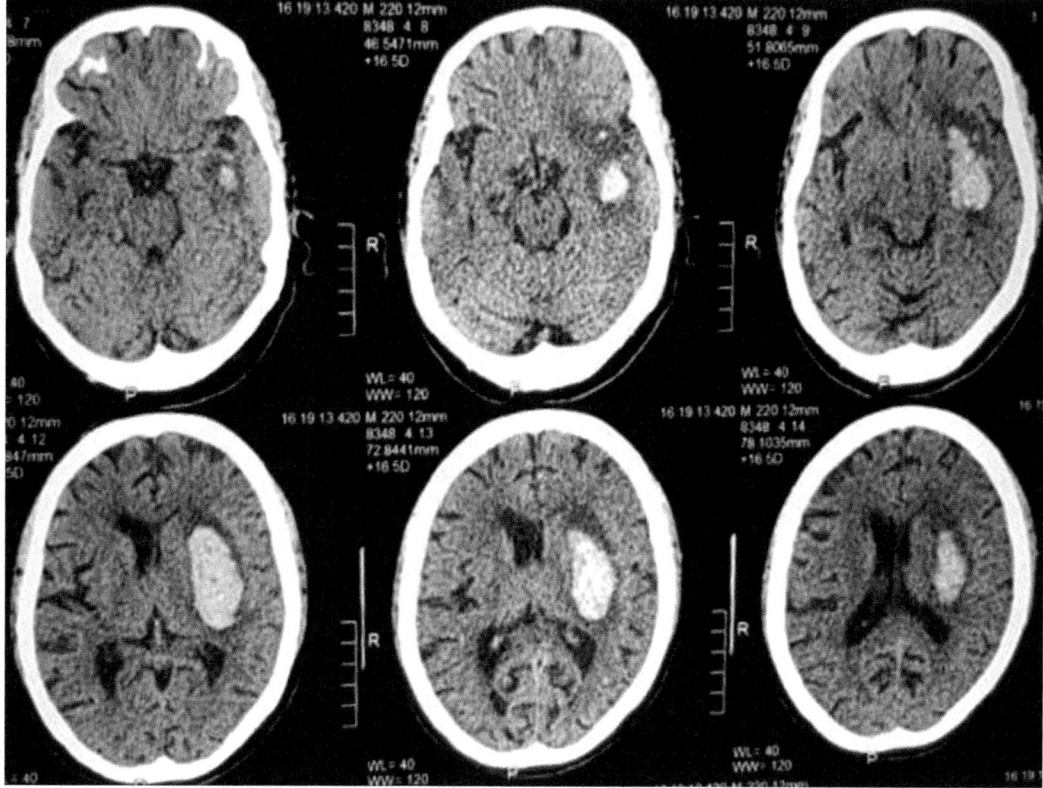

Fig. 12.1 Plain CT of the head reveals a large intracerebral hemorrhage (ICH) in left putamen region with effacement of ventricle

12.1 Introduction

Stroke can be broadly divided into ischemic and hemorrhagic forms. Hemorrhagic strokes can be further classified as intracerebral hemorrhage (ICH) and subarachnoid hemorrhage (SAH). ICH is one of the most life-threatening subtypes of stroke with high morbidity and mortality. There are various causes of ICH, the major ones in adults being hypertension and bleeding diathesis. Rupture of AV malformations is one of the most common causes of ICH in children. The management and prognosis of these patients depends upon various factors like the location of bleed, volume of blood, age of the patient and neurological status at presentation.

12.2 Epidemiology

Though ICH is responsible for only 10–15% of all forms of stroke, it carries a remarkably high risk of mortality or long-term disability. There are various advancements in the management of ischemic stroke and subarachnoid hemorrhage; however, limited progress has been made in ICH management. There is variability in the care of these patients from aggressive management to palliative care.

ICH is more common in Asians for two main reasons: limited primary care for hypertension (HTN) and non-compliance with treatment [1]. Spontaneous ICH can be either primary or secondary based on the underlying cause. Primary

ICH comprises about 70–80% of total ICH cases. It is mainly caused by spontaneous rupture of small arteries involved in HTN or amyloid angiopathy. According to location, primary ICH can be either lobar or non-lobar and supratentorial or infratentorial.

The most common cause of lobar ICH is cerebral amyloid angiopathy (CAA). CAA is caused by deposition of amyloid in small to medium-sized cortical perforators which are very likely to rupture in the elderly population. Long-standing hypertension may increase in lipohyalinosis of small perforating vessels of the basal ganglia, thalamus, pons and cerebellum. Rupture of these vessels can result in deep hemorrhages which may even extend to ventricles. Hypertensive ICH is most commonly seen in the putamen, thalamus, pons, cerebellum and subcortical white matter. Arteriovenous malformations (AVM), tumors, thrombophilias, antiplatelets or anticoagulants, vasculitis, drug or substance abuse, and cerebral venous sinus thrombosis are commonly associated with secondary ICH.

Early and aggressive management of ICH patients during the initial "golden hour" is essential for better outcomes. Due to perceived poor outcome and lack of timely proper treatment, ICH patients are usually vulnerable to undertreatment. There are often do-not-resuscitate (DNR) orders and trends towards palliative care treatment. In a prospective multicenter study which included 109 patients from 5 centers, avoidance of early DNR and aggressive management as per the ICH guidelines were associated with substantially lower mortality than predicted by ICH score (30-day mortality: predicted 50% versus observed 20.2%) [2].

The principles of management of ICH during the initial "golden hour" are as follows:

1. Stabilising patient's airway, breathing, and circulation (ABCs) and regular reassessment
2. Timely brain imaging for proper diagnosis
3. Proper assessment regarding ICH manifestations and patient's clinical condition

4. Evaluation for potential early interventions including:
   (a) Proper blood pressure management
   (b) Coagulopathy correction
   (c) Need for early surgical intervention

12.3 Diagnosis

Multiple etiologies may result in the development of ICH. About 60% of ICH cases occur secondary to chronic hypertension. CAA, coagulopathies secondary to anticoagulants, sympathomimetic drugs like cocaine, and arteriovenous malformations (AVMs) or cavernous malformations are a few other common causes of ICH. Vasculitis, infections and rupture of a saccular or mycotic aneurysm less commonly result in ICH. In some cases of ischemic stroke and venous infarct, hemorrhagic transformation or symptomatic hemorrhage can be present. Other important risk factors for ICH are advancing age, obesity and inactivity, heavy alcohol consumption, black population, smoking and some genetic associations.

The most common clinical feature associated with ICH is the development of sudden-onset focal neurological deficit. Neuroimaging with either a non-contrast CT of the head or an MRI of the brain is the most reliable imaging modality to distinguish ICH from ischemic stroke. Persistent cephalgia, altered sensorium and stuporous state, sudden rise in blood pressure, and rapid neurological deficits are common features of ICH. Non-contrast computed tomography (CT) is the gold standard (very high sensitivity and specificity) and the most common neuroimaging modality for the diagnosis because of its availability, and it can be quickly carried out in comparison to MRI [3].

12.3.1 Interpreting the CT Scan

Hypertensive ICH commonly bleeds at typical areas such as basal ganglia, thalamus, pons

Table 12.1 ICH score

Components	ICH score points
GCS	
3–4	2
5–12	1
13–15	0
ICH volume	
>30 mL	1
<30 mL	0
Presence of IVH	
Yes	1
No	0
Age	
>80	1
>80	0
Infratentorial origin of hemorrhage	
Yes	1
No	0
Total score	0–6

(brainstem) and cerebellum. ICH secondary to CAA or AVM is usually located in the lobar area. The amount of hematoma in various brain areas can help to prognosticate the patient's clinical outcome, which can be calculated from the baseline CT scan. The calculation of hematoma volume can be done using automated CT software algorithms or manually by using the ABC/2 formula, which approximates the volume of an ellipsoid. In this formula, A means longest diameter of hematoma, B is the diameter perpendicular to A, and C is the number of CT slices. Thus the formula is simple, popular in clinical practice and also comparable to computerised methods [4].

The ICH score is a commonly used tool for prognosticating the outcome of ICH patients. It includes five components assessed at the time of hospital admission (Table 12.1) [5]. Any acute fall in the neurological status or need for a follow-up of any underlying lesion or vascular anomaly warrants a repeat imaging.

12.4 Management of BP

Many patients with ICH have high blood pressure, which can lead to hematoma expansion or worsening of edema. Adequate control of blood pressure with lifestyle modification and antihypertensive treatment can decrease the chances of hypertensive bleed. The exact blood pressure target remains controversial. INTERACT II and ATACH II trials have shown that rapid lowering of blood pressure is safe and does not lead to ischemia. The recently published American Heart Association guidelines recommend lowering of systolic blood pressure (SBP) to a target of 140 mmHg and maintaining that within 130 to 150 mmHg thereafter if the initial BP is in the range of 150 to 220 mmHg to improve functional outcomes [6]. Optimal BP targets remain elusive for patients presenting with an initial systolic BP of >220 mmHg and this warrants further research. For patients presenting with an initial SBP >220 mmHg, BP should not be lowered to <140 mmHg as this has the potential to cause harm [7–9].

The treatment should be done using a rapidly acting and titratable agent like beta blockers and calcium channel blockers. Intravenous labetalol, which is a nonselective alpha and beta antagonist, is the most preferred agent as it is widely available. In ATACH II, which is one of the largest trials on ICH, the calcium channel blocker nicardipine was used as the first-line antihypertensive at a starting dose of 5 mg/h as continuous IV infusion, which was up-titrated by 2.5 mg/h every 15 min as needed, up to a maximum dose of 15 mg/h. Achieving a target systolic blood pressure of 110–139 mmHg didn't result in reduction of mortality rate or disability in comparison to standard reduction to a target of 140–179 mmHg. Nitroprusside and nitroglycerine should be avoided if possible as these agents can cause cerebral vasodilation and elevation of intracranial pressure (ICP) [7].

12.4.1 Correction of Coagulopathy

The presence of coagulopathy is associated with a higher incidence of hematoma expansion and hence needs to be corrected quickly (Table 12.2). Routine coagulopathy evaluation in ICH should include complete blood count including platelets, prothrombin time (international normalised ratio)

Table 12.2 Reversal agents for various anticoagulants-related ICH

Anticoagulant agent	Reversal agent
Vitamin K antagonist (VKA) and INR ≥2	• Prothrombin complex concentrate (PCC) in preference to fresh frozen plasma (FFP) • Vitamin K
VKA and INR 1.3–1.9	• PCC in preference to FFP
Factor Xa inhibitors	• Andexanet alfa • 4-F PCC or activated PCC (aPCC) may be considered to improve hemostasis
Direct thrombin inhibitors (dabigatran)	• Idarucizumab • When Idarucizumab is not available, aPCC or PCCs may be considered to improve hemostasis • Renal replacement therapy
Unfractionated heparin (UFH)	• Intravenous protamine
Low-molecular weight heparin (LMWH)	• Intravenous protamine

(PT(INR)) and activated partial thromboplastin time. Patients on warfarin with INR >1.4 should receive reversal agents like fresh frozen plasma (FFP), Vitamin K or prothrombin complex concentrate (PCC). FFP comprises various components such as factors I (fibrinogen), II, V, VII, IX, X, XI, and XIII, and antithrombin. Large volumes of blood products, especially FFP (10–15 mL/kg) for reversal of coagulopathy, should be cautiously transfused, due to increase in the risk for volume overload [10]. Alternatively, PCCs contain factors II, VII, IX and X (vitamin K-dependent coagulation factors) which contain concentrated clotting factors, and the transfusion volume is significantly lower than FFP. Thus, correction of INR is faster with far fewer cardiopulmonary complications when PCC is used over FFP for reversal [11].

Current recommendations for reversal of warfarin-induced coagulopathy include the administration of intravenous vitamin K 5–10 mg, along with FFP or PCC. Though the onset of action of Vitamin K is longer, it has a longer-lasting effect than PCC or FFP [12]. For patients taking acetylsalicylic acid (ASA), clopidogrel or other anti-platelet agents, platelet transfusion may be required. Additionally, desmopressin which promotes the release of von Willebrand factor may be added for patients taking clopidogrel. Protamine sulfate can be administered for reversal of unfractionated heparin (UFH) at a dose of 1 mg for every 100 U of intravenous UFH received in the previous 2 h [13].

If the last dose of UFH was administered more than 4 h prior to ICH onset, reversal may not be necessary because of its short half-life. Protamine sulfate can also be used in an attempt to reverse the effect of low-molecular weight heparin (LMWH) that was given within the previous 8 h. However, this reversal may be incomplete.

12.4.2 Surgical Management

Most patients with ICH are managed conservatively without surgical intervention. Intraventricular hemorrhagic extension is seen in about 45% of patients, which is a poor prognostic marker. External ventricular drain (EVD) is the management option in case of overt hydrocephalus, large IVH, poor GCS or signs of herniation. Few patients will need a VP shunt in the long term due to communicating hydrocephalus as a result of absorption failure. rt-PA to clear the clots early has been increasingly used. However, a CLEAR III (Clot Lysis: Evaluation of Accelerated Resolution of Intraventricular Hemorrhage) trial failed to show convincing benefits in improving outcomes [14]. There are some groups of patients who could benefit from evacuation of hematoma. Theoretically, hematoma evacuation decreases ICP and midline shift and prevents secondary injury from blood degradation products. This shows that surgery is beneficial in reducing the volume of intracerebral hemorrhage. Evidence suggests that hematoma removal reduces nervous tissue damage and ICP secondary to a reduction in local ischemia and removal of noxious chemicals. Large surgically accessible clots with mass effect might benefit from early surgery. On the other hand, deep clots involving speech and motor regions generally do not improve with the surgical approach.

The STICH trial is one of the largest trials in the surgical management of ICH in good and poor prognosis groups. The trial aims to investigate the effectiveness of early surgery within 24 h versus initial conservative medical treatment. Patient on conservative treatment if requires evacuation can be done later. This trial showed no benefit in outcome from early surgery over initial conservative management [15]. The STICH II trial reveals that early intervention does not increase mortality or disability at 6-month follow-up in comparison to the initial conservative group [16]. Cerebellar ICH, unlike supratentorial bleed, is an emergency, and emergent evacuation is advised. Large hematoma size (>3 cm), hydrocephalus and decreasing GCS are indications for surgery. Placement of EVD alone is not sufficient as this can lead to upward herniation and clinical deterioration.

In the minimally invasive catheter evacuation followed by thrombolysis (MISTIE) III trial, patients were randomised to image-guided MISTIE treatment (1.0 mg alteplase every 8 h for up to nine doses) or standard medical care. Though the minimally invasive procedure was safe, there was no difference in functional recovery between the surgical and the medical groups. Clinical outcome was found to be better in patients with residual post-operative clot volume lower than 15 mL [14].

12.4.3 Ancillary Management

Perihematoma edema is the cause of worsening neurological status and can occur between 48 and 72 h of the ictus. If clinically significant, it has to be managed with hypertonic saline or mannitol. There is no role for prophylactic decongestants for asymptomatic small hematoma. Seizures can occur in 16% of patients, especially in patients with hematoma extending up to the cortex. Routine anti-seizure prophylaxis is not warranted [17, 18]. Both hyperglycemia and hypoglycemia are associated with poorer outcome. The target should be in the range of 140 to 180 mg/dL. Fever is common after ICH especially in patients with intraventricular hemorrhage. Prolonged hyperthermia is associated with poorer outcome. However, therapeutic hypothermia has not shown to improve outcome [19]. There is significant risk (1–5%) of deep vein thrombosis (DVT) in patients with ICH as they are often hemiparetic and bed ridden. Mechanical methods like intermittent pneumatic compression should be initiated as soon as possible. Pharmacological methods like LMWH or unfractionated heparin can be started after 48 h of ictus once the hematoma is stable. This has not shown to significantly increase the chances of bleeding.

12.5 Prognosis

ICH is considered a debilitating disease with high economic and social burden. Many patients die during their first hospitalisation because of care withdrawal due to the nature of the disease. Many factors such as location of blood, volume, age and intraventricular extension are considered in ICH score to predict 30-day mortality. However, ICH score cannot accurately predict outcome and is not reliable. Those patients who survive the initial onslaught may need prolonged ventilation, intensive physiotherapy and rehabilitation. Recent advances in neurocritical care and minimally invasive surgical interventions look promising to improve outcomes.

References

1. van Asch CJ, Luitse MJ, Rinkel GJ, van der Tweel I, Algra A, Klijn CJ. Incidence, case fatality, and functional outcome of intracerebral haemorrhage over time, according to age, sex, and ethnic origin: a systematic review and meta-analysis. Lancet Neurol. 2010;9(2):167–76.
2. Morgenstern LB, Zahuranec DB, Sánchez BN, Becker KJ, Geraghty M, Hughes R, et al. Full medical support for intracerebral hemorrhage. Neurology. 2015;84(17):1739–44.
3. Chalela JA, Kidwell CS, Nentwich LM, Luby M, Butman JA, Demchuk AM, et al. Magnetic resonance imaging and computed tomography in emergency assessment of patients with suspected acute stroke: a prospective comparison. Lancet. 2007;369(9558):293–8.

4. Kothari RU, Brott T, Broderick JP, Barsan WG, Sauerbeck LR, Zuccarello M, et al. The ABCs of measuring intracerebral hemorrhage volumes. Stroke. 1996;27(8):1304–5.

5. Hemphill JC III, Bonovich DC, Besmertis L, Manley GT, Johnston SC. The ICH score: a simple, reliable grading scale for intracerebral hemorrhage. Stroke. 2001;32(4):891–7.

6. Greenberg SM, Ziai WC, Cordonnier C, Dowlatshahi D, Francis B, Goldstein JN, et al. 2022 guideline for the management of patients with spontaneous intracerebral hemorrhage: a guideline from the American Heart Association/American Stroke Association. Stroke. 2022;53(7):e282–361.

7. Hemphill JC III, Greenberg SM, Anderson CS, Becker K, Bendok BR, Cushman M, et al. Guidelines for the management of spontaneous intracerebral hemorrhage: a guideline for healthcare professionals from the American Heart Association/American Stroke Association. Stroke. 2015;46(7):2032–60.

8. Qureshi AI, Huang W, Lobanova I, Barsan WG, Hanley DF, Hsu CY, et al. Outcomes of intensive systolic blood pressure reduction in patients with intracerebral hemorrhage and excessively high initial systolic blood pressure: post hoc analysis of a randomized clinical trial. JAMA Neurol. 2020;77(11):1355–65.

9. Anderson CS, Heeley E, Huang Y, Wang J, Stapf C, Delcourt C, et al. Rapid blood-pressure lowering in patients with acute intracerebral hemorrhage. N Engl J Med. 2013;368(25):2355–65.

10. Hanley JP. Warfarin reversal. J Clin Pathol. 2004;57(11):1132–9.

11. Sarode R, Milling TJJ, Refaai MA, Mangione A, Schneider A, Durn BL, et al. Efficacy and safety of a 4-factor prothrombin complex concentrate in patients on vitamin K antagonists presenting with major bleeding: a randomized, plasma-controlled, phase IIIb study. Circulation. 2013;128(11):1234–43.

12. Guidelines on oral anticoagulation: third edition. Br J Haematol. 1998;101(2):374–87.

13. Schulman S, Bijsterveld NR. Anticoagulants and their reversal. Transfus Med Rev. 2007;21(1):37–48.

14. Hanley DF, Lane K, McBee N, Ziai W, Tuhrim S, Lees KR, et al. Thrombolytic removal of intraventricular haemorrhage in treatment of severe stroke: results of the randomised, multicentre, multiregion, placebo-controlled CLEAR III trial. Lancet. 2017;389(10069):603–11.

15. Mendelow AD, Gregson BA, Fernandes HM, Murray GD, Teasdale GM, Hope DT, et al. Early surgery versus initial conservative treatment in patients with spontaneous supratentorial intracerebral haematomas in the International Surgical Trial in Intracerebral Haemorrhage (STICH): a randomised trial. Lancet. 2005;365(9457):387–97.

16. Mendelow AD, Gregson BA, Rowan EN, Murray GD, Gholkar A, Mitchell PM. Early surgery versus initial conservative treatment in patients with spontaneous supratentorial lobar intracerebral haematomas (STICH II): a randomised trial. Lancet. 2013;382(9890):397–408.

17. De Herdt V, Dumont F, Hénon H, Derambure P, Vonck K, Leys D, et al. Early seizures in intracerebral hemorrhage: incidence, associated factors, and outcome. Neurology. 2011;77(20):1794–800.

18. Schwarz S, Häfner K, Aschoff A, Schwab S. Incidence and prognostic significance of fever following intracerebral hemorrhage. Neurology. 2000;54(2):354–61.

19. Lord AS, Karinja S, Lantigua H, Carpenter A, Schmidt JM, Claassen J, et al. Therapeutic temperature modulation for fever after intracerebral hemorrhage. Neurocrit Care. 2014;21(2):200–6.

Cerebral Sinus and Venous Thrombosis

13

Reema Rajbhandari and Niraj Gautam

Case Scenario

A 54-year-old male patient presented with a history of headache for 8 days which was acute on onset, located over the occipital and nape of the neck region, throbbing in character, without any radiation, associated with mild blurring of vision without diplopia, aggravated with strenuous activities, and in supine position. Headache was progressively increasing in severity over the days, associated with nausea and vomiting. He also had three episodes of generalized tonic-clonic movements lasting for 1 min for 1 day. Following the last seizure episode, he developed weakness of right upper and lower limbs. There was no history of fever, ear discharges, loose stool, trauma, diplopia, dysphagia, or dysarthria. There was no history of smoking, alcohol, or any chronic illness. His vitals were stable. On examination, he was found to be plethoric. Fundus examined was normal. His higher mental function was intact, no meningeal signs, and normal cranial nerves.

His motor examination revealed power of 4−/5 over the right upper and lower limbs across all the joints, reflexes of 3+ and an upgoing planter over the right. All sensory modalities were normal. Coordination and gait were intact and normal. His investigations revealed hemoglobulin of 18.6 g/dL and a hematocrit of 51%, and the rest of his routine blood parameters were normal. Chest X-ray, ultrasonography abdomen and pelvis, echocardiography, and arterial blood gas were normal. His contrast tomography (CT) head plain showed a hyperdense lesion over the left parietal deep white matter, and hyperdensities were present over the straight sinus and superior sagittal sinus region (Fig. 13.1a, b). His magnetic resonance imaging (MRI) showed T2 high-signal changes with central hypointensity over the left frontal and parietal cortical areas, suggestive of acute hemorrhage (Fig. 13.1c). His magnetic resonance venogram (MRV) revealed a filling defect over the superior sagittal sinus (Fig. 13.1d).

R. Rajbhandari (✉) · N. Gautam
Department of Neurology, Tribhuvan University
Institute of Medicine, Maharajgunj Medical Campus,
Kathmandu, Nepal

© Springer Nature Singapore Pte Ltd. 2024
K. K. Oli et al. (eds.), *Case-based Approach to Common Neurological Disorders*,
https://doi.org/10.1007/978-981-99-8676-7_13

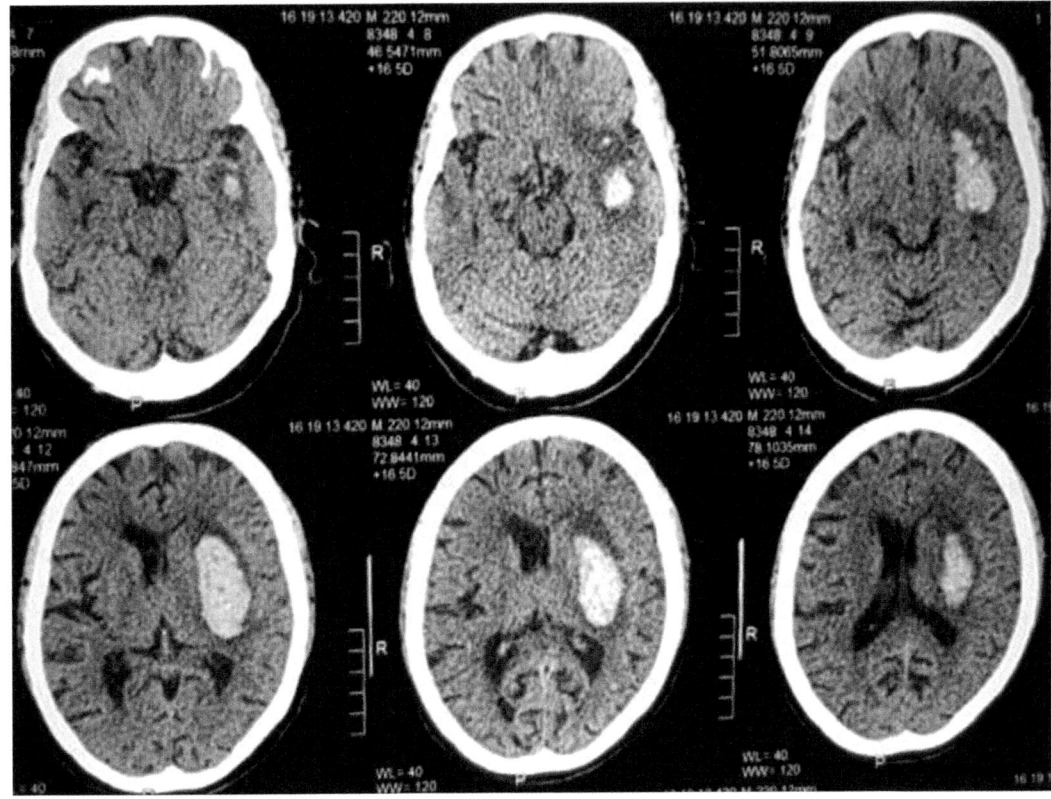

Fig. 13.1 CT head plain showed a hyperdense lesion over left parietal deep white matter, and hyperdensities were present over the straight sinus and superior sagittal sinus region (**a** and **b**); MRI T2 shows high signal changes with central hypointensity over left frontal and parietal cortical areas, suggestive of acute hemorrhage (**c**); MRV of the brain revealed a filling defect over the superior sagittal sinus, suggestive of thrombosis (**d**)

13.1 Introduction

Cerebral venous thrombosis (CVT) is a less common cause of cerebrovascular disease, with a prevalence of 0.5%, female predominance, and can occur at any age [1]. It can present in various spectrums but usually has a favorable outcome with a low mortality rate. CVT patients may present to multiple specialties: otorhinologist, pediatrician, obstetrician, ophthalmologist, and physicians, with symptoms of recurrent ear infections, headache and vomiting, complicated pregnancy or puerperium, blurring of vision, and vague symptoms, respectively. There is usually 1 week of delay in the diagnosis from the onset of symptoms.

A newer approach with widespread use of imaging techniques allows for early diagnosis and proper understanding of CVT and, therefore, has been found to be more frequently diagnosed in recent days. MRI sequences with T1, T2, fluid-attenuated inversion recovery, and a venogram are the best diagnostic methods; however, diagnosis may still be difficult sometimes [2].

Most of the CVT patients have raised D-dimer level, but normal D-dimers can be present, particularly in CVT patients with isolated headache symptom. Heparin is the first line of treatment; however, aggressive treatments such as intravenous thrombolysis, mechanical thrombectomy, and decompressive surgery may be needed in certain cases [3].

13.2 Relevant Anatomy

Cerebral veins have no valves and muscular layer in their thin walls. They arise from the brain tissues and remains within the subarachnoid space. Cerebral veins pierce the arachnoid and dura mater, which then drain into the cranial venous sinuses. Dural sinuses are endothelial-lined channels forming the terminal part of the cerebral venous system that drain into the internal jugular vein [4]. Cerebral venous system comprises superficial and deep venous system. Sagittal sinuses and cortical veins are part of the superficial venous system, which drains the superficial surfaces of the bilateral cerebral hemispheres. Lateral sinuses, straight sinuses, and sigmoid sinuses, along with deep cortical veins, are part of the deep venous system. Finally, blood from these systems drain into internal jugular veins. The venous drainage system of the brain does not follow the similar course as the arterial system. In contrast, venous blood drains to the nearest venous sinus, except deep veins which drain into deeper structure. Superior sagittal sinus (SSS) receives venous blood from the superior convexity veins of the lateral and medial cortex. SSS is connected to sylvian vein by the largest anastomotic channel called vein of Trolard. Temporal, occipital, and few areas of parietal cortex drain into the transverse sinus via temporo-occipital veins. Vein of Labbe connects the sylvian vein to the transverse sinus. Sylvian veins drain part of the frontal and temporal areas to the cavernous sinus and pterygoid plexus [4]. Ophthalmic veins drain into the cavernous sinus, which drains to the sigmoid sinus via the superior petrosal sinus and to the internal jugular vein via the inferior petrosal sinus. The deep venous system consists of the septal vein, which combines with thalamostriate veins and caudate veins to form the internal cerebral vein, which in turn combines with basal vein of Rosenthal to form the vein of Galen, which together with the inferior sagittal sinus forms a straight sinus to drain into the confluence.

13.3 Pathophysiology

Virchow's triad underlying CVT comprises state of hypercoagulability, stasis of flow, and endothelial injury [5]. Thus, intracellular vessel wall damage may result in the activation of the coagulation cascade and thrombus formation. Occlusion of cerebral veins results in raised venous pressure, which subsequently causes pooling of blood in the venous compartment. This will cause blood brain barrier disturbance and further leads to vasogenic edema. In CVT, cytotoxic edema also occurs due to impairment of NA/K-ATPase pump function.

13.4 Etiology

The common causes are inherited and acquired thrombophilia [6, 7]. In some patients even with extensive investigations no cause may be found. The major lists of causes that are associated with CVT are shown in the Table 13.1.

Table 13.1 Causes associated with cerebral venous thrombosis

Local	Systemic	Drugs	Blood dyscrasias	Coagulopathy
(a) Head injury	(a) Dehydration	(a) Oral contraceptives	(a) Leukemia	(a) Protein S, protein C, antithrombin III deficiency
(b) Neurosurgery	(b) Septicemia	(b) Hormone replacement therapy	(b) Myeloproliferative disorders	(b) Factor V Leiden mutation
(c) Meningitides	(c) Pregnancy and puerperium	(c) Androgens	(c) Thrombocythemia	(c) Antiphospholipid antibodies
(d) Arterio-venous malformation	(d) Inflammatory bowel disease	(d) L-asparaginase	(d) Sickle-cell trait	
(e) Sepsis (sinusitis, mastoiditis, cellulitis)	(e) Malignancy	(e) Ecstasy	(e) Paroxysmal nocturnal hemoglobinuria	
(f) Space-occupying lesions	(f) Sarcoidosis		(f) Thrombotic thrombocytopenic purpura	
(g) Jugular catheterization	(g) Collagen disease (Behcet's syndrome, SLE, Sjögren's syndrome)		(g) Heparin-induced thrombocytopenia	
	(h) Hyperhomocysteinemia			
	(i) Nephrotic syndrome			
	(j) Autoimmune thyroiditis			

13.5　Clinical Features

The clinical features of CVT usually have symptoms and signs of increased intracranial pressure (ICP), a focal parenchymal lesion, or both. Headache is the most common symptom usually with acute onset and throbbing in character. CVT can also present with pain around the auricular or mastoid region with or without discharge, suggestive of transverse sinus thrombosis secondary to mastoiditis. Seizure is also a common clinical presentation, of which early symptomatic seizures can be found in 44.3% and status epilepticus may be present in 12.8% [8]. Other focal neurological symptoms and signs may also be there with motor weakness, visual field impairment, sensory symptoms, inattention, or neglect, which may secondarily be due to infarction or hemorrhage. Patients may also have acute cognitive dysfunction causing drowsiness or stupor, suggestive of a deep venous infarction of the thalamus [9]. Cranial nerves that can be involved are III, IV, V, VI, VII, VIII, IX, X, and XI; either single or multiple cranial nerve involvement is possible. Cranial nerves such as III, IV, V, and VI can be involved in anterior cavernous sinus thrombosis. Moreover, other atypical presentation of CVT can be subarachnoid hemorrhage, psychiatric symptoms, parkinsonism, visual blurring, micrographia and hypophonia, migraine-like symptoms, hearing impairment, ocular flutter, or even sometimes asymptomatic.

13.6　Diagnosis

The clinical manifestation is diverse and not specific; hence, a high index of clinical suspicion should be made in a patient presenting with this myriad of symptoms; however, certain clinical features of new-onset severe throbbing headache, seizure, focal neurological deficit, and sometimes cognitive abnormality to sensorium disturbances should be suspected to be as a result of CVT. Imaging plays a major role in the diagnosis of CVT.

A non-contrast CT head of the patient may show the cord or dense vein sign, which is a direct visualization of the fresh thrombus in the occluded sinus. It may be present in 2–25% of patients [10]. A CT contrast head may show a central hypodense core with an outer bright triangle, called an empty delta sign. This sign is due to enhanced contrast of the dilated collaterals around the clot, seen in 25–52% of CVT patients involving sagittal, straight, and lateral sinus [11]. The most specific MRI finding is the loss of expected signal flow void on standard spin echo T1W and T2W sequences. MRV has evolved as the most popular technique to confirm the diagnosis of CVT and can be performed with non-contrast, i.e., time of flight (TOF) or phase contrast techniques (PCT).

13.7　Management

The treatment should be a good balance between decreasing intracranial hypertension and decreasing the chance of hemorrhage by treating with anticoagulation and trying to avoid ICP-lowering medications, which tend to increase viscosity and thus increase coagulability. A good management strategy would be to address the underlying pathophysiology and complications, while the primary aim is to anticoagulate the patient.

13.7.1　Anticoagulations

The role of anticoagulation in CVT treatment is suggested, regardless of the associated ICH. Anticoagulation could significantly alleviate the neurological deficits with venous recanalization [12]. Therefore, intravenous heparin is the choice of early CVT therapy, even in associated hemorrhagic changes. Following the acute therapy, heparin is replaced with oral anticoagulation (warfarin or dabigatran). Anticoagulation therapy helps to prevent thrombus growth or formation, promote recanalization, and further prevent from deep vein thrombosis of limbs or pulmonary embolism.

13.7.2 Management of Early Complications

Seizure is one of the common complications of CVT, and antiepileptic drugs should be initiated even after a single episode of seizure [13]. Both obstructive and communicating hydrocephalus can be present in the patient with CVT [14]. Neurosurgical interventions such as ventriculostomy can be done in such a scenario, or a ventriculoperitoneal shunt can be an option if the condition is persistent. Thrombolytic therapy, CSF removal with lumbar drainage, and the use of acetazolamide are possible therapeutic alternatives for the treatment of raised intracranial pressure associated with CVT [15].

Long-term treatment with heparin or warfarin for 3–6 months after resolution of initial symptoms is advocated. The management also includes the investigation of the underlying cause of the CVT, as failure to address this issue results in recurrent thrombosis or a more serious diagnosis. A careful, systematic approach to looking for local causes, thrombophilia screening, and screening for underlying collagen vascular disease, malignancy, and offending drugs should be done meticulously.

13.8 Prognosis

Most patients with CVT have a good prognosis as compared to those with arterial stroke in terms of mortality. The reasons for this may be improvements in treatment, risk assessment, an increased recognition of mild cases, and advancements in diagnostic technologies [16]. The short-term benefit of available injectable and oral anticoagulants cannot be ignored.

References

1. Bousser MG, Ferro JM. Cerebral venous thrombosis: an update. Lancet Neurol. 2007;6:162–70.
2. Coutinho JM, Ferro JM, Canhão P, Barinagarrementeria F, Cantú C, Bousser MG, et al. Cerebral venous and sinus thrombosis in women. Stroke. 2009;40:2356.
3. Coutinho J, de Bruijn SF, deVeber G, Stam J. Anticoagulation for cerebral venous sinus thrombosis. Cochrane Database Syst Rev. 2011;2011:CD002005.
4. Uddin MA, Haq TU, Rafique MZ. Cerebral venous system anatomy. J Pak Med Assoc. 2006;56:516.
5. Esmon CT. Basic mechanisms and pathogenesis of venous thrombosis. Blood Rev. 2009;23:225.
6. Martinelli I, De Stefano V, Mannucci PM. Inherited risk factors for venous thromboembolism. Nat Rev Cardiol. 2014;11:140.
7. Ferro JM, Canhão P, Stam J, Bousser MG, Barinagarrementeria F. Prognosis of cerebral vein and dural sinus thrombosis: results of the International Study on Cerebral Vein and Dural Sinus Thrombosis (ISCVT). Stroke. 2004;35:664.
8. Teh CM, Go T, Askalan R, De Veber G, MacGregor D, Moharir M, et al. Predictors of early symptomatic seizures in children with cerebral sino-venous thrombosis. Ann Neurol. 2011.
9. Behrouzi R, Punter M. Diagnosis and management of cerebral venous thrombosis. Clin Med J R Coll Physicians Lond. 2018;18:75.
10. Rao KCVG, Knipp HC, Wagner EJ. Computed tomographic findings in cerebral sinus and venous thrombosis. Radiology. 1981;140:391.
11. Virapongse C, Cazenave C, Quisling R, Sarwar M, Hunter S. The empty delta sign: frequency and significance in 76 cases of dural sinus thrombosis. Radiology. 1987;162:779.
12. Xu W, Gao L, Li T, Shao A, Zhang J. Efficacy and risks of anticoagulation for cerebral venous thrombosis. Medicine (United States). 2018;97:e10506.
13. Masuhr F, Busch M, Amberger N, Ortwein H, Weih M, Neumann K, et al. Risk and predictors of early epileptic seizures in acute cerebral venous and sinus thrombosis. Eur J Neurol. 2006;13:852.
14. Kersbergen KJ, De Vries LS, Van Straaten HLM, Benders MJNL, Nievelstein RAJ, Groenendaal F. Anticoagulation therapy and imaging in neonates with a unilateral thalamic hemorrhage due to cerebral sinovenous thrombosis. Stroke. 2009;40:2754.
15. Ferro JM, Canhão P. Acute treatment of cerebral venous and dural sinus thrombosis. Curr Treat Options Neurol. 2008;10:126.
16. Luo Y, Tian X, Wang X. Diagnosis and treatment of cerebral venous thrombosis: a review. Front Aging Neurosci. 2018;10:2.

Large Hemispheric Stroke

14

Bikram Prasad Gajurel

Case Scenario

A 72-year-old female was brought to the emergency with a history of right-sided weakness and inability to speak which was discovered at 5 pm when her family members returned from work. She was well when she had breakfast with them at 7 am. The family said that she had not cooked the morning meal that day. She did not have a significant medical history except that she was on losartan 50 mg once daily for hypertension. On examination, her vital signs were stable. She had global aphasia, right homonymous hemianopia, forced eye deviation to the left side, right upper motor neuron-type facial nerve palsy, and complete plegia of the right upper and lower limbs. Her National Institutes of Health Stroke Scale (NIHSS) score was 22. Her computed tomography (CT) scan done at presentation did not show any abnormality (Fig. 14.1). Due to the lack of facility for mechanical intervention, she was managed conservatively. However, on day 2, her level of consciousness deteriorated. Her repeat CT scan of the head then showed a large hemispheric infarct with significant mass effect (Fig. 14.2). The next day, her level of consciousness further deteriorated and she had to be intubated to maintain airway and prevent aspiration. Further, CT scan of the head was repeated which showed massive midline shift (Fig. 14.3). She underwent decompressive hemicraniectomy the same day, and subsequently improved to a modified Rankin Score (mRS) of 5 after a long stay in the intensive unit care (Fig. 14.4).

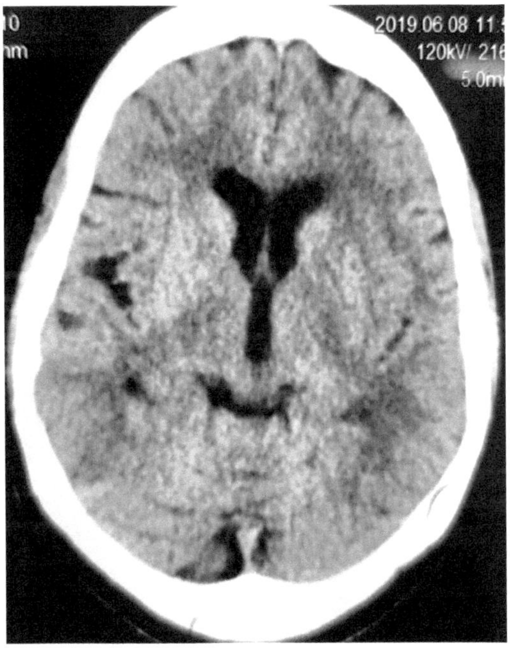

Fig. 14.1 CT head of the patient at presentation

B. P. Gajurel (✉)
Department of Neurology, Tribhuvan University Institute of Medicine, Maharajgunj Medical Campus, Kathmandu, Nepal
e-mail: bikram_gajurel@iom.edu.np

K. K. Oli et al. (eds.), *Case-based Approach to Common Neurological Disorders*,
https://doi.org/10.1007/978-981-99-8676-7_14

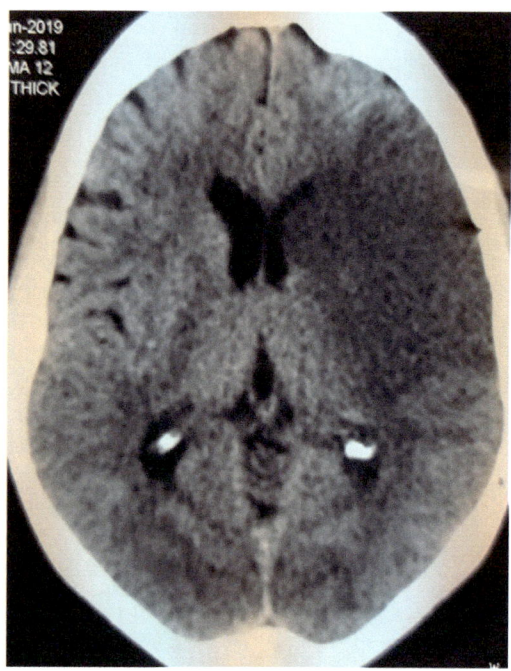

Fig. 14.2 CT of the head of the patient the next day. Note the mass effect in the left MCA territory

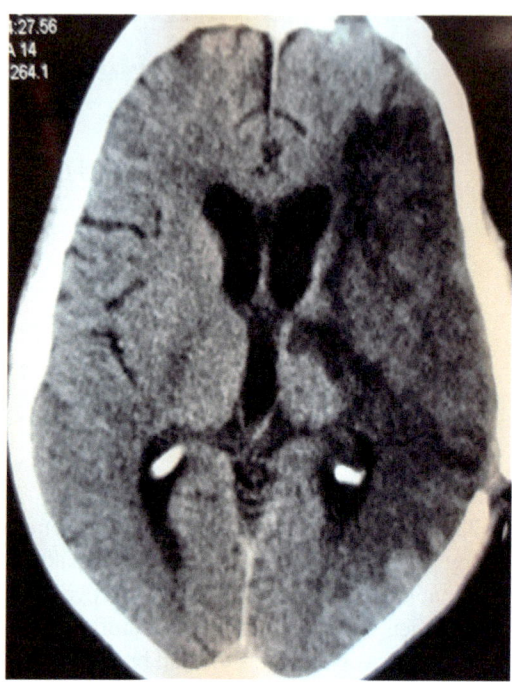

Fig. 14.4 CT of the head of the patient weeks after decompressive hemicraniectomy

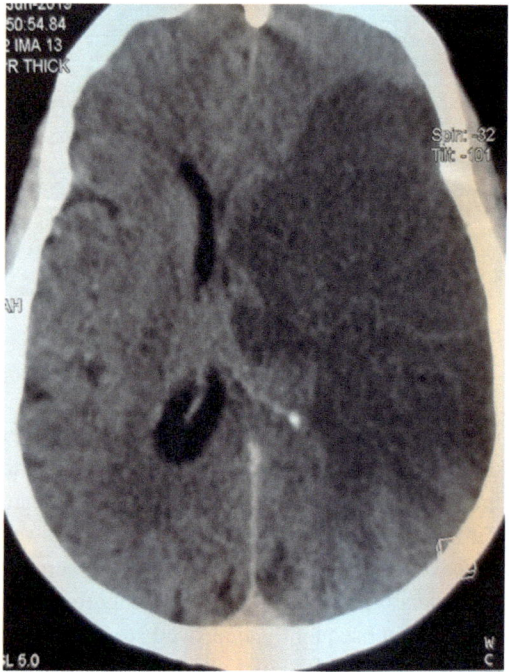

Fig. 14.3 CT of the head of the patient on day 3. Note malignant cerebral edema on the left side

14.1 Introduction

Large hemispheric stroke (LHS) is a severe type of brain infarction which occurs when the middle cerebral artery (MCA) or the internal carotid artery gets occluded. It usually involves a major portion of the basal ganglia as well and, in addition, may be associated with anterior or posterior cerebral artery territory infarction [1]. The most likely cause of large hemispheric stroke is an embolus that arises from the heart or in-situ atherothrombosis of the internal carotid artery. Patients who are younger than 45 years of age may develop such infractions when the major cervical arteries are affected by dissections. The diagnosis of LHS is established based on a constellation of signs and symptoms.

When the blood supply to the brain is suddenly cut off, a small area of brain in which basic metabolic activities cannot be sustained gets infarcted within a few minutes (infarct core). The surrounding area which is also involved to a lesser degree (penumbra) remains viable for several hours due to collateral blood supply from adjacent vessels. This collateral circulation will eventually fail if the blood supply to the penumbra is not established within a certain but variable time window by either chemical or mechanical means.

The incidence of LHS is less than 10% of all ischemic strokes [2]. It is associated with higher rates of morbidity and mortality because of the development of massive cerebral edema, or malignant cerebral edema (MCE). MCE leads to dangerous local mass effect which can result in herniation of the medial temporal lobe into the brainstem. This subsequently gets compressed leading to dysfunction of vital brainstem structures. It is also associated with many significant systemic complications like hyperglycemia, hyperpyrexia, deep venous thrombosis, and chest infections. Most patients with LHS develop malignant MCE after 2–3 days of onset of symptoms. This will manifest itself by neurological deterioration which can be very rapid and progressive. The mortality rate in patients in MCE who are only medically treated can reach up to 80% [3].

14.2   Pathophysiology

The breakdown of the blood brain barrier (BBB) is the key pathophysiological mechanism behind the development of cerebral edema in LHS [4*]. Cerebral edema starts developing after a few hours of interruption of blood supply to the brain. The first event is the development of cytotoxic edema, which starts within minutes of ischemia and is characterized by intact BBB. It is caused by failure of the Na/K pump in the brain cells and usually declines within the first few days. This is simultaneously accompanied by ionic edema, which occurs when decrease in solutes in the brain cells creates an osmotic gradient which extracts ions from the endothelium into the brain parenchyma [5]. This is accompanied by shifts of water across the endothelium leading to brain edema. However, the BBB remains intact. The BBB ultimately fails, and the endothelial junc-

tions give way allowing the movement of proteins, solutes, and plasma into the parenchymal space. The brain parenchymal cells also rupture, adding more solutes to the brain parenchyma which will extract more water into it. This vasogenic edema peaks around 24–48 h of onset of ischemia [6]. The mass effect thus produced and the resultant rise of the intracranial pressure is the reason behind the neurological deterioration in patients with LHS and MCE with significant shifts of intracranial contents. If left untreated, this will ultimately lead to brainstem compression and death.

14.3   Clinical Features

Patients who have infarctions of the large portion of cerebral hemispheres present with sudden onset of hemiplegia, hemisensory loss, global aphasia (dominant hemisphere), hemineglect, anosognosia and asomatognosia (non-dominant hemisphere), forced eye deviation, complete hemianopia, hemisensory loss, and decrease in level of consciousness [7*]. These signs and symptoms are also known by the term "hemispheric syndrome." The development of MCE is heralded by worsening of the presenting symptoms, headache, vomiting, and further impairment of consciousness. In patients who are more likely to develop MCE and worsen, the NIHSS score is very high, more than 20 when the dominant side is involved and more than 15 when the non-dominant side is involved. Some patients with MCE deteriorate neurologically when there is confluent hemorrhagic transformation at the site of infarction.

14.4   Imaging

Computed tomography (CT) of the head without contrast is the primary imaging modality for the initial evaluation of patients with acute ischemic stroke. It is cheap, readily available, reliably excludes hemorrhage, and can be carried out rapidly. Depending on availability and local expertise, CT of the head findings can be substantiated with CT angiogram of the head and neck, CT perfusion, MRI of the head with MR angiogram, and perfusion studies. Certain early signs in CT of the head are highly suggestive of large infarcts with potential for MCE and poor prognosis. These signs are attenuation of the lentiform nucleus, loss of the insular ribbon, effacement of sulci in the affected hemisphere, and the dense MCA sign [8]. The 10-point Alberta Stroke Program Early CT Score (ASPECTS) is a grading system for assessment of early ischemic changes in CT of the head. The ASPECTS value of <6 is highly suggestive of a large lesion size and potential for MCE. Important predictors of progression to LHS are hypodensity in >50% of the MCA territory in CT of the head, diffusion-weighted imaging lesion volume >145 mL within 14 h of onset, CT perfusion study demonstrating perfusion deficit in >66% of the MCA territory within 6 h of stroke onset, and cerebral blood flow map showing an infarct core of >27.9% [9].

14.5 Management

The 2018 American Heart Association/American Stroke Association guidelines for the early management of acute ischemic stroke recommends that for patients with acute ischemic stroke who meet the standard eligibility criteria and present within 4.5 h of onset of symptoms, the standard of care is intravenous thrombolysis with recombinant tissue plasminogen inhibitor alteplase [10*]. All patients with acute ischemic stroke should also undergo imaging of the arterial anatomy from the arch of the aorta to the vertex to look for large vessel occlusion. Patients who have large vessel occlusion on their angiogram should be evaluated for mechanical thrombectomy if the onset of symptoms is within 24 h. Rapid and successful brain reperfusion can limit the size of the affected area of the brain and can significantly reduce the chances of MCE. Mechanical thrombectomy is undertaken for patients whose ASPECT is ≥6. Currently trials of mechanical thrombectomy are including patients who have more extensive infarct size (ASPECT <6) and also those who present late in the time window.

Other important aspects of management of all patients with acute ischemic stroke are airway control and ventilation (if necessary), adequate control of blood pressure (less than 180 mmHg systolic after reperfusion established and less than 220 mmHg/120 mmHg in other patients unless hypertensive emergency), maintenance of adequate fluid volume with isotonic solutions, maintenance of appropriate blood glucose level (140–180 mg/dL) with insulin, avoidance of hyperthermia, prevention of deep venous thrombosis, and control of brain edema [10*].

Patients with LHS or suspected LHS based on clinical features should be admitted in an intensive care unit or a dedicated stroke unit because of the monitoring needed as the development of MCE and neurological deterioration can be fairly rapid and need to be attended to as early as possible. Neurological monitoring should be carried out every hour for the first 48 h. Level of consciousness, pupillary diameter, and new or progressive neurological deficits should be actively monitored to identify patients who would benefit from urgent medical and surgical interventions in a timely manner and avoid irreversible brain insults. Patients who deteriorate due to cerebral edema with significant mass effect can effectively respond to osmotic agents like hypertonic saline and mannitol, or invasive means like hyperventilation (in those who are already intubated). These interventions should not be considered for prolonged use and are best used as bridging therapy to decompressive hemicraniectomy [11*].

The surgical procedure of choice for patients who have LHS and are deteriorating with significant midline shift (≥5 mm) is decompressive hemicraniectomy. Decompressive hemicraniectomy is a surgical treatment which allows room for edematous brain to expand, ultimately reversing the mass effect and controlling the shifting of brain parenchyma. In 2015, a meta-analysis of six important clinical trials of surgical interventions for LHS concluded that patients who undergo decompressive hemicraniectomy have significantly lower mortality compared to patients who are managed medically [12*]. In this same analysis, surgery significantly increased the proportion of patients with slight disability. However, significantly more patients, especially those older than 60 years of age, remained moderately to severely disabled after decompressive hemicraniectomy. In order for decompressive hemicraniectomy to be beneficial, it has to be undertaken within 48 h of the onset of symptoms [7*]. There is some evidence that even if surgery is done later (48–96 h), it may still have better outcomes [13]. The American Heart Association/American Stroke Association guidelines state that decompressive hemicraniectomy is reasonable in individuals ≤60 years of age with LHS and neurological deterioration within 48 h despite medical treatment, and can be considered within 48 h for patients >60 years of age with neurological deterioration despite receiving medical therapy. The wishes of the patient and the family should always be taken into consideration when deciding to treat patients aggressively after LHS and MCE. Decompressive hemicraniectomy is not an appropriate treatment for many older people with other significant comorbidities. It should be avoided in patients who do not wish to live with severe disability. These recommendations are irrespective of the side of the brain that is involved.

14.6 Prognosis

The mortality rate in patients with MCE who are not aggressively treated can be up to 80% [3]. Many factors are associated with poor outcome after LHS. Younger age, female sex, severe disability (NIHSS >20), low Glasgow Coma Scale at presentation, and horizontal pineal displacement >4 mm are frequently associated with poor outcome [14*]. Mortality is significantly increased in patients who develop decreased level of consciousness at 3 h after admission and those who stop reacting to pain within the first 24 h of admission [15]. Patients who have good collateral flow on pretreatment CT angiography of the brain tend to have smaller final infarct volumes, better response to treatment, and less disability [16].

14.7 Future Directions

Recent advances in LHS research are focusing on various molecules which get upregulated because of the ischemic insult to brain cells and vascular endothelium [4*]. Some of these targets are aquaporins and SUR1-TRPM4 (sulfonylurea receptor 1-transient receptor potential melastatin protein 4). Both molecules are found to have important roles in the development and perpetuation of cytotoxic edema. Trials of prevention of cerebral edema targeting these molecules are currently underway and are expected to provide insights into novel approaches to mitigate the development of brain edema before becoming evident both clinically and by neuroimaging.

References

1. Wijdicks EFM, Sheth KN, Carter BS, Greer DM, Kasner SE, Kimberly WT, Schwab S, Smith EE, Tamargo RJ, Wintermark M, on behalf of the American Heart Association Stroke Council. Recommendations for the management of cerebral and cerebellar infarction with swelling: a statement for healthcare professionals from the American Heart Association/American Stroke Association. Stroke. 2014;45:1222–38.
2. Hao Z, Chang X, Zhou H, Lin S, Liu M. A cohort study of decompressive craniectomy for malignant middle cerebral artery infarction: a real-world experience in clinical practice. Medicine (Baltimore). 2015;94:e1039.
3. Hartmann F, Juettler E, Singer OC, Lehnhardt FG, Köhrmann M, Kersten JF, Sobesky J, Gerloff C, Villringer A, Fiehler J, Neumann-Haefelin T, Schellinger PD, Röther J, Thomalla G, Clinical Trial Net of the German Competence Network Stroke. Prediction of malignant middle cerebral artery infarction by magnetic resonance imaging within 6 hours of symptom onset: a prospective multicenter observational study. Ann Neurol. 2010;68:435–45.
4. Liebeskind DS, Jüttler E, Shapovalov Y, Yegin A, Landen J, Jauch EC. Cerebral edema associated with large hemispheric infarction. Stroke. 2019;50(9):2619–25.
5. Kahle KT, Simard JM, Staley KJ, Nahed BV, Jones PS, Sun D. Molecular mechanisms of ischemic cerebral edema: role of electroneutral ion transport. Physiology (Bethesda). 2009;24:257–65.
6. Dostovic Z, Dostovic E, Smajlovic D, Ibrahimagic OC, Avdic L. Brain edema after ischaemic stroke. Med Arch. 2016;70:339–41.

7. Kimberly WT, Sheth KN. Approach to severe hemispheric stroke. Neurology. 2011;76(7 Suppl 2):S50–6.
8. Moulin T, Cattin F, Crépin-Leblond T, Tatu L, Chavot D, Piotin M, Viel JF, Rumbach L, Bonneville JF. Early CT signs in acute middle cerebral artery infarction: predictive value for subsequent infarct locations and outcome. Neurology. 1996;47:366–75.
9. Oppenheim C, Samson Y, Manaï R, Lalam T, Vandamme X, Crozier S, Srour A, Cornu P, Dormont D, Rancurel G, Marsault C. Prediction of malignant middle cerebral artery infarction by diffusion weighted imaging. Stroke. 2000;31(9):2175–81.
10. Powers WJ, Rabinstein AA, Ackerson T, Adeoye OM, Bambakidis NC, Becker K, Biller J, Brown M, Demaerschalk BM, Hoh B, Jauch EC, Kidwell CS, Leslie-Mazwi TM, Ovbiagele B, Scott PA, Sheth KN, Southerland AM, Summers DV, Tirschwell DL, on behalf of the American Heart Association Stroke Council. Guidelines for the early management of patients with acute ischemic stroke: a guideline for healthcare professionals from the American Heart Association/American Stroke Association. Stroke. 2018;2018(49):e46–99.
11. Torbey MT, Bösel J, Rhoney DH, Rincon F, Staykov D, Amar AP, Varelas PN, Jüttler E, Olson D, Huttner HB, Zweckberger K, Sheth KN, Dohmen C, Brambrink AM, Mayer SA, Zaidat OO, Hacke W, Schwab S. Evidence-based guidelines for the management of large hemispheric infarction: a statement for health care professionals from the Neurocritical Care Society and the German Society for Neurointensive Care and Emergency Medicine. Neurocrit Care. 2015;22(1):146–64.
12. Back L, Nagaraja V, Kapur A, Eslick GD. Role of decompressive hemicraniectomy in extensive middle cerebral artery strokes: a meta-analysis of randomised trials. Intern Med J. 2015;45(7):711–7.
13. Vahedi K, Hofmeijer J, Juettler E, Vicaut E, George B, Algra A, Amelink GJ, Schmiedeck P, Schwab S, Rothwell PM, Bousser MG, van der Worp HB, Hacke W, DECIMAL, DESTINY, and HAMLET investigators. Early decompressive surgery in malignant infarction of the middle cerebral artery: a pooled analysis of three randomised controlled trials. Lancet Neurol. 2007;6(3):215–22.
14. Jaramillo A, Góngora-Rivera F, Labreuche J, Hauw JJ, Amarenco P. Predictors for malignant middle cerebral artery infarctions: a postmortem analysis. Neurology. 2006;66:815–20.
15. Cucchiara BL, Kasner SE, Wolk DA, Lyden PD, Knappertz VA, Ashwood T, Odergren T, Nordlund A, CLASS-I Investigators. Early impairment in consciousness predicts mortality after hemispheric ischemic stroke. Crit Care Med. 2004;32(1):241–5.
16. Elijovich L, Goyal N, Mainali S, Hoit D, Arthur AS, Whitehead M, Choudhri AF. CTA collateral score predicts infarct volume and clinical outcome after endovascular therapy for acute ischemic stroke: a retrospective chart review. J Neurointervent Surg. 2016;8:559–62.

Childhood Absence Epilepsy

15

Ethan Rosenberg, Janice Rodriguez Hernandez, and Theresa M. Czech

Case Scenario

A 5-year-old girl presented with a 1-year history of staring spells. She initially had fleeting episodes of staring off that her parents noted sporadically. Recently, these episodes had become more frequent, now occurring multiple times a day. The staring spells often interrupted activities, and during the episodes, she was unresponsive to touch and voice. There were no associated abnormal movements of the extremities or the face during these events. Her parents estimated that the spells could last up to 10 s. Nothing apparently triggered these episodes.

Prior to this presentation, she had an unremarkable prenatal history, birth and development. She had no other medical conditions. Her pediatrician referred her for an electroencephalogram (EEG). With hyperventilation, she had clinical absence seizures characterized by behavioral arrest and inability to recall verbal prompts. Her EEG (Fig. 15.1) demonstrated runs of generalized, frontally predominant 3 Hz spike-and-wave discharges lasting up to 10 s. She was referred to Neurology for further management.

E. Rosenberg · J. R. Hernandez · T. M. Czech (✉)
Department of Neurology, Ann & Robert H. Lurie Children's Hospital of Chicago, Chicago, IL, USA
e-mail: tczech@luriechildrens.org

© Springer Nature Singapore Pte Ltd. 2024
K. K. Oli et al. (eds.), *Case-based Approach to Common Neurological Disorders*,
https://doi.org/10.1007/978-981-99-8676-7_15

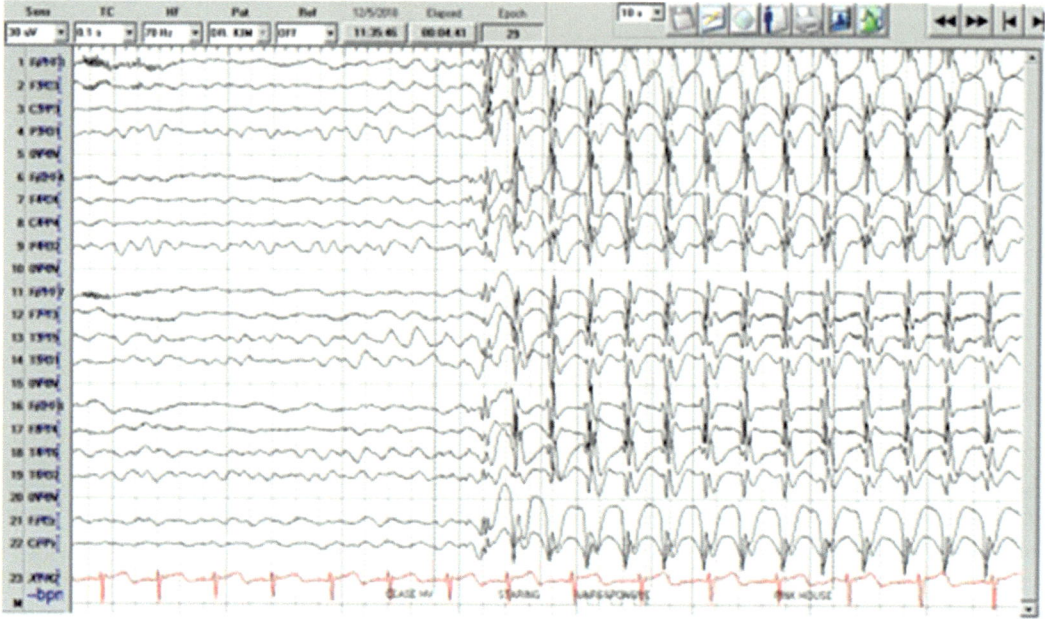

Fig. 15.1 This EEG demonstrates an absence seizure that was triggered by hyperventilation. There is abrupt onset of generalized, frontally predominant 3 Hz spike-and-wave discharges with associated clinical change, which is described as staring and unresponsiveness. Patient is unable to recall the words "Pink House" which are spoken to her during the event, indicating a loss of awareness. The recording is displayed in a longitudinal bipolar montage set at a sensitivity of 30 μV

15.1 Introduction

The patient in the vignette has childhood absence epilepsy (CAE). CAE is a common genetic generalized epilepsy that presents in early school-aged children. Without treatment, children with CAE have dozens of seizures each day. The frequent interruptions can potentiate a decline in school performance at a critical period in a child's development. For this reason, it is important to be able to recognize the signs of CAE in order to initiate prompt and appropriate treatment.

15.2 Epidemiology

CAE is a common generalized epilepsy syndrome, but it remains a rare disease. The annual incidence of CAE is estimated to be between 5.8 and 7.1 cases per 100,000 [1]. Incidence and prevalence of rare diseases are generally difficult to estimate due to migratory populations and a general lack of centralized records. One way to overcome these limitations is to study a single healthcare region. A study of a single healthcare region in Sweden from 1978 to1982 found the mean annual incidence of absence epilepsy with absence seizures alone or with generalized tonic-clonic seizures (GTC) to be 6.3/100,000 in children 0–15 years of age [2]. A recent study from Sweden demonstrated that CAE had a prevalence of 0.20/1000 among children and adolescents which accounted for approximately 6% of all pediatric epilepsies [3]. In a study from Israel, absence epilepsy accounts for 7% of all childhood epilepsies with a mean age of onset of 6 years (range 2–13 years) [4]. This group was unable to reliably report incidence, because their population was particularly mobile. While various epidemiological studies have demonstrated similar incidence and prevalence estimates, it is important to note that these studies are limited because they are primarily confined to European/Caucasian populations.

15.3 Pathophysiology

Absence seizures are characterized by 3–4 Hz spike-wave complexes on electroencephalogram (EEG). Most investigations into how these spike-wave complexes are generated have been performed in animal models. Based on these models, both the thalamus and the cortex are needed to generate spike-wave discharges. Removal of the cortex, the thalamus, or the interconnections between the two will abolish the spike-wave discharges. There is, however, no agreement on how these discharges are generated [5]. The importance of the thalamus in the pathogenesis of absence seizures can also be inferred by the efficacy of ethosuximide, a seizure medication which acts upon t-type calcium channels found in the thalamus [6].

15.4 Genetics

CAE is considered a genetic generalized epilepsy, but the inheritance is not fully understood. There have been several genes implicated in CAE, including those that encode the subunits of gamma-aminobutyric acid (GABA) receptors and glucose transporter 1 (GLUT1). Copy number variants, particularly deletions in chromosome 15, are also associated with absence epilepsy. Despite these discoveries, a genetic cause for most cases of CAE cannot be found [7]. The search continues, and our understanding of CAE inheritance continues to evolve.

15.5 Diagnosis

Patients with CAE often present between 4 and 10 years of age with a history of episodic behavioral arrest and a decline in school performance. Behavioral arrest in CAE can be perceived as inattention; however, elucidating a complete history of these episodes can make one more or less suspicious of underlying epilepsy. Seizures in CAE interrupt activities. Parents may describe that their children pause mid-sentence then pick up again a few seconds later as if nothing has happened. Seizures can also be associated with a flattening of the child's affect and eyelid fluttering. Rarely, children can have hand automatisms or habitually repeat sounds during their seizures. Seizures in CAE are typically brief, lasting 5–10 s each. When uncontrolled, children can have dozens of seizures each day [1].

The differential diagnosis for CAE includes focal seizures with altered awareness, non-epileptic staring spells, juvenile absence epilepsy, and Jeavon's syndrome. The patient's history may help one narrow this differential, but EEG is necessary to complete the evaluation. The background EEG in CAE is often normal. The classic EEG finding seen in CAE is generalized, frontally predominant bursts of 3-Hz spike-and-wave discharges. These discharges can be provoked by hyperventilation. The interictal and ictal EEG findings of CAE are similar, differing only in duration and association with a clinical change [8]. CAE is also associated with the EEG finding of occipital intermittent rhythmic delta activity (OIRDA). This pattern appears as short runs of bilateral, occipital rhythmic delta activity in the range of 2–4 Hz. OIRDA can occur in either awake or drowsy states with eye closure. OIRDA is found in nearly 30% of patients with CAE [9].

15.6 Treatment

Childhood absence epilepsy is often treated with ethosuximide or a broad-spectrum anti-seizure medication. The best evidence for ethosuximide as the treatment of choice comes from a double-blind randomized control trial conducted across 32 sites in the United States [10, 11]. This study compared the efficacy of ethosuximide, valproic acid, and lamotrigine as monotherapy for newly diagnosed epilepsy. The study measured seizure freedom in 446 patients at 4 months [10] and then at 12 months [11]. Ethosuximide and valproic acid were found to be equally effective (seizure freedom of 45% vs. 44% respectively, $p = 0.82$), while lamotrigine was found to be inferior to both other treatments (seizure freedom of 21%, $p < 0.001$ when compared to either ethosuximide or valproic acid). Valproic acid use led to more treatment-related side effects (intolerable adverse events in 33% of subgroup, $p < 0.037$) and more side effect-related discontinuation than either ethosuximide or lamotrigine. The study ultimately supports ethosuximide as the initial medication of choice for CAE because of its high efficacy and low side effect profile. Since ethosuximide works via T-type calcium channels in the thalamus, its use is limited to the treatment of absence seizures [6]. In patients with other seizure types, such as generalized tonic-clonic or myoclonic seizures, ethosuximide monotherapy is not an appropriate treatment choice.

Absence status epilepticus can be provoked if patients with CAE are exposed to the "wrong" medications. Agents that tend to worsen CAE are the medications used commonly in focal epilepsies: carbamazepine and phenytoin [12]. Typical signs of absence status epilepticus include confusion, fluctuating level of consciousness, and myoclonia [13]. An EEG can confirm the diagnosis by showing continuous 3 Hz spike-and-wave discharges. Treatment for absence status epilepticus includes benzodiazepines and removal of the offending agent.

15.7 Outcomes

A majority of children with CAE will achieve remission on an anti-seizure medication. Remission rates have been reported between 56% and 84% [1], and a significant positive predictive factor for remission is early control with the first seizure medication chosen. A minority of patients will progress to another epilepsy syndrome such as juvenile myoclonic epilepsy (JME). In a Canadian cohort of CAE patients, 15% progressed to have JME. Factors that predicted who would progress to JME included lack of response to anti-seizure medications in the first year of treatment, absence status epilepticus, a slow EEG background, and a history of generalized tonic-clonic seizures in a first-degree relative [14, 15].

Psychosocial comorbidities exist in CAE and are often underestimated. Regardless of seizure control, patients with CAE can have attention deficit hyperactivity disorder (ADHD), depression, and anxiety [1]. The incidence of psychosocial comorbidities also appears to be greater than what is seen with other chronic diseases. Compared to age-matched controls with juvenile rheumatoid arthritis, those with CAE had significantly higher rates of high school dropout, unplanned pregnancy, and substance abuse [15]. It is not understood whether epilepsy leads to these issues or is correlated with them through common pathophysiologic processes.

References

1. Matricardi S, Verrotti A, Chiarelli F, Cerminara C, Curatolo P. Current advances in childhood absence epilepsy. Pediatr Neurol. 2014;50(3):205–12.
2. Olsson I. Epidemiology of absence epilepsy. I. Concept and incidence. Acta Paediatr Scand. 1988;77(6):860–6.
3. Larsson K, Eeg-Olofsson O. A population based study of epilepsy in children from a Swedish county. Eur J Paediatr Neurol. 2006;10(3):107–13.
4. Kramer U, Nevo Y, Neufeld MY, Fatal A, Leitner Y, Harel S. Epidemiology of epilepsy in childhood: a cohort of 440 consecutive patients. Pediatr Neurol. 1998;18(1):46–50.
5. Blumenfeld H. Cellular and network mechanisms of spike-wave seizures. Epilepsia. 2005;46(Suppl 9):21–33.
6. Broicher T, Seidenbecher T, Meuth P, Munsch T, Meuth SG, Kanyshkova T, et al. T-current related effects of antiepileptic drugs and a Ca^{2+} channel antagonist on thalamic relay and local circuit interneurons in a rat model of absence epilepsy. Neuropharmacology. 2007;53(3):431–46.
7. Mullen SA, Berkovic SF, ILAE Genetics Commission. Genetic generalized epilepsies. Epilepsia. 2018;59(6):1148–53.
8. Sadleir LG, Farrell K, Smith S, Connolly MB, Scheffer IE. Electroclinical features of absence seizures in childhood absence epilepsy. Neurology. 2006;67(3):413–8.
9. Seneviratne U, Cook M, D'Souza W. The electroencephalogram of idiopathic generalized epilepsy. Epilepsia. 2012;53(2):234–48.
10. Glauser TA, Cnaan A, Shinnar S, Hirtz DG, Dlugos D, Masur D, et al. Ethosuximide, valproic acid, and lamotrigine in childhood absence epilepsy. N Engl J Med. 2010;362(9):790–9.
11. Glauser TA, Cnaan A, Shinnar S, Hirtz DG, Dlugos D, Masur D, et al. Ethosuximide, valproic acid, and lamotrigine in childhood absence epilepsy: initial monotherapy outcomes at 12 months. Epilepsia. 2013;54(1):141–55.

12. Thomas P, Valton L, Genton P. Absence and myoclonic status epilepticus precipitated by antiepileptic drugs in idiopathic generalized epilepsy. Brain. 2006;129(Pt 5):1281–92.

13. Kaplan PW. Behavioral manifestations of nonconvulsive status epilepticus. Epilepsy Behav. 2002;3(2):122–39.

14. Wirrell EC, Camfield CS, Camfield PR, Gordon KE, Dooley JM. Long-term prognosis of typical childhood absence epilepsy: remission or progression to juvenile myoclonic epilepsy. Neurology. 1996;47(4):912–8.

15. Wirrell EC. Natural history of absence epilepsy in children. Can J Neurol Sci. 2003;30(3):184–8.

Laxmi Dhakal and William O. Tatum

Case Scenario

EMM is a 67-year-old female presented to an outlying hospital with unresponsiveness for 2 h. At the emergency department she had generalized tonic-clonic seizure lasting 60 min. She was treated with intravenous (IV) lorazepam, levetiracetam, and fosphenytoin. Recurrent seizures did not respond to anti-seizure medication and subsequently she was intubated and begun on a propofol infusion. She was also noted to have a temperature of 104 °F, neck rigidity, and leukocytosis. Lumbar puncture was performed which drained purulent CSF. CSF white blood cell count (WBC) was 15,315/μL with 96% neutrophils and 3% lymphocytes. Gram stain was 2+ for gram-positive cocci representing streptococcus pneumoniae. CT of the head did not reveal an acute structural abnormality. She was started on ceftriaxone, vancomycin, and dexamethasone. When she presented to our facility she was intubated and sedated with propofol. Her neurological exam was unremarkable except for subtle horizontal nystagmus and meningismus. Status epilepticus (SE) with bacterial meningitis was her initial diagnosis and she was monitored with continuous EEG (CEEG). CEEG demonstrated nonconvulsive status epilepticus (NCSE). She was reloaded with fosphenytoin and levetriacetam and continued with propofol for 24 h with a CEEG target of 2–3 bursts per 15 s epoch on a suppressed background. During the next 24 h she was seizure-free. A slow taper of the propofol infusion with CEEG monitoring was done. After 3 days of hospitalization, she was awake and followed commands. Following spontaneous breathing trial, she was subsequently extubated without complications. After 1 week she was transferred to a rehabilitation facility because of generalized weakness. Three months later she was seen in the neurology clinic and appeared neurologically intact except for a mild cognitive deficit. She was able to return to full-time employment with steady improvement.

L. Dhakal (✉)
Neuroscience Intensive Care Department, Wesley Medical Center, Wichita, KS, USA

Department Neurology, Kansas University and Department of Internal Medicine-Wichita, KS, USA

Department of Internal Medicine-Wichita, KS Wesley Medical Center, Wichita, KS, USA

W. O. Tatum
Department of Neurology, Mayo Clinic, Jacksonville, FL, USA

16.1 Introduction

The WHO estimates that there are approximately 25 million people with epilepsy in the Southeast Asian region [1]. In the paper by Rajbhandari et al., the estimated prevalence of epilepsy in Nepal was 7.3/1000 [2]. The estimated incidence of status epilepticus (SE) in developing countries

© Springer Nature Singapore Pte Ltd. 2024
K. K. Oli et al. (eds.), *Case-based Approach to Common Neurological Disorders*,
https://doi.org/10.1007/978-981-99-8676-7_16

is largely unknown, while in the United States it is estimated to be between 10 and 40 per 100,000, with the highest mortality among the elderly population [3].

16.2 Etiology and Pathophysiology

Seizures are a manifestation of imbalance between abnormal excitation and ineffective inhibition of neuronal activity [4]. Therefore, excitatory states like pre-existing epilepsy, structural brain lesions including tumor, stroke, traumatic brain injury, and focal cortical dysplasia can increase the risk of seizures. Anti-seizure medication discontinuation, substance abuse, drug overdose, and CNS infection in the form of meningitis and encephalitis, as well as toxic metabolic state, may initiate a sustained mechanism of abnormal neuronal electrical discharge and recruitment of surrounding brain regions. Autoimmune and paraneoplastic etiologies are increasingly recognized as a cause for refractory seizures and SE. As the seizure goes into a prolonged state, changes occur in neurotransmitters mainly involving the gamma-amino butyric acid receptors, which are endocytosed, in addition to glutamate receptors that are recruited. This can result in a continuous excitatory state which if it continues for a prolonged period of time can cause neuronal damage.

16.3 Definition/Classification

In 2015, the Commission on Epidemiology of the International League Against Epilepsy (ILAE) proposed a twofold definition of status epilepticus [5].

1. After time point T1—Status epilepticus is a condition resulting either from the failure of the mechanisms responsible for seizure termination or from the initiation of mechanisms, which lead to abnormally, prolonged seizures. Multiple studies have shown that a seizure lasting more than 5 min can eventually lead to abnormal prolonged seizure.

2. After time point T2—This is a condition which can have long-term consequences including neuronal death, neuronal injury, and alteration of neuronal networks, depending on the type and duration of seizures. Animal studies have shown that after 30 min of seizures there is irreversible neuronal damage.

A newer definition of SE reflects seizures lasting more than 5 min. Prolonged seizures should be treated in an emergent fashion. The traditional definition of SE was continuous seizure activities or multiple seizures without return to baseline in between seizures, for more than 30 min. This definition was changed in order to ensure earlier management in an effort to prevent irreversible damage to the neurons associated with continuous seizure activity.

Refractory status epilepticus (RSE) by definition occurs when seizures continue despite treatment with properly selected first- and second-line anti-seizure drugs (ASDs). Super-refractory status epilepticus (SRSE) occurs after SE fails to be controlled following addition of a third-line agent involving anesthetic infusions.

Status epilepticus can be classified as convulsive and nonconvulsive. Typical convulsive SE can manifest as generalized tonic-clonic seizures which may evolve over time to subtle or absent motor activity leading to nonconvulsive SE (NCSE). Generalized convulsive status epilepticus (GCSE) can occur without focal features or evolve from a focal onset. It may also present with myoclonic SE. Epilepsia partialis continua (EPC) is a rare form of focal motor SE. By definition NCSE is devoid of motor phenomena except perhaps subtle twitching of the face, eye, or extremity. NCSE may also present as a prolonged state of altered mental status or persisting coma in patients with toxic-metabolic encephalopathy (e.g., hepatic failure, sepsis, etc.).

Newly recognized categories of SE such as new-onset refractory status epilepticus (NORSE), febrile infection-related epilepsy syndrome (FIRES), and acute encephalitis with refractory, repetitive partial seizures have been increasingly recognized. These syndromes are due to acute infections or inflammatory processes without clear etiology.

16.4 Diagnosis

Clinically diagnosing GCSE is usually easy when seizures manifest as episodes of generalized tonic stiffness followed by rhythmic jerking with impaired consciousness. The diagnosis is usually straightforward, although unusual motor manifestations with atypical non-anatomic spread of movements and comorbid psychiatric condition could suggest psychogenic nonepileptic events or an abnormal dystonic or choreiform movement disorder. Focal status epilepticus may present as progressive jerking that spreads from one body part to another propagating in the form of "Jacksonian march." EPC is a drug-resistant focal motor seizure that can last for days or months [6]. Myoclonic status epilepticus is most commonly seen in juvenile myoclonic epilepsy. Status myoclonus may exhibit myoclonus that is secondary due to anoxic brain injury or a toxic-metabolic-systemic source. It is characterized by frequent rhythmic or arrhythmic myoclonic jerks. Diagnosing NCSE (illustrated on Figs. 16.1, 16.2, and 16.3) is often a challenge faced by neurocritical care as well as in the medical and surgical ICU. There needs to be a high degree of suspicion for seizures in a patient with a persistent altered level of consciousness when a reasonable causative explanation is absent. Claassen et al. showed that 19% of critically ill comatose patients who underwent diagnostic continuous EEG (CEEG) had seizures present, and 95% were nonconvulsive, including 54% with NCSE [7]. Establishing the etiological nature of status epilepticus requires neuroimaging modalities involving MRI/MRA of the brain, CT scanning, and ultrasound, for example. In addition, an array of laboratory tests including those for metabolic and autoimmune etiologies and cerebrospinal fluid analysis is necessary to address infectious and inflammatory etiologies.

16.4.1 Continuous EEG Monitoring

Continuous video-EEG monitoring is an essential tool in the management of patients with SE. In order to establish an accurate diagnosis and quantification of the seizure burden in patients, electrographic evidence of seizures identified by CEEG is essential in detecting nonconvulsive events. These patients frequently require more than 24 h of CEEG to detect the first electrographic seizure. Neurocritical care guidelines strongly recommend CEEG monitoring at for least 48 h for comatose patients being evaluated for NCSE [8]. The American Clinical Neurophysiology Society has proposed a standardized terminology for CEEG in critically ill patients to describe electrographic features of the EEG for clinical and research use [9]. Lateralized periodic discharges (LPD) (Fig. 16.2), LPD plus fast activity (Fig. 16.3), bilateral independent periodic discharges (BiPD), generalized periodic discharges (GPD), stimulus-induced rhythmic, periodic, or ictal discharges (SIRPID), lateralized rhythmic delta activity (LRDA), and generalized rhythmic delta activity (GRDA) are abnormal findings present along the "Ictal–interictal continuum." This area is currently a rapidly evolving field of research to distinguish patterns that require more aggressive therapy. Periodic discharges include LPD Plus, LPD, SIRPIDs, BiPDs, and triphasic waves associated with ictal patterns. Therefore, the periodic patterns in EEG are recommended to have CEEG considered to address their association with seizures and SE [10]. Critical care CEEG has been increasingly utilized not only for seizure detection but also for ischemia in patients with altered mental state.

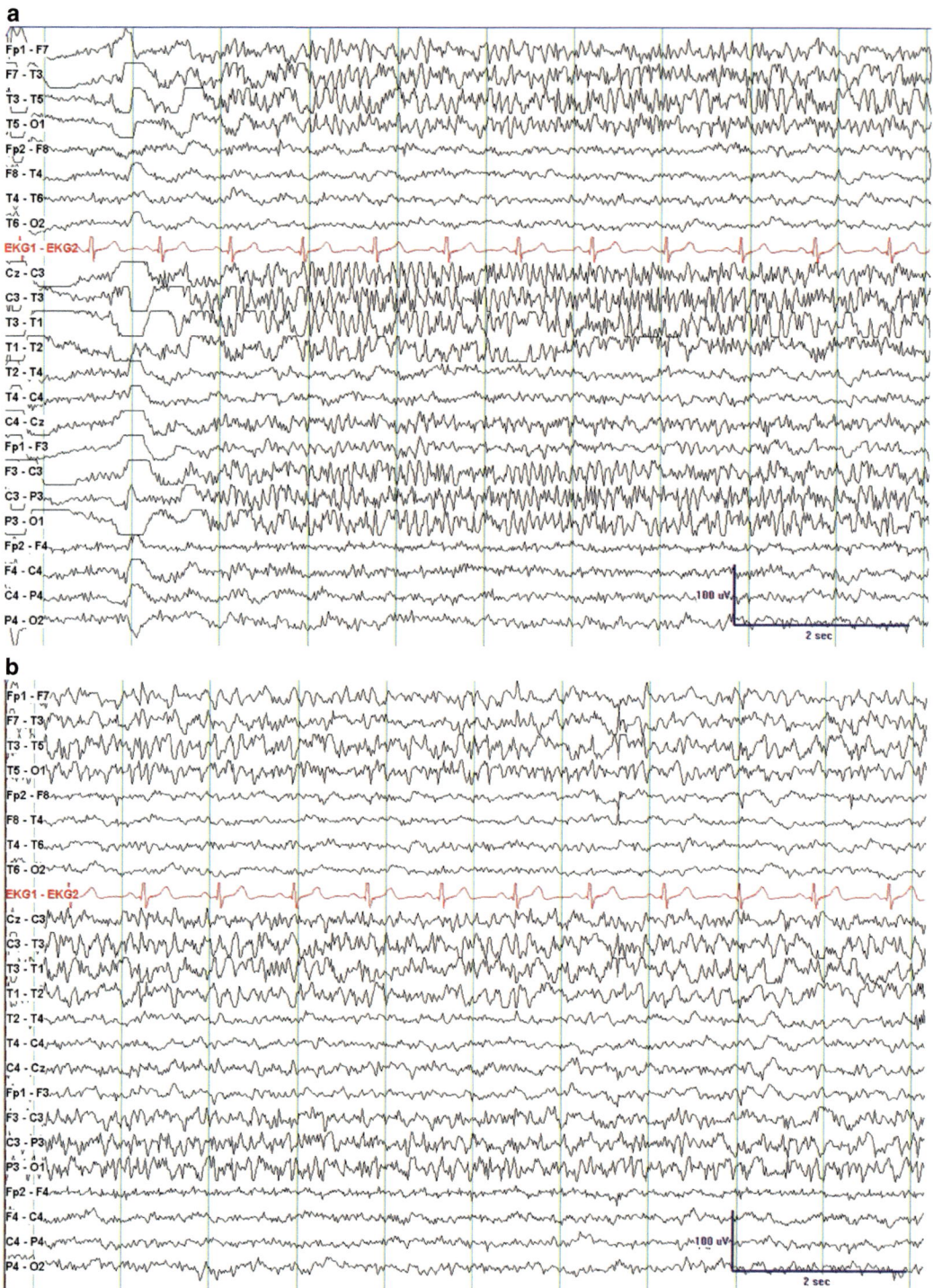

Fig. 16.1 (**a–c**) Discrete left hemispheric seizure captured during stat EEG in an unresponsive patient in the ICU following a series of generalized tonic-clonic sei- zures. Serial non-convulsive seizures were subsequently captured on continuous EEG monitoring. Sensitivity 7 µV/mm, display speed 30 mm/s, filter settings 1–70 Hz

c

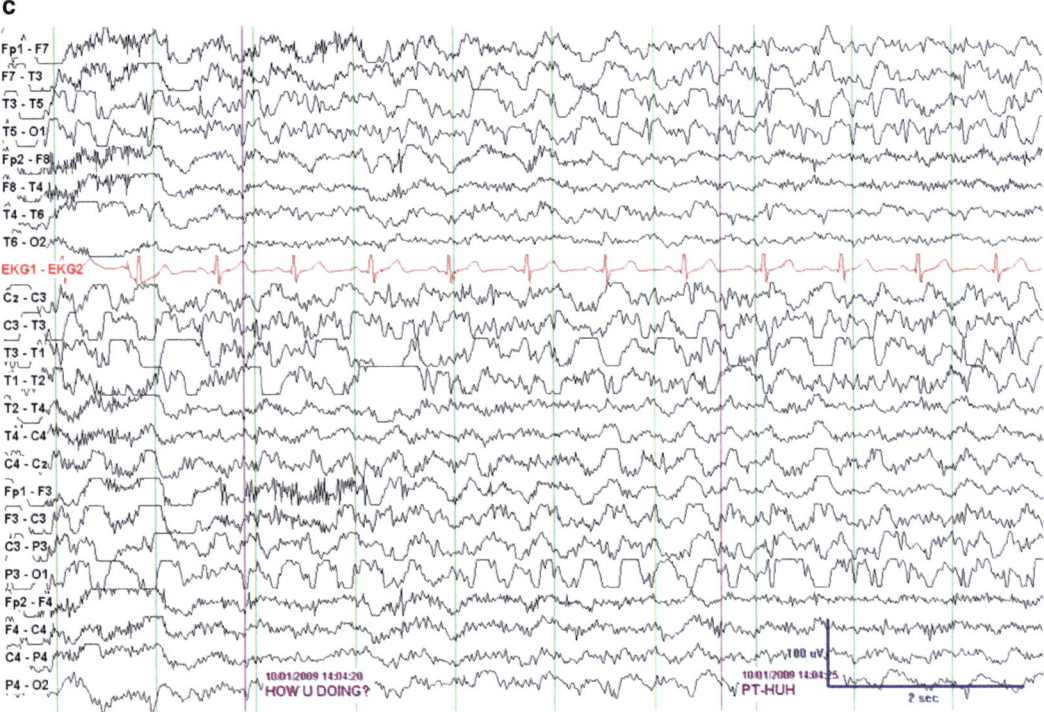

Fig. 16.1 (continued)

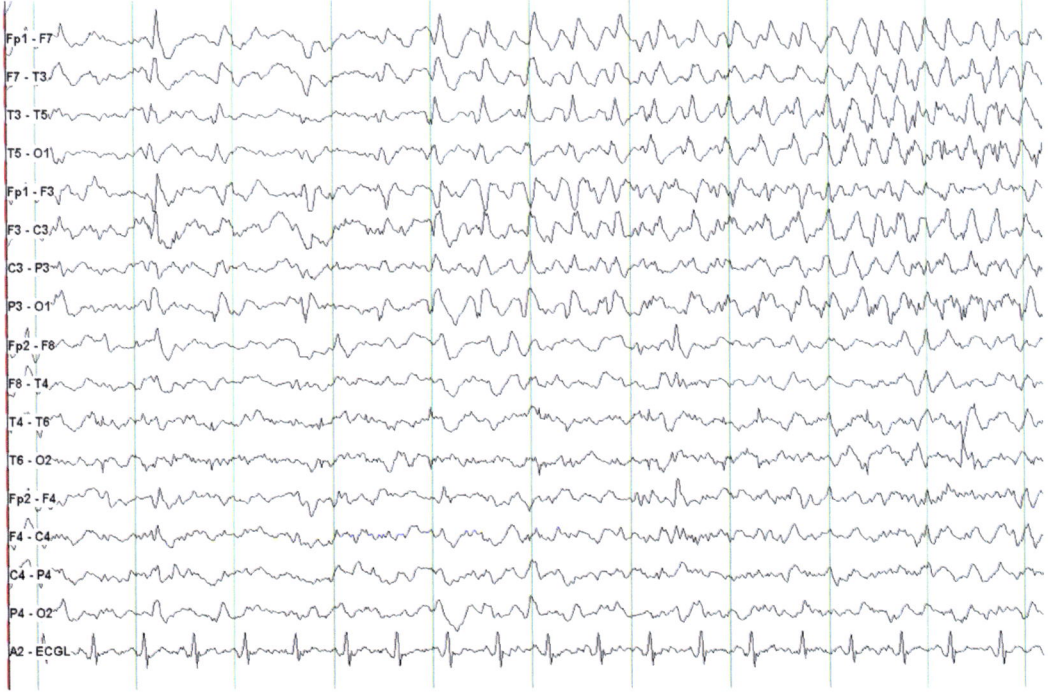

Fig. 16.2 Left hemispheric periodic discharges with frontal predominance evolving into an electrographic seizure. Note the right parasagittal field of the LPD in second 2 and the spatial propagation during the seizure at the end of the epoch. Sensitivity 7 μV/mm, display speed 30 mm/s, filter settings 1–70 Hz

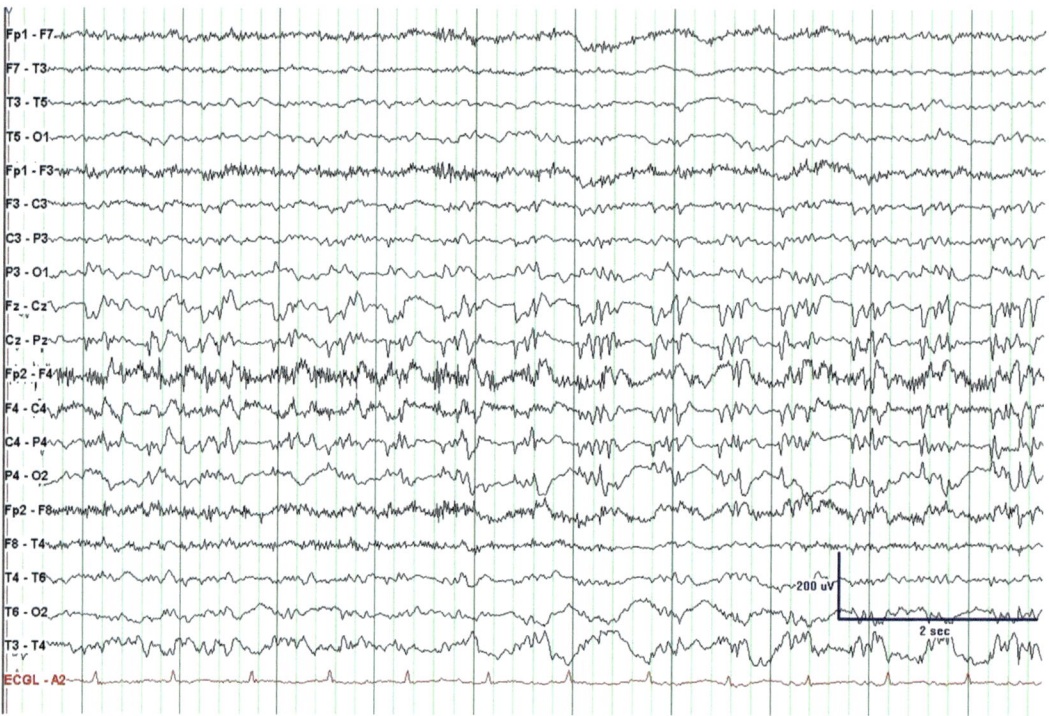

Fig. 16.3 Right central-parietal lateralized periodic discharges with fast activity and a restricted parasagittal field in a patient with a glioblastoma multiforme. Sensitivity 7 µV/mm, display speed 30 mm/s, filter settings 1–70 Hz

16.5 Treatment

Initial treatment of SE involves rapid assessment of airway, breathing, and circulation similar to other medical emergencies. Supportive care is similar to other acute resuscitation measures. Patients should be evaluated for toxic-metabolic-systemic etiologies and structural brain abnormalities. When securing the airway during intubation in patients with SE particular attention has to be paid using neuromuscular blockade as this could make convulsive SE appear non-convulsive. If absolutely necessary a neuromuscular block with the shortest half-life should be used. Alternatively, one should always try to use agents like ketamine or midazolam with the ability to rapidly titrate and taper medication [4]. Intramuscular benzodiazepines are recommended to abort prolonged seizures in the prehospital setting [10]. There have been multiple trials using intramuscular midazolam in adults as well as children with efficacy in controlling ongoing seizures [11–13].

Inpatient SE may be treated with a three-tier approach to medication management. This is summarized in Table 16.1 [4, 8, 14, 15].

Addressing the underlying etiology for SE is also a major concern in its management. Patients presenting with an underlying structural lesion such as a brain tumor, trauma-related brain injury (e.g., subdural hematoma), subarachnoid hemorrhage with/without hydrocephalus, stroke, or central nervous system infection (e.g., empyema) may need surgical intervention. Patients presenting with a metabolic encephalopathy due to sepsis or organ failure require therapy directed toward treating the underlying etiology. Meningoencephalitis needs to be evaluated and treated in an emergent fashion. More recently, autoimmune and paraneoplastic etiologies have been increasingly recognized as an etiology responsive to immunomodulation including steroids and immunosuppressant agents like intravenous immunoglobulin and plasmapheresis. Continuous EEG monitoring helps to assess patients effectively to modify usage of medication in SE, and stage the

Table 16.1 Antiepileptic drugs used in Status Epilepticus

Drugs	Doses, route	Relevant pharmacokinetics	Side effects and interaction and special considerations
1. Prehospital			
(a) IM midazolam	10 mg	Onset 5 min	
(b) IV lorazepam	2–4 mg	Onset 10 min	
2. Inhospital (ER/ICU)			
First line			
(a) IV lorazepam	0.1 mg/kg max rate 2 mg/min		Hypotension
(b) IV diazepam	0.15–0.2 mg/kg rate of 5 mg/min		
Second line			
(a) IV Fosphenytoin	Loading dose 20 mg PE/kg IV (can reload another 10 mg PE/kg if needed) followed by 100 mg IV every 6–8 h		Cardiac arrhythmia and hypotension. The maximum rate of infusion for fosphenytoin 150 mg PE/min
(b) IV Levetiracetam	1500–3000 mg loading dose followed by 10–15 mg/kg q12h	Lower does with renal failure	Commonly used as first agent nowadays
(c) IV Valporate	20–40 mg/kg load then 4–6 mg/kg q6h	Liver metabolized	
(d) IV Lacosamide	200–400 mg load followed by 200–300 mg q12h		
Third line (anesthetics—continuous drip)			
(a) Propofol	Loading dose of 1–2 mg/kg followed by 2–10 mg/kg per hour		Hypotension, bradycardia, propofol infusion syndrome
(b) Midazolam	Loading dose 0.2 mg/kg followed by 0.1–2 mg/kg per hour		Tachyphylaxis
(c) Pentobarbital	Loading dose 5–10 mg/kg followed by 0.5–5 mg/kg per hour	Prolong half-life	Hypotension, ileus, metabolic acidosis
(d) Ketamine	Loading dose 1.5 mg/kg up to 4.5 mg/kg loading dose followed by 2–5 mg/kg per hour		NMDA antagonist—inhibits glutamic excitotoxicity—increasingly used
Super-refractory status			
(a) Iso/desflurane			Needs to involve anesthesiologist
(b) Topiramate	Per tube 300–600 mg		Metabolic acidosis
(c) Magnesium	4 g bolus follow be infusion 2–6 g/h		Keep serum magnesium <6 mEq/L
(d) Pyridoxine	IV or tube 100–600 mg/day		For inborn error of pyridoxine metabolism
(e) Steroid	IV methylprednisolone 1 g/day for 5 days followed by prednisone 1 mg/kg/day for a week		For autoimmune encephalitis, EPC, NORSE, AERPPS
(f) IVIG, plasmapheresis	For five doses/sessions		For autoimmune encephalitis, EPC, NORSE
(g) Hypothermia		33–35 °C	
(h) Ketogenic diet, ECT, VNS, TMS, and neurosurgical resection			Electrolyte imbalance, bleeding and infection risk

Note: *AERPPS* acute encephalitis with refractory, repetitive partial seizures, *NORSE* new-onset refractory status epilepticus, *ECT* electroconvulsive therapy, *VNS* vagal nerve stimulator, *TMS* transcranial magnetic stimulation, *IVIG* intravenous immunoglobulin timing of anesthetic drug implementation in addition to guiding titration and de-escalation of anti-seizure medications. When third-line anesthetics medications are required, patients are usually maintained in a suppression-burst pattern on CEEG for 12–24 h. During that time, second-line ASDs could be optimized.

16.6 Outcome

Patients with SE are prone to complications common to the ICU, namely multiple organ failure, deep venous thrombosis, pulmonary embolism, and sepsis. Critical illness polyneuropathy and myopathy is also a common complication in patients who have prolonged hospitalizations. Medication interactions and adverse effects are also common and need to be actively determined and eliminated when possible. Adverse drug reactions including Steven-Johnson syndrome, toxic epidermal necrosis, are propofol infusion syndrome are some of the serious complications that may occur during the course of treating patients with SE, and a heightened index of suspicion should be maintained.

Both GCSE and NCSE carry a high risk for morbidity and mortality [8]. Inappropriate dosing, delays in initiating therapy, lack of EEG monitoring, older age, and higher acuity of patient can contribute to increased mortality and morbidity [8]. Some reports suggest a relationship between the duration of electrographic SE and outcome with higher risks for subsequent epilepsy, cognitive dysfunction, and overall disability [16].

References

1. Mac TL, Tran D-S, et al. Epidemiology, aetiology, and clinical management of epilepsy in Asia: a systematic review. Lancet Neurol. 2007;6:533–43.
2. Rajbhandari KC. Epilepsy in Nepal. Neurol J Southeast Asia. 2003;8:1–4.
3. Dham BS, Hunter K, et al. The epidemiology of status epilepticus in the United States. Neurocrit Care. 2014;20(3):476–83.
4. Hantus S. Epilepsy emergencies. Continuum. 2016;22(1):173–90.
5. Trinka E, Cock H, et al. A definition and classification of status epilepticus—report of the ILAE Task Force on Classification of Status Epilepticus. Epilepsia. 2015;56(10):1515.
6. Cockerell OC, Rothwell J, et al. Clinical and physiological feature of epilepsia partialis continua: cases ascertained in the UK. Brain. 1996;119(2):393–407.
7. Claassen J, et al. Detection of electrographic seizures with continuous EEG monitoring in critically ill patients. Neurology. 2004;62(10):1743–8.
8. Brophy G, Bell R, et al. Guidelines for the evaluation and management of status epilepticus. Neurocrit Care. 2012;17:3–23.
9. Hirsh LJ, LaRoche SM, et al. American Clinical Neurophysiology Society's standardized critical care EEG terminology: 2012 version. J Clin Neurophysiol. 2013;30:1–27.
10. Emily J, Peter K. Population of ictal-interictal zone: the significance of periodic and rhythmic activity. Clin Neurophysiol Pract. 2017;2:107–18.
11. Silbergleit R, Lowenstein D, et al. The Neurological Emergency Treatment Trials (NETT) Investigators. RAMPART (Rapid Anticonvulsant Medication Prior to Arrival Trial): a double-blind randomized clinical trial of the efficacy of intramuscular midazolam versus intravenous lorazepam in the prehospital treatment of status epilepticus by paramedics. Epilepsia. 2011;52(Suppl 8):45–7.
12. Silbergleit R, Durkalski V, et al. Intramuscular versus intravenous therapy for prehospital status epilepticus. N Engl J Med. 2012;366(7):591–600.
13. Chamberlain JM, Altieri MA, et al. A prospective, randomized study comparing intramuscular midazolam with intravenous diazepam for the treatment of seizures in children. Pediatr Emerg Care. 1997;13(2):92–4.
14. Cuero MR, Varelas PN. Curr Neurol Neurosci Rep. 2015;15:74.
15. Rossetti A, Lowenstein D. Management of refractory status epilepticus in adults still more questions than answers. Lancet Neurol. 2011;10(10):922–30.
16. Young GB, Jordan KG, et al. An assessment of nonconvulsive seizures in the intensive care unit using continuous EEG monitoring: an investigation of variables associated with mortality. Neurology. 1996;47(1):83–9.

Myasthenia Gravis

17

Babu Ram Pokharel

Case Scenario

A 57-year-male was admitted with difficulty in swallowing, breathing, and speaking for 2 months, which increased in the evenings. The onset was insidious and gradually progressive. Clinical examination revealed diplopia on horizontal gaze and wasting of muscles: intercostal, sternocleidomastoid, and flexors of the neck. There was no history of chest or cardiac disease and his oxygen saturation was low and respiratory rate was high. The patient was intubated and a nasogastric tube was inserted. He was started on high-dose methylprednisolone and tab pyridostigmine with other supportive measures. Serum acetylcholine receptor antibody was positive. MRI of the brain and CT of the chest were normal. After 7 days, tracheotomy and percutaneous endoscopic gastrostomy insertion were done. The patient gradually improved and was shifted to the ward. He was discharged in stable condition after 3 weeks of hospital admission with closed tracheostomy and in situ percutaneous endoscopic gastrostomy. He was on a tapering dose of steroid and pyridostigmine (60 mg 5 times daily) at first follow-up. Six months after admission his percutaneous endoscopic gastrostomy tube was removed.

17.1 Introduction

Myasthenia gravis (MG) is an autoimmune disorder of the neuromuscular junction (NMJ) involving post-synaptic membrane. The first reported case was by Thomas Willis (1672) where he described a patient female who temporarily lost her power of speech and became "as mute as a fish" [1]. Similarly, other scientists who contributed are the field of myasthenia gravis are Samuel Wilkes, Wilhelm Erb of Heidelberg, Samuel Goldflam of Warsaw, and Frederick Jolly.

The prevalence is about 2 of every 100,000 and can occur at any age [2]. Age of onset of myasthenia gravis follows a bimodal distribution. The early type (age <50 years) has a female preponderance and the later predominant group (age >60 years) male. Between the ages of 50 and 60, there is similarity in the frequency of male and female distribution [3]. Myasthenia gravis commonly affects the eyes, face, pharyngeal muscles and limbs. Around 80% of myasthenia gravis are generalized type and clinical features are limited to the eyes in 15–20% [4].

17.2 Pathophysiology

In myasthenia gravis, autoantibodies are formed against the acetylcholine receptor (AChR) antibodies of post-synaptic membrane of the neuromuscular junction. Autoantibodies in the

B. R. Pokharel (✉)
Department of Neuroscience, Nepal Mediciti
Hospital, Kathmandu, Nepal

post-synaptic membrane lead to a number of changes including compromise of end plate potential, downregulation of receptors, and reduction of safety factor synaptic transmission. The antibodies cause the destruction of post-synaptic membrane. Another target receptor found in the post-synaptic membrane is muscle-specific kinase (MuSK), believed to have a role in clustering of AChRs. The other newer targets are low-density lipoprotein receptor-related protein 4 (LRP-4) and argin.

The process of antibody binding to the AChR initiates autoimmune response targeting the end plate region. AChR destruction of the post-synaptic region is dependent on complement activation. The stimulation of the post-synaptic membrane subsequently leads to the simplification of its typically intricate and folded surface, which is accompanied by a decrease in the quantity and concentration of AChR. A muscle-specific kinase is a recently identified antigenic target in MG patients with negative AChR antibodies. Activated T cells play a central role in autoantibody production in MG, but the mechanism of tolerance breakdown is unclear. It is likely that T-lymphocyte tolerance to self-antigens occurs in the thymus, and thymic abnormalities are common in MG. In about 10% of MG patients, thymomas are present, and thymic hyperplasia has been reported in about 65% of MG [5].

17.3 Clinical Presentation

The hallmark of MG is that muscles become fatigued and weaker with repeated usage. The involved muscles will have fluctuating weakness involving ocular, bulbar, and limb muscles [4]. MG can be classified into pure ocular myasthenia and generalized myasthenia with severity ranging from mild to moderate to severe [6]. Ptosis is initially unilateral, to gradually involve the bilateral eyelid. If bilateral, it is likely to be asymmetric; ptosis is also known as "plus minus ptosis." MG patients also often complain of difficulty in seeing bright lights.

In speech evaluation of MG patients, initial sound production is usually as loud as normal. However, repeated production of sound causes the voice to become gradually quieter [4, 5]. Patients may experience chewing difficulty, and may need to manually open and close their jaw. Jaw weakness may be pronounced in some patients causing the jaw to hang open, for which the patient may need chin support with the hand.

Difficulty swallowing is another manifestation of MG. Patients often have more difficulty swallowing liquid than solid food, causing coughing and aspiration. Exacerbation of symptoms can occur when individuals are exposed to high temperatures, stress, or infections, or suffer from any systemic disease [6]. Patients sometimes are unable to hold flatus and often complain of cramps in limb muscles.

17.4 MuSK Myasthenia

MuSK myasthenia primarily affects females, with symptoms typically arising during the fourth decade. Common clinical presentation includes pronounced faciobulbar weakness, leading to challenges in both speech and swallowing abilities. Patients may even experience atrophy in their facial and tongue muscles, which resembles amyotrophic lateral sclerosis [6]. The majority of patients with MuSK-positive myasthenia gravis exhibit limited or negligible ocular manifestations [7].

This group of patients has severe faciopharyngeal weakness with bulbar symptoms and have few or minimal associated ocular symptoms. Facial and tongue atrophy in MuSK myasthenia usually mimics **amyotrophic lateral sclerosis** [6].

17.5 MGFA Classification of Myasthenia Gravis

The Medical Scientific Advisory Board (MSAB) of the Myasthenia Gravis Foundation of America (MGFA) was established in May 1997 with the purpose of addressing the matter of universally recognized classifications, grading systems, and analytical methods for the management of patients receiving therapy and for application in therapeutic research trials [8]. According to MGFA classification, patients have weakness limited to the eyes in Class I. Class II encompasses ocular muscle involvement with mild weakness of other muscles. Similarly, Class III and IV encompass moderate and severe generalized muscle weakness.

Different provocative maneuvers used in suspected MG are:

1. Fatigable ptosis if sustained upgaze for 60–180 s.
2. Hering's Law of equal innervation elicits manually elevating the more ptotic eyelid and may result in worsening of ptosis in the opposite eyelid.
3. The presence of a "peek sign" is observed when the eyelids are tightly closed for an extended period, resulting in fatigue of the orbicularis oculi. This will slowly result in prominence of white sclera of the eye.
4. There will be fatigable diplopia with images appearing sideways in sustained lateral gaze for 60 s.
5. The patient experiences weakness on sustained abduction of the arms for a duration of 120 s, resulting in an inability to maintain arm elevated.
6. Counting aloud from 1 to 50 enhances progressive change in the voice causing dysarthria or dyspnea.

17.6 Investigations

Edrophonium challenge (neostigmine challenge) test: Edrophonium, also known as tensilon, is a short-acting acetylcholinesterase (AChE) inhibitor which helps to ameliorate muscle weakness in individuals with MG. The Patient is given IV/IM neostigmine/edrophonium along with inj. atropine. The result is considered positive if there is improvement in subjective response (e.g., improvement in ptosis).

The anti-AChR antibody test has demonstrated a high degree of reliability in the diagnosis of MG. The specificity of the phenomenon is reported to be remarkably high, reaching up to 100% [9]. Antibody tests are positive in about 90% of patients with generalized MG. However, only 50–70% with ocular MG have positive antibodies to AChR.

Patients with anti-AChR Ab negative (seronegative) should be considered for the MuSK antibody test [10]. Approximately 10% of people with MG are considered seronegative. Sometimes antibodies for other proteins such as agrin or low-density lipoprotein receptor-related protein 4 (LRP4) are present, signaling that these autoantibodies may be biomarkers of MG [11]. As newer antibodies are discovered for MG, a smaller number of patients are likely to be classified as seronegative. Other antibody tests are being increasingly recognized.

17.7 Electrophysiological Test

Repetitive nerve stimulation (RNS) and single-fiber electromyography (SFEMG) are specific tests performed for the diagnosis of myasthenia gravis. RNS is done at 2–3 Hz which is used to diagnose and differentiate various NMJ disorders. A decremental response (a gradual reduction in action potential with each repetitive stimulus) is an abnormal finding of MG. In 1895, Friedrich Jolly, a German neurologist, first described the test [12]. RNS is abnormal in about 50–70% of patients with generalized MG and is often normal in Class I or ocular MG.

The performance of SFEMG generally necessitates the utilization of a specifically designed single-fiber EMG needle electrode or facial concentric needle electrode featuring a small recording surface measuring 25 μm. This recording surface is exposed at a designated port located on the side of the electrode, positioned 3 mm away from the tip. SFEMG aims at evaluating neuromuscular block, jitter, and fiber density. An SFEMG test has higher diagnostic sensitivity than other investigations like tensilon, RNS, and AChR antibody test [13].

17.8 Thymus and Myasthenia

The thymus gland has been known to be associated with pathogenesis of seropositive MG. It acts to enhance autoimmune reaction involving autoantigens, AChR-specific T cells, and plasma cells. Pathologic changes in the thymus such as hyperplastic or tumoral can be seen in most AChR-positive patients. Chest CT with contrast scan is mandatory to look for thymoma or thymic enlargement in patients with MG. MRI/CT of the head may be required to rule out cranial pathology in case of ocular myasthenia gravis.

17.9 Management

MG is an autoimmune disorder and requires both symptomatic and disease-modifying treatment. Its management has been divided into the following areas.

17.9.1 Pharmacological Treatment

Acetylcholine esterase is the enzyme present at the neuromuscular junction. This enzyme is responsible for the breakdown of acetylcholine into acetyl and choline terminating action potential. A cholinesterase inhibitor, physostigmine, was used as the first effective medication for MG in a published report in 1934 [14]. Acetylcholine esterase inhibitors like neostigmine and pyridostigmine block the enzyme and prolong the action of acetylcholine.

Pyridostigmine is a commonly used acetylcholine esterase inhibitor for maintenance therapy in MG [15]. Tablets of pyridostigmine of 30–120 mg are given at various intervals during the day. Its effectiveness lasts for about 3–4 h in the daytime and may even have a longer effect of 6 h at night. The total daily dose varies depending on the severity of the weakness, usually in the range of 5–20 tablets.

The common side effects of pyridostigmine are abdominal cramps and increase frequency of urination. The increase in the drug level may give rise to clinical condition of cholinergic crisis lower dosages may be required in patient of renal failure.

17.9.2 Autoimmune Treatment

Corticosteroid and azathioprine are the most important drugs and have long been used in myasthenia gravis as immune modulators. The effectiveness of corticosteroids usually starts earlier, even within days, and in most patients, benefits may be observed in about 2 weeks [16]. Steroid treatment in MG may require periods of 3–4 months. Common side effects of steroids are acne, glaucoma, cataract, increased blood pressure, blood sugar changes, peptic ulcer, osteoporosis, and easy bruising. To lessen the side effects of corticosteroids, azathioprine-like drugs should be started concomitantly.

Azathioprine is a cytotoxic antimetabolite that inhibits DNA and RNA synthesis, resulting in impairment of purine metabolism. The usual starting dose for azathioprine is 50 mg/day and dosing can be increased by 50 mg in 2–4 weeks to a target dose of 2–3 mg/kg/day. Complete blood analysis and liver function test should be done at baseline and then regularly in order to monitor the adverse effects of azathioprine.

Mycophenolate mofetil was initially used as an immunosuppressor in organ transplantation and was only later introduced in treatment of MG [17]. Mycophenolate mofetil is teratogenic and is contraindicated in pregnancy. Due to its excretion in breast milk, mycophenolate mofetil is also contraindicated in lactation. The common side effects of mycophenolate are diarrhea, asthenia, thrombocytopenia, leukopenia, and herpes simplex infection.

Cyclophosphamide is commonly used as an anti-cancer drug and works as an alkylating agent, interfering with DNA of white blood cells that produce autoantibodies. Cyclophosphamide is considered in the treatment of myasthenia when it becomes refractory to other modalities of treatment. Rituximab is a monoclonal antibody directed against the CD20 antigen, a transmembrane protein expressed on the surface of B cells which usually causes long-lasting effects on immune response [18].

17.9.3 Plasma Exchange and Intravenous Immunoglobulin

Plasma exchange (PLEX) has been widely used as an effective treatment for MG since 1970 [19]. PLEX has usually been used in myasthenic crisis and in patients undergoing thymectomy. In this procedure, patient plasma that contains pathogenic antibodies is removed and replaced by donated plasma along with crystalloids and albumin. The procedure is done through peripheral or central venous access points.

Intravenous immunoglobulin (IVIG), which is derived from plasma of donors, is a safe and effective immunosuppressive and anti-inflammatory therapy for MG [20]. The effectiveness of IVIG can be observed in about a week and lasts for about 4–6 weeks, making it a good treatment option in myasthenia crisis and for patients not responding to other acute therapies. IVIG is given over 2–5 days at a total dose of 2 g/kg, with caution in patients with associated renal impairment and heart failure and in the elderly population. In comparison to PLEX, IVIG was found to have less serious adverse effects, and better response rate was observed in the PLEX treatment group [21].

17.9.4 Newer Treatments

Eculizumab is a recombinant monoclonal antibody that targets the C5 complement protein and inhibits the activation of the C5b-9 membrane attack complex. It was approved in 2017 for the treatment of refractory generalized myasthenia gravis [22]. Moderate to severe myasthenia patients who have already received adequate trials for other immunotherapies are candidates for eculizumab. It is given in infusions of 900 mg weekly for 4 weeks, followed by 1200 mg for the fifth week, and 1200 mg every 2 weeks.

17.10 Thymectomy

Thymectomy is the beneficial treatment for AChR-positive generalized MG that can improve the clinical status of MG and also might be helpful in reducing the maintenance dose. Although the optimal time for thymectomy is not clear, it should be scheduled when the patient's symptoms are well controlled in the preoperative period. Thymectomy in patients with antibodies such as MuSK, LRP4, and agrin-positive MG is not found to be beneficial [23].

References

1. Hughes T. The early history of myasthenia gravis. Neuromuscul Disord. 2005;15:878–86.
2. Li Y, Arora Y, Levin K. Myasthenia gravis: newer therapies offer sustained improvement. Cleve Clin J Med. 2013;80(11):711–2.
3. Alkhawajah NM, Oger J. Late onset myasthenia gravis: a review when incidences in older adults keeps increasing. Muscle Nerve. 2013;48(5):705–10.
4. Juel VC, Massey JM. Myasthenia gravis. Orphanet J Rare Disord. 2007;2:44.
5. Namba T, Brunner NG, Grob D. Myasthenia gravis in patients with thymoma, with particular reference to onset after thymectomy. Medicine. 1978;57:411–33.
6. Sieb JP. Myasthenia gravis: an update for the clinician. Clin Exp Immunol. 2014;175:408–18.
7. Guptill JT, Sanders DB, Evoli A. Anti-MuSK antibody myasthenia gravis: clinical findings and response to treatment in two large cohorts. Muscle Nerve. 2011;44:36–40.
8. Jaretzki A, Barohn RJ, Ernstoff RM, et al. Myasthenia gravis: recommendations for clinical research standards. Task Force of the medical Scientific Advisory Board of the Myasthenia Gravis Foundation of America. Neurology. 2000;55:16–23.
9. Padua L, Stalberg E, LoMonaco M, Evoli A, Batocchi A, Tonali P. SFEMG in ocular myasthenia gravis diagnosis. Clin Neurophysiol. 2000;111:1203–7.
10. Hoch W, McConville J, Helms S, Newsom-Davis J, Melms A, Vincent A. Auto-antibodies to the receptor tyrosine kinase MuSK in patients with myasthenia gravis without acetylcholine receptor antibodies. Nat Med. 2001;7:365–8.
11. Higuchi O, Hamuro J, Motomura M, Yamanashi Y. Auto antibodies to low-density lipoprotein receptor-related protein 4 in myasthenia gravis. Ann Neurol. 2011;69:418–22.
12. Ropper AH, Samuels MA. Adams and Victor's principles of neurology. 9th ed. New York: McGraw Hill; 2009. p. 1241–2.
13. Sarrigiannis PG, Kennett RP, Read S, Farrugia ME. Single fiber EMG with a concentric needle elec-

trode validation in myasthenia gravis. Muscle Nerve. 2006;33:61–5.

14. Walker MB. Treatment of myasthenia gravis with physostigmine. Lancet. 1934;223:1200–1.

15. Saperstein DS, Barohn RJ. Management of myasthenia gravis. Semin Neurol. 2004;24:41–8.

16. Pascuzzi RM, Coslett HB, Johns TR. Long-term corticosteroid treatment of myasthenia gravis: report of 116 patients. Ann Neurol. 1984;15:291–8.

17. Simmons WD, Rayhill SC, Sollinger H. Preliminary risk-benefit assessment of mycophenolate mofetil in transplant rejection. Drug Saf. 1997;17:75–92.

18. Tandan R, Hehir MK 2nd, Waheed W, Howard DB. Rituximab treatment of myasthenia gravis: a systematic review. Muscle Nerve. 2017;56:185–96.

19. Dau PC, Lindstrom JM, Cassel CK, Denys EH, Shev EE, Spitler LE. Plasmapheresis and immunosuppressive drug therapy in myasthenia gravis. N Engl J Med. 1977;297:1134–40.

20. Gajdos P, Outin H, Elkharrat D, et al. High-dose intravenous gamma globulin for myasthenia gravis. Lancet. 1984;1:406–7.

21. Ipe TS, Davis AR, Raval JS. Therapeutic plasma exchange in myasthenia gravis: a systematic literature review and meta-analysis of comparative evidence. Front Neurol. 2021;12:662856.

22. Howard JF Jr, Barohn RJ, Cutter GR, Freimer M, Juel VC, Mozaffar T, MG Study Group, et al. A randomized, double-blind, placebo-controlled phase II study of eculizumab in patients with refractory generalized myasthenia gravis. Muscle Nerve. 2013;48:76–84.

23. Sanders DB, Wolfe GI, Benatar M, Evoli A, Gilhus NE, et al. International consensus guidance for management of myasthenia gravis: executive summary. Neurology. 2016;87:419–25.

Amyotrophic Lateral Sclerosis

18

Seena Vengalil, Saraswati Nashi,
Veeramani Preethish-Kumar, Kiran Polavarapu,
and Atchayaram Nalini

Case Scenario

A 65-year-old man presented with progressive weakness and wasting of right hand for 2 years followed by proximal weakness of right upper limb for 1½ years. He also had distal weakness of right lower limb for 1 year and bulbar symptoms with difficulty in swallowing and speaking for 2 months. He had a history of muscle cramps and fasciculations in his extremities. He also experienced fatigue and had weight loss of around 3 kg over the past few months. He had no sensory, cerebellar, extrapyramidal, autonomic, behavioral, or memory disturbances. There was no positive family history. On examination, the eye movements were normal; there was an atrophic, weak flabby tongue with fasciculations and slow movements. There was a mixed type of dysarthria, and the jaw jerk was brisk. There was asymmetric wasting of small muscles of hands, predominantly of the thenar eminence (ape thumb deformity). The shoulder girdle muscles were wasted. Minipolymyoclonus was prominently present. He had proximal and distal weakness of all four limbs with spasticity and exaggerated tendon reflexes. There was no Babinski's sign, and

abdominal reflexes were elicited. Sensory system examination was normal. He had a pure motor syndrome with a clinical diagnosis of amyotrophic lateral sclerosis (ALS). Blood investigations like hemogram, renal, liver, and thyroid function tests were normal. Nerve conduction study showed a decrease in compound muscle action potential (CMAP) amplitudes with normal distal latency and velocity in tested nerves of upper and lower limbs. Sensory conductions were normal. Electromyography (EMG) confirmed a diagnosis of ALS by showing changes of denervation and partial re-innervation in sampled muscles of the upper and lower limbs and the cranial musculature. Workup for other secondary causes like endocrinopathy, paraproteinemia, and neoplasm was negative. The patient fulfilled the criteria for a clinically definite case of ALS by modified Airlie House El Escorial criteria.

18.1 Introduction

Amyotrophic lateral sclerosis (ALS) is a progressive neurodegenerative disease of the motor system. It was first described by Jean Martin Charcot in 1869 and became well known when Lou Gehrig, a famous US baseball player, was diagnosed with the disease [1*]. Most of the cases are sporadic; however, 5–10% may be familial with an autosomal dominant, recessive, or X-linked inheritance pattern. Recent advances in under-

S. Vengalil (✉) · S. Nashi · A. Nalini
Department of Neurology, National Institute of
Mental Health and Neurosciences, Bangalore, India

V. Preethish-Kumar · K. Polavarapu
Department of Clinical Neurosciences, National
Institute of Mental Health and Neurosciences,
Bangalore, India

© Springer Nature Singapore Pte Ltd. 2024
K. K. Oli et al. (eds.), *Case-based Approach to Common Neurological Disorders*,
https://doi.org/10.1007/978-981-99-8676-7_18

standing the pathogenesis of ALS may improve the diagnosis and treatment of ALS and result in extended longevity for the patients.

18.2 Epidemiology

Incidence is about 1.5–2.7/100,000, while prevalence is around 0.32/100,000. Male-to-female ratio is 1.5:1, and it is almost the same for familial cases [2*]. Lifetime risk of ALS is 1:400 for women and 1:350 for men [2]. Peak age of onset is 58–63 years for sporadic cases and 47–52 years for familial cases [2]. Around 5% of cases can have an age of onset less than 30 years. In Asia, the highest incidence is noted in Japan, while China and India have a low incidence [3]. A large study on 1153 patients with ALS in India found that the mean age of onset is a decade earlier, progression is slower, and survival is longer compared to Caucasian patients with ALS [4].

18.3 Phenotypes and Clinical Features

Around two-thirds of cases present with spinal-onset ALS (classical Charcot ALS) [5], and they usually have focal muscle weakness or wasting of the distal upper limbs as the initial symptom which may be associated with cramps and fasciculations. Weakness is asymmetrical and insidious in onset and later spreads to other limbs and later involves bulbar and respiratory musculature too. Bulbar-onset ALS presents with dysarthria or dysphagia, and they may have sialorrhea and pseudobulbar symptoms like emotional lability or excessive yawning.

About 5% of patients have respiratory muscle weakness at onset without much limb weakness or bulbar symptoms and hence present with symptoms of type 2 respiratory failure like nocturnal dyspnea, orthopnea, daytime somnolence, morning headaches, decreased concentration, irritability, etc. Classically the findings include a combination of upper motor neuron (UMN) and lower motor neuron (LMN) signs in affected segments. UMN findings include spasticity, loss of dexterity of affected limbs, weakness, brisk reflexes, or retained reflexes in an atrophic limb, and presence of primitive reflexes due to loss of inhibitory UMN control (to be interpreted as pathologic only in the presence of associated UMN signs) [6]. A study by Okuda et al. found that corneomandibular reflex may be a sensitive indicator of ALS [7]. LMN signs include weakness, wasting, fasciculations, hyporeflexia, and cramps (Figs. 18.1, 18.2, 18.3 and 18.4). Intrinsic muscles of hand are wasted early with a split-hand phenomenon, wherein muscles of lateral aspect of hand are wasted early and more severe compared to those in medial aspect. Palpable flaccidity of muscles and trophic joint changes with pain and pericapsulitis may occur rarely.

UMN syndrome in bulbar palsy presents with spastic dysarthria, slowness of tongue movements, dysphagia more to liquids, pseudobulbar affect, hyperactive gag, and brisk jaw jerk, while LMN findings include weakness of face, palate, and tongue muscles with hypoactive gag reflex

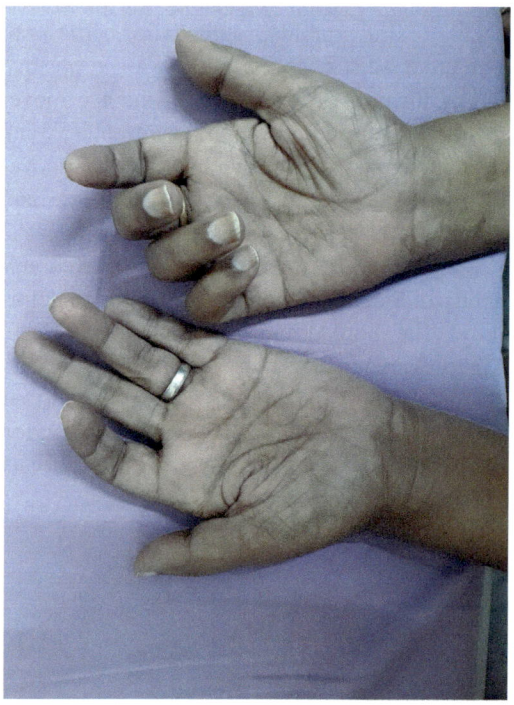

Fig. 18.1 Wasting of small muscles of hand, especially those of thenar muscles with partial clawing

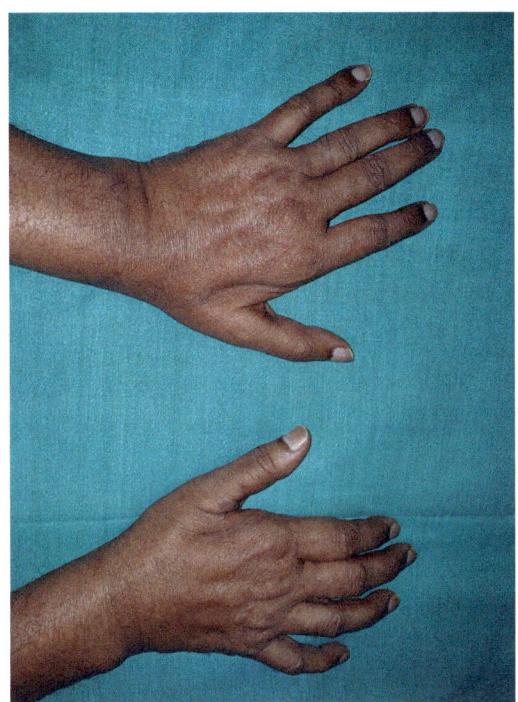

Fig. 18.2 Wasting of interossei, especially the first dorsal interossei

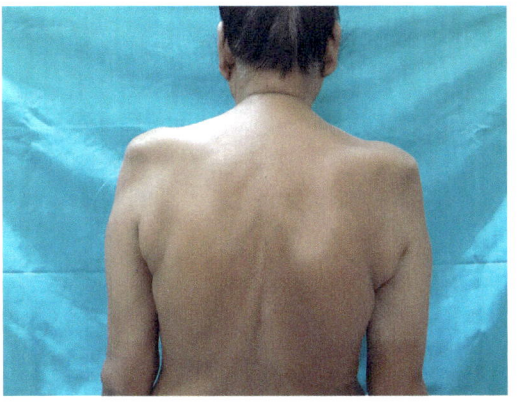

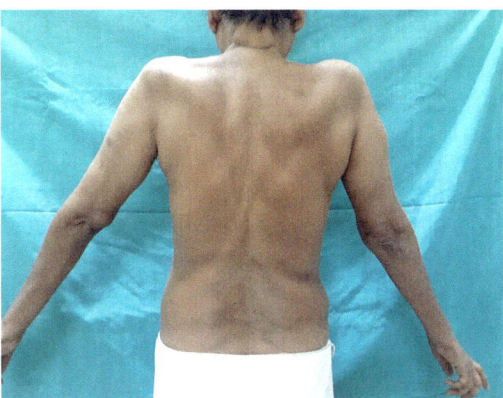

Fig. 18.4 Proximal muscle weakness with severe inability in raising arm

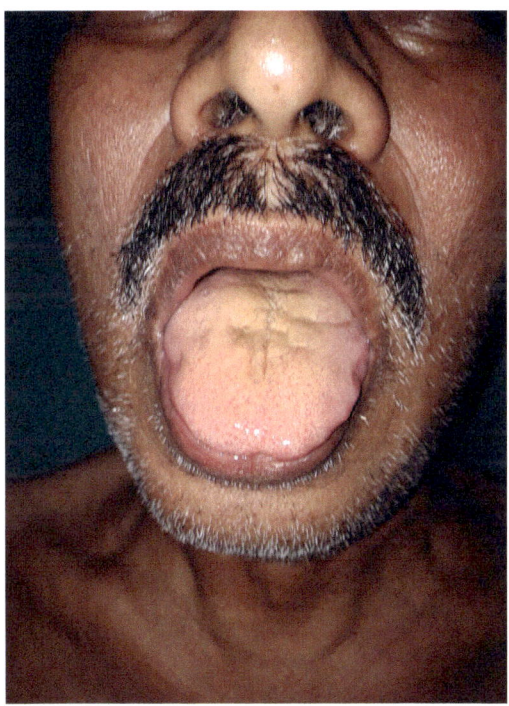

Fig. 18.3 Wasting of shoulder girdle muscles—supraspinatus and infraspinatus with flattening of shoulder contour

Fig. 18.5 Atrophic and flabby tongue in a patient with ALS

and absent jaw jerk. Tongue is atrophic and flaccid and shows fasciculation in resting position in the floor of the mouth (Fig. 18.5). Involvement of paraspinal muscles causes head drop, bent spine, and camptocormia. Survival in ALS is around 20–48 months; however, 10–20% of patients with ALS may survive 10 years or more.

Other variant presentations include the following.

(a) Progressive muscular atrophy (PMA, Duchenne-Aran muscular atrophy): PMA present as pure LMN syndrome, characterized by asymmetrical flaccid weakness with wasting, fasciculations, and hyporeflexia, usually of distal limb onset. PMA accounts for 2.5–11% of motor neuron disease. Age of onset is older than for ALS, mean being 63.4 +/− 11.7 years. About 20% may have symmetrical proximal limb onset. Bulbar muscles are spared initially though 40% may subsequently develop bulbar involvement. Those who develop bulbar weakness are more likely to progress to ALS. It is rare to find axial or respiratory muscle involvement at onset. Around 22–35% may later develop UMN features in a span of 8 months to 5 years [8]. PMA is usually slowly progressive, and median survival is 48 months, about 12 months longer than those with ALS [8].

(b) Flail arm syndrome (Vulpian–Bernhardt syndrome or brachial amyotrophic diplegia, man-in-the-barrel syndrome)—their frequency is about 2–11% of MND. Age of onset is 53–57 years, begins in upper limb proximal muscles, and may be asymmetric in onset. Unlike ALS with limb onset, where distal muscles are involved initially, proximal muscles are involved more in flail arm syndrome. Reflexes are sluggish to absent. Disease remains confined to a single spinal region for 12–18 months. Prognosis is generally better than for ALS with mean survival being 76–79 months with 52% having more than 5-year survival [9].

(c) Flail leg syndrome (leg amyotrophic diplegia, pseudopolyneuritic form, Marie–Patrikios form, peroneal form)—their frequency is about 2.5–6.3% of MND. Age of onset is around 55–57 years with an asymmetric pelviperoneal pattern or distal leg weakness and remains confined to the lumbosacral segment for more than 12–24 months. Prognosis is better than ALS with a mean survival of 76–87 months and a 5-year survival rate of 64–77% [9].

(d) Primary lateral sclerosis (PLS)—PLS is a progressive UMN dysfunction in the absence of LMN involvement and absence of history; it even sometimes mimics hereditary spastic paraplegia. Patients present with stiffness, mild weakness, and clumsiness and may develop spastic dysarthria and emotional labiality. Stiffness as a presenting symptom is more common in PLS than ALS. PLS accounts for 1–3% of MND and remains a diagnosis of exclusion and requires presence of symptoms for more than 3 years (Pringle criteria) or more than 4 years (Singer criteria). Symptoms are usually of lower limb onset and spreads from one side to other and then ascends up, averaging 3.5 years from onset to upper limb involvement and 5 years to bulbar involvement. Prognosis is better than for ALS, and those patients who do not develop LMN findings after 4 years of disease onset have an almost normal life span [10].

(e) Mills hemiplegic variant—progressive ascending or descending hemiplegia [5, 9, 10] in the absence of sensory involvement. Due to unilateral corticospinal tract involvement, this entity is now debatable with some considering it to be a variant of PLS.

(f) Isolated bulbar amyotrophic lateral sclerosis (IBALS)—their frequency is about 4% of MND, and the age of onset is slightly older, mean being 61 years and more common in females. Patients may have flaccid, spastic, or mixed dysarthria with one-third having tongue wasting and about a half developing emotional lability. Initial EMG shows confinement to the bulbar area, and respiratory muscles are uninvolved at onset. Percutaneous endoscopic gastrostomy (PEG) tube placement may be needed early in disease due to severe swallowing difficulties and risk of aspiration. IBALS also has a more benign prognosis compared to classic ALS with 75% being alive at 2–8 years of follow-up [9].

A variety of sleep abnormalities have been described in ALS including insomnia, sleep-disordered breathing, and restless leg syndrome. Patients with ALS have increased sleep latency, a shorter duration of sleep, with poor quality of sleep, resulting in daytime somnolence [11].

Fatigue and depression are also seen in patients with ALS; profound weight loss and "ALS cachexia" unrelated to calorie intake occurs in some patients. In the sacral cord, motor neurons of Onufrowicz which control bladder muscles are typically spared in ALS. However, in patients with severe spasticity, urgency of micturition and urinary retention can occur, which correlates with the Ashworth scale [12]. Though extraocular muscles are usually not involved in ALS, studies have found a variety of abnormalities ranging from reduction of saccadic velocities and smooth pursuits to voluntary upgaze restriction and eye-lid-opening apraxias in subjects with ALS [6, 13]. There are case reports of patients on ventilator for long time, who develop a supranuclear type of progressive external ophthalmoplegia and who died in a totally locked-in state [14]. Sensory system is spared though patients may report vague sensory complaints. Extrapyramidal involvement is seen in 5%, and impairment of postural reflexes may be seen [6]. Cognitive impairment though not universal is increasingly being recognized in ALS. Various cognitive abnormalities ranging from anomia and executive dysfunction to frank frontotemporal dementia have been described.

18.4 Pathogenesis

Numerous genes have been identified which contribute to pathogenesis of ALS. Other precipitating factors debated include repeated head trauma, pesticides, toxins and heavy metals, smoking, physical exertion, electrical injury, etc., but causation is not clear. Various pathogenetic mechanisms proposed are defects in RNA processing, intra-neuronal aggregation of various abnormal proteins leading to oxidative stress, mitochondrial dysfunction, glutamate excitotoxicity, inflammation, defects in axoplasmic flow, and protein misfolding [15].

18.5 Diagnostic Criteria of ALS

World Federation of Neurology Subcommittee on Motor Neuron Disease conducted a 3-day workshop on "Clinical limits of ALS" in El Escorial, Spain, in 1990, where the El Escorial criteria (EEC) was developed. If there were clear-cut upper and lower motor neuron findings in two to three regions, EMG was not considered essential (Box 18.1). In 1998, Western ALS group modified this criterion, which required the presence of LMN findings in two limbs and UMN findings in one area and EMG findings of fibrillation potentials for LMN involvement and also allowed the use of electrodiagnosis, neuroimaging, and laboratory studies for ruling out ALS mimics. In 2006, a group of researchers met in Awaji-Shima in Japan to refine the criteria to improve sensitivity. EMG findings of denervation were considered equivalent to clinical LMN findings, and the term "laboratory-supported probable ALS" was replaced by "probable ALS." Fasciculations in EMG were counted as depictive of denervation even in the absence of fibrillations and positive sharp waves (PSW). Thus, Awaji-Shima criteria improved the sensitivity of electrodiagnostic criteria of ALS (Box 18.2) [16].

Box 18.1 Summary of Revised El Escorial Research Diagnostic Criteria for Amyotrophic Lateral Sclerosis [14]

Diagnosis of amyotrophic lateral sclerosis requires

1. Evidence of LMN degeneration by clinical, electrophysiological, or neuropathological examination.
2. Evidence of UMN degeneration by clinical examination.
3. Progressive spread of symptoms or signs within a region or to other regions, as determined by history or examination.

Together with the absence of

1. Electrophysiological and pathological evidence of other disease that might explain the signs of LMN and/or UMN degeneration.
2. Neuroimaging evidence of other disease processes that might explain the observed clinical and electrophysiological signs.

Categories of clinical diagnostic certainty on clinical criteria alone.
Definite amyotrophic lateral sclerosis.
- UMN signs and LMN signs in three regions.

Probable amyotrophic lateral sclerosis.
- UMN signs and LMN signs in two regions with at least some UMN signs rostral to LMN signs.

Probable amyotrophic lateral sclerosis—laboratory supported.
- UMN signs in one or more regions, and LMN signs defined by EMG in at least two regions.

Possible amyotrophic lateral sclerosis
- UMN signs and LMN signs in one region (together).
- UMN signs in two or more regions.
- UMN and LMN signs in two regions with no UMN signs rostral to LMN signs.
- UMN signs: Clonus, Babinski sign, absent abdominal skin reflexes, hypertonia, loss of dexterity.
- LMN signs: Atrophy, weakness. If only fasciculation, search with EMG for active denervation.
- Regions: Bulbar, cervical, thoracic, and lumbosacral.

Box 18.2 Awaji Criteria
Clinically definite:
UMN and LMN signs in bulbar region and two spinal regions; or UMN and LMN signs in three spinal regions.
Clinically probable:
UMN + LMN signs in two spinal regions and "with some UMN signs necessarily rostral to the LMN signs."

Clinically possible:
UMN and LMN signs in one spinal region; or UMN signs in two spinal regions.
LMN signs are found rostral to UMN signs—appropriate neuroimaging and laboratory tests to be performed to exclude other possible differential diagnosis that may mimic ALS.

18.6 Investigations

18.6.1 Nerve Conduction Studies (NCS)

NCS is essential to exclude peripheral nerve disorders and other ALS mimics. Motor conductions may show normal compound muscle action potential (CMAP), CMAPs with decreased amplitude, asymmetric side-to-side CMAP differences, prolonged distal latency, and reduced velocity consistent with axon loss (never below 70% of expected). "F" wave latencies and chronodispersion are increased, and F-wave persistence is decreased in patients with ALS [17]. Sensory conductions are usually normal unless entrapment neuropathies are associated. However, few studies have found sensory abnormalities on NCS, suggesting ALS to be a multisystem disorder. Initial insult in sensory system is in dorsal root ganglion followed by progressive axonal atrophy, secondary demyelination and remyelination changes, and later axonal loss [18].

18.6.2 Electromyography (EMG)

EMG is of utmost importance in detecting LMN involvement when clinical signs may not be apparent. Clinical and electrophysiological abnormalities are of equal importance as per revised EEC. EMG must be done in muscles innervated by cranial nerves (facial, tongue, and jaw muscles), thoracic muscles (paraspinals, rectus abdominis, and external oblique), and cervical and lumbar roots (at least two muscles with different innervations). As trapezius and sternocleidomastoid have dual innervation from cranial nerves and upper cervical roots, their sampling may confound results in those with cervical degenerative changes. EMG findings of chronic and acute denervation should be looked for and include spontaneous activity like fibrillations, fasciculations, and positive sharp waves (PSW), large amplitude, long duration, polyphasic MUPs, and decreased motor unit recruitment with rapid firing of reduced motor units [17].

18.6.3 Repetitive Nerve Stimulation and Single-Fiber EMG

Abnormalities of neuromuscular transmission are known in ALS and result from collateral nerve terminal sprouting. Slow RNS at 3 Hz stimuli may show decrements of more than 10% in CMAP amplitude. Single-fiber EMG may also show increased jitter, blocking, and fiber density paralleling muscle atrophy and weakness. However, in the presence of appropriate clinical and electrodiagnostic findings consistent with ALS, the presence of these abnormalities should not hinder one from making a diagnosis of ALS.

Motor unit number estimation (MUNE) assesses the number of motor units in a muscle and can be serially followed for estimating motor neuron loss. MUNE is measured by dividing the size of maximum CMAP amplitude by the size of the average surface-detected MUP [17].

18.6.4 Neuroimaging Findings in ALS

Hyperintensity of corticospinal tracts on MRI is seen, though it is not specific for ALS. Cerebral atrophy detection using voxel-based morphometry correlates to cognitive impairment. Magnetic resonance spectroscopy (MRS) shows a reduced N-acetyl aspartate-to-creatine ratio in the primary motor cortex and is a sensitive indicator of UMN dysfunction, and helps distinguish those with

PMA from those with ALS. Diffusion-tensor imaging exhibits reduced fractional anisotropy within corticospinal tracts in patients with ALS. Functional imaging using PET studies may show frontal deficits correlating with neuropsychological impairment. Molecular imaging using ^{11}C-flumazenil have shown reduced GABA-ergic inhibition supporting the role of cortical hyperexcitability as a pathophysiological mechanism of ALS. Reduced serotonergic receptor ligand binding in frontotemporal areas in patients with FTD-ALS is also seen. DTI has revealed early changes in the posterior limb of the internal capsule in patients with the superoxide dismutase 1 (SOD1) mutation compared to healthy controls and thus may serve as a pre-symptomatic biomarker of the disease [2].

18.6.5 Other Investigations

Muscle enzymes like creatine kinase (CK) is elevated two to three times above normal limit. Serum protein and immunoelectrophoresis, thyroid function tests, paraneoplastic profile, serum calcium and phosphorus, hexosaminidase B levels (where deficiency is more prevalent), and heavy metal screening (if toxicity is suspected) may be done to rule out other differentials of ALS [1].

18.7 Familial ALS (FALS)

In 1993, the superoxide dismutase 1 (SOD1) gene was identified, which was a breakthrough in considering the genetic etiology of ALS. With newer genetic technology like genome-wide association studies (GWAS) and next-generation sequencing, more than 50 ALS-associated genes have been identified. Extramotor features associated with gene variants of ALS include FTD, extrapyramidal features, and inclusion body myopathy. FALS is mostly adult onset though some genes may also have juvenile onset of disease. Inheritance is mainly autosomal dominant, but autosomal recessive and X-linked dominant forms are also seen [18]. Criteria for diagnosing familial ALS are given in Box 18.3.

Box 18.3 Criteria for the Diagnosis of FALS

Classification	Family history
Definite	More than two first- or second-degree relatives with ALS More than one relative with ALS and gene-positive co-segregation
Probable	One first- or second-degree relative with ALS
Possible	Distant relative (third degree or beyond) with ALS Patient with sporadic ALS and no family history of ALS, but positive for an FALS gene More than one first- or second-degree relative with confirmed frontotemporal dementia

18.8 ALS Management and Multidisciplinary Approach

The treatment of ALS has changed drastically in the past few years. A multidisciplinary approach helps in dealing with complex issues of ALS like respiratory involvement, bulbar symptoms and nutrition, depression, and other psychosocial issues. The only FDA-approved oral drug for the treatment of ALS is riluzole, which helps in prolonging the survival of patients with ALS. The mechanism of action includes inhibition of glutamate release and inactivation of voltage-gated sodium channels. It is also an NMDA receptor antagonist and is recommended at a dose of 50 mg twice daily for those with a duration of <5 years, forced vital capacity of more than 60%, and no tracheostomy [1]. Intravenous edaravone is a recently approved medication for early-stage ALS to slow the progression.

Symptomatic management includes the following:

1. Sialorrhea: It is a troublesome symptom reported by more than 50% of patients with ALS, due to pharyngeal weakness, and can lead to aspiration pneumonia. It can be treated with anticholinergic medications, atropine, glycopyrrolate, transdermal scopolamine, or non-pharmacological approaches like suctioning. For those with medically refractory sialorrhea, botulinum toxin injection or low-dose radiation therapy for salivary glands may be helpful [19].

2. Pseudobulbar affect: Selective serotonin reuptake inhibitors (SSRI), serotonin–norepinephrine reuptake inhibitors, or tricyclic antidepressants (TCA) can be used to manage pseudobulbar effect. A novel combination of dextromethorphan/quinidine (20/10 mg) has been found to be effective in a phase III randomized trial [19].

3. Sleep disruption: It may be due to a variety of causes like anxiety, depression, nocturnal hypoventilation, or limited mobility. Electric beds or air mattresses can be used to enhance mobility or decrease discomfort due to limited mobility. Non-invasive pressure ventilation can improve sleep quality, and the use of anxiolytics and antidepressants like zolpidem and mirtazapine is beneficial.

4. Respiratory insufficiency: Supine forced vital capacity (FVC) and maximum inspiratory pressure (MIP) may be monitored, and non-invasive ventilation must be initiated if FVC falls to less than 50% of normal or if MIP is less than 60 cm. Other parameters which can be monitored to detect respiratory insufficiency include sniff nasal pressure, sniff transdiaphragmatic pressure, and nocturnal desaturation (<90% for more than 1 cumulative minute). Centers for Disease Control and Prevention (CDC) also recommends pneumococcal vaccine and yearly influenza vaccine for patients with significant neuromuscular illness [19].

5. Nutritional management: Initially it consists of altering food consistencies or maneuvers like chin tuck or head tilt to facilitate swallowing. When weight loss exceeds 10% of pre-diagnostic evaluations or problems of aspiration and dehydration occur, percutaneous endoscopic gastrostomy (PEG) is indicated.

6. Fatigue—Modafinil, 100–300 mg daily has been found to decrease fatigue and improve the quality of life.

7. Spasticity—Spasticity restricts mobility and also contributes to pain experienced by many patients with ALS. Moderate exercises and medications like baclofen, tizanidine, dantrolene, and benzodiazepines may be of help. In medically refractory cases, intrathecal baclofen pump has been found to reduce Ashworth spasticity score.

8. Autonomic dysfunction: Constipation and urinary urgency are reported in 29% of patients and may be due to involvement of intermediolateral columns or Onuf's nucleus. Increasing fiber intake, hydration, prune juices, stool softeners, fiber laxatives, and osmotic agents like lactulose and polyethylene glycol are recommended. Patients with ALS may have high urinary frequency and urgency and may need to void every 1–2 h, which may affect their social activities.

18.8.1 Dietary Supplements

Antioxidants like vitamin E have been found to delay the onset and slow the progression of ALS. However, significant benefit has not been found on the survival of these patients. Chinese studies have also shown that Pu-erh tea extract may prevent abnormal protein accumulation and hence prevent the progression of ALS. Further in vivo studies may be needed to ascertain its beneficial effects [1].

References

1. Zarei S, Carr K, Reiley L, et al. A comprehensive review of amyotrophic lateral sclerosis. Surg Neurol Int. 2015;6:171.
2. Kiernan MC, Vucic S, Cheah BC, et al. Amyotrophic lateral sclerosis. Lancet. 2011;377(9769):942–55.
3. Shahrizaila N, Sobue G, Kuwabara S, et al. Amyotrophic lateral sclerosis and motor neuron syndromes in Asia. J Neurol Neurosurg Psychiatry. 2016;87(8):821–30.
4. Nalini A, Thennarasu K, Gourie-Devi M, et al. Clinical characteristics and survival pattern of 1153 patients with amyotrophic lateral sclerosis: experience over 30 years from India. J Neurol Sci. 2008;272(1–2):60–70.
5. Wijesekera LC, Leigh PN. Amyotrophic lateral sclerosis. Orphanet J Rare Dis. 2009;4:3.
6. Katirji B, Kaminski HJ, Ruff RL, editors. Neuromuscular disorders in clinical practice. 2nd ed. Springer Science: New York; 2014.
7. Okuda B, Kodama N, Kawabata K, Tachibana H, Sugita M. Corneomandibular reflex in ALS. Neurology. 1999;52(8):1699–701.
8. Liewluck T, Saperstein DS. Progressive muscular atrophy. Neurol Clin. 2015;33(4):761–73.
9. Jawdat O, Statland JM, Barohn RJ, Katz J, Dimachkie MM. ALS regional variants (brachial amyotrophic diplegia, leg amyotrophic diplegia, isolated bulbar ALS). Neurol Clin. 2015;33(4):775–85.
10. Statland JM, Barohn RJ, Dimachkie MM, Floeter MK, Mitsumoto H. Primary lateral sclerosis. Neurol Clin. 2015;33(4):749–60.
11. Panda S, Gourie-Devi M, Sharma A. Sleep disorders in amyotrophic lateral sclerosis: a questionnaire-based study from India. Neurol India. 2018;66:700–8.
12. De Carvalho L, Motta R, Battaglia MA, Brichetto G. Urinary disorders in amyotrophic lateral sclerosis subjects. Amyotroph Lateral Scler. 2011;12(5):352–5.
13. Leveille A, Kiernen J, Goodwin A, et al. Eye movements in amyotrophic lateral sclerosis. Arch Neurol. 1982;39:684–6.
14. Mizutani T, Sakamaki S, Tsuchiya N, Kamei S, Kohzu H, Horiuchi R, Ida M, Shiozawa R, Takasu T. Amyotrophic lateral sclerosis with ophthalmoplegia and multisystem degeneration in patients on long term use of respirators. Acta Neuropathol. 1992;84:372–7.
15. Morgan S, Orrell RW. Pathogenesis of amyotrophic lateral sclerosis. Br Med Bull. 2016;119:87–97.
16. Statland JM, Barohn RJ, McVey AL, Katz JS, Dimachkie MM. Patterns of weakness, classification of motor neuron disease, and clinical diagnosis of sporadic amyotrophic lateral sclerosis. Neurol Clin. 2015;33(4):735–48.
17. Joyce NC, Carter GT. Electrodiagnosis in amyotrophic lateral sclerosis. PM&R. 2013;5(5):S89–95.
18. Isaacs JD, Dean AF, Shaw CE, Al-Chalabi A, Mills KR, Leigh PN. Amyotrophic lateral sclerosis with sensory neuropathy: part of a multisystem disorder? J Neurol Neurosurg Psychiatry. 2007;78:750–3.
19. Jackson CE, McVey AL, Rudnicki S, Dimachkie MM, Barohn RJ. Symptom management and end-of-life care in amyotrophic lateral sclerosis. Neurol Clin. 2015;33(4):889–907.

Myotonic Dystrophy

19

Hrishikesh Kumar and Purba Basu

Case Scenario

A 31-year-old gentleman presented with gait imbalance since childhood. He was unable to run in school sports and playground and used to fall recurrently. Gradually he started developing difficulty in walking. He was lethargic and had subnormal intelligence in academics. He also had difficulty in gripping objects, mild slurring of speech, low appetite, and recurrent pain and swelling of legs (left > right). He has three maternal uncles who have similar problems. His mother died at the age of 50 years; she was bedridden and had loss of speech during last few years of her life. One of his brothers was also affected with similar problem who died because of head injury.

On examination, he was found to have frontal balding and a bradykinesia score of 2/4 on both sides. He had myoclonus in both hands along with some polyminimyoclonus. There was delayed relaxation of small muscles of hand. His gait was ataxic, and deep tendon reflexes were diminished in all four limbs. Urea, creatinine, complete blood count, and other routine tests were normal, but creatinine phosphokinase (CPK) was abnormally high (1102 U). ECG was suggestive of occasional supraventricular tachycardia. Eye examination was normal.

Electromyography (EMG) of biceps, tibialis anterior, and extensor digitorum communis showed waxing and waning type of myotonic discharge which also had "dive bomber" sound. MRI brain was normal. The result of genetic testing for myotonic dystrophy was positive. Diagnosis of myotonic dystrophy was made, and patient had been put on phenytoin sodium along with vitamin and neurotrophic factor supplements.

19.1 Introduction

Myotonic dystrophy (DM) is an inherited disorder of muscle characterized by weakness and sustained muscle contractions [1]. Myotonia signifies inability to relax muscles at will. Wasting and shrinkage of muscles, a degenerative process known as dystrophy, accompany the disease. This illness is also referred by its Greek name "dystrophia myotonica." DM is a multi-system disease with core features of myotonia, muscle weakness, cataract, and cardiac conduction abnormalities. The disorder is characterized by specific abnormalities in muscle biopsy from patients. Cytopathology of muscle specimen derived from biopsy usually shows variation of muscle fiber size, muscle fiber necrosis, scar tissue formation, and inflammation.

H. Kumar (✉) · P. Basu
Department of Neurology, Institute of Neurosciences, Kolkata, Kolkata, India

19.2 Epidemiology

The incidence of DM is estimated to be 1 in 8000 births, and its worldwide prevalence ranges from 2.1 to 14.3/100,000 inhabitants [2, 3]. But these statistics may represent the tip of the iceberg, as the florid signs and symptoms may evolve over a period of one to two decades. DM is the most common adult-onset muscular dystrophy and occurs equally in men and women. Fleischer recognized in 1918 the tendency of the disease to become more severe with successive generation especially when the disorder is passed on from mother. This tendency is known as "anticipation" [4]. The disease is lesser severe when passed on from father. There are rare sporadic cases of myotonic dystrophy. There are two main types of dystrophia myotonica, DM type 1 and type 2 [5]. DM type 1 is sub-classified as mild DM1, classic DM1, and congenital DM1. It is caused by an alteration in the *DMPK* gene [6]. DM type 2 does not cause congenital disease and is a lesser evil form, though its symptoms are similar to those of DM type 1. DM2 is caused by an alteration in the *CNBP* gene [7]. Both DM1 and DM2 are inherited as autosomal dominant pattern.

19.3 Pathogenesis

The structural defect in the affected gene results in defective transport of messenger RNA (for serine threonine protein kinase) to the cytoplasm. This protein kinase may have a role in the normal function of skeletal muscle sodium channels. In DM type 1 the responsible gene is located on chromosome 19. The disease is characterized by abnormal repeat expansion of CTG on the DMPK (dystrophia myotonica protein kinase) gene. In healthy people, the repeats are between 5 and 37, whereas in disease states, these repeats can be anywhere from 50 to more than 4000 repeats of the CTG sequence [7].

The genes responsible for DM2 are found on chromosome 3. Four nucleotide CCTG on Znf9 DNA stretch are repeated, and the disease occurs when the repeat exceeds a particular threshold. People with DM type 2 has more than 75 repeats, which can be anywhere between 75 and 11,000 repeats [7].

Histopathology findings are the presence of type 1 fiber atrophy, often clumped in pyknotic longitudinal chains and substantial central nucleation noted in DM1 in light microscopy. Electron microscopy may show central nuclei in muscle biopsies. Light microscopic characteristics observed in myotonic dystrophy type 2 include central nucleation, prevalence of pyknotic nuclear clumps, and predominance of type 2 muscle fibers. Muscle fibers look severely atrophied along with lipofuscin accumulation while characterizing ultrastructural abnormalities. The presence of internal nuclei is also a consistent finding in electron microscopy [8].

19.4 Clinical Manifestations

Myotonic dystrophy type 1 is the most common form of the disease. Though the disease is chiefly characterized by muscle weakness, it may affect other systems of the body. There may be associated cardiac, hormonal, respiratory, digestive, and mental disorders that accompany the disease symptoms. Typically, the initial symptoms develop in early teen years in the form of hand weakness or a tendency toward foot drop. There may be noticeable difficulty in releasing a firm grasp during cold weather. Fine motor movements of hands like handling keys, hammer, or buttoning can be problematic. Gradual wasting of facial muscles can give rise to the characteristic appearance of a "haggard" or "mournful" face. Frontal hair loss, drooping eyelids, and an open mouth may soon follow. In middle age, patient may experience frequent falls resulting from sudden movement producing sustained muscle contractions leading to loss of balance. Difficulty in swallowing, voice changes, and recurrent jaw dislocations may gradually ensue. Muscle atrophy sometimes becomes pronounced, and there may be early infertility. In milder form the disease progresses slowly, and many patients can have normal life span [9]. The disease has a severe form where it progresses rapidly and patient becomes disabled over 10–20 years from the onset of illness. Death may ensue by the sixth decade, usually from respiratory failure. Congenital DM1 is the most severe form of the disease. Signs and symptoms of muscle weakness and hypotonia may present since birth. Infants grow up as floppy and may have facial diplegia and clubfoot. Child can have abnormal visual acuity, farsightedness, and impaired curving of the lenses of the eye (astigmatism) contributing to poor quality of vision. Mild to moderate intellectual disabilities are frequent accompaniment of the disease. Learning and behavioral disabilities may become apparent as children grow older [9]. The patients may also present with varied degree of myoclonus.

Children often fail to thrive because of poor feeding. Gastroparesis, a condition consistent with sluggish emptying of solid food (rarely, liquid nutrients) from the stomach, may become symptomatic. This can result in persistent digestive symptoms, especially nausea. Infants and children with congenital DM1 may have breathing difficulties due to muscle weakness. This can be so severe that it may lead to respiratory failure, a common cause of mortality in congenital DM1. Surviving infants and children with congenital DM1 develop severe complications when grown up. Cardiac issues can begin as early as the second decade of life. Severely affected newborns may develop cardiac abnormalities in early neonatal period, though incidence is relatively rare.

The symptomatic appearance of DM2 can be anywhere between the second and sixth decades of life, though onset in the third decade is more prevalent. The signs and symptoms are highly variable. Cognitive impairment, mental retardation, and attention deficits are commonly seen neuropsychiatric manifestations. Cardiac involvement in this disease is significant and should be always looked for. Other systemic manifestations are listed in Table 19.1.

19.4.1 Diagnosis

Standard evaluation of myotonic dystrophy includes neurological examination, blood biochemistry, EMG evaluation, MRI findings, and

Table 19.1 Other system manifestations

Various system	Manifestations
Eye	Cataract
Endocrine system	Diabetes, thyroid dysfunction, hypogonadism
Gastrointestinal system	Dysphagia, constipation, gallbladder stones, pseudo-obstruction
Cardiovascular system	Atrio-ventricular block, supraventricular arrhythmias, ventricular dysfunction, ischemic heart disease, mitral valve prolapse

genetic testing. Findings on examination are uniquely characteristic and can often lead to the diagnosis of myotonic dystrophy. A marked transient increase in muscle tone, often elicited by percussion or precipitated by the use of a muscle, is the key diagnostic feature. "Haggard" facies, muscle weakness, muscle atrophy, and testicular atrophy in males are other characteristic features. Distal muscle involvement precedes proximal muscle involvement, and increased muscle tone becomes less prominent in late stage of the disease.

19.4.2 EMG

Abnormal spontaneous muscle fiber discharge is observed on the needle EMG. This is known as electrical myotonia, which appears as repetitive muscle fiber potential discharges (e.g., positive waves or fibrillation potentials). These discharges have a typical waxing and waning pattern and amplitude, with a firing rate between 20 and 80 Hz. The auditory representation of these myotonic discharges has the characteristic sound of a dive bomber or, in the modern day, an accelerating and decelerating motorcycle engine [10]. Electrical myotonia must be distinguished from neuromyotonia. Neuromyotonia produces a pinging sound in audio player as the frequency of repetitive muscle discharge is greater than 150 Hz. Less frequently, it can have a waning pattern with a machine-like sound. Neuromyotonia is a form of peripheral nerve hyperactivity resulting in spontaneous discharge of skeletal muscle fibers [11].

Many individuals with DM may have mild to moderately elevated creatine phosphokinase or CPK, a muscle enzyme found in blood serum. Some individuals have low levels of immunoglobulin G. Liver function tests may show elevated levels of liver enzymes in some people. MRI findings commonly show cerebellar degeneration. Diffuse cortical atrophy and white matter hyperintensities may be associated signs.

Genetic testing is confirmatory, with the expanded cytosine–thymine–guanine (CTG) repeat in the dystrophia myotonica protein kinase (DMPK) gene in DM1 and the cytosine–cytosine–thymine–guanine (CCTG) repeat in the ZNF9 gene in DM2. By combining the restriction fragment length polymorphism (RFLP) method with the polymerase chain reaction (PCR) method, the gene defect was characterized. Both myotonic dystrophy type 1 and type 2 are autosomal dominant. Muscle function gets affected by microsatellite repeat expansion disorders.

In DM1 and DM2, the DNA repeat expansions connected with the gene actually do not affect the gene. Instead, they work through a genetic mechanism called "RNA gain of function" in which they interfere with the coding of several other more distant genes such as a muscle chloride channel, an insulin receptor, and a cardiac muscle protein gene. This explains the systemic effects of the disease on skeletal muscle, the risk for diabetes, and heart problems.

19.4.3 Differential Diagnosis

Paramyotonia congenita and hyperkalemic periodic paralysis are associated with clinical paramyotonia and electrical myotonia. Acid maltase deficiency often produces myotonic potentials without clinical evidence of myotonia or paramyotonia. Muscle stiffness produced by increased activity of muscle in myotonia actually improves with repeated activity. Paramyotonia produces a similar symptom, but the stiffness paradoxically increases with activity. The waxing and waning patterns of myotonic discharges are easily recognized by electrodiagnostic testing.

19.4.4 Treatment and Prognosis

A complete cure is yet to come on the horizon for the management of myotonic dystrophy, though partial help is available through research studies. Current treatment is individualized toward the specific symptoms that are apparent.

There is no specific treatment for muscle weakness. Physical and occupational therapy can be of benefit. Braces, ankles support, or walkers can benefit some individuals. Wheelchair seems necessary in severe instances. Children with skeletal malformations may require orthopedic surgery. Ankle-foot orthotics (AFOS) are used for foot drop, and wrist braces can be recommended for wrist weakness.

Often myotonia is not severe and does not require treatment. Sodium channel blockers showed promising results in some small sample research studies. The most commonly used among those is mexiletine, which has been shown to have some effect in DM [12]. Phenytoin is another drug found to be effective in some patients [13].

Surgery for cataract may be done in relevant cases. Regular cardiac evaluation with electrocardiogram and Holter monitoring is important as cardiac arrhythmias are well-known complications. Pulmonary hygiene should be maintained with breathing exercises and postural drainage. Hormonal support is relevant in special cases with hormonal imbalance. Patients with myotonic dystrophy should be aware of their special vulnerability while undergoing general anesthesia. Genetic counseling is also an important part of medical management and the prevention of this disease.

References

1. Timchenko L, Monckton DG, Caskey CT. Myotonic dystrophy: an unstable CTG repeat in a protein kinase gene. In: Seminars in cell biology. Elsevier; 1995.
2. Passos-Bueno MR, Cerqueira A, Vainzof M, Marie SK, Zatz M. Myotonic dystrophy: genetic, clinical, and molecular analysis of patients from 41 Brazilian families. J Med Genet. 1995;32(1):14–8.

3. Mathieu J, De Braekeleer M, Prévost C, Boily C. Myotonic dystrophy clinical assessment of muscular disability in an isolated population with presumed homogeneous mutation. Neurology. 1992;42(1):203.
4. McInnis MG. Anticipation: an old idea in new genes. Am J Hum Genet. 1996;59(5):973.
5. Mankodi A, Urbinati CR, Yuan Q-P, Moxley RT, Sansone V, Krym M, et al. Muscleblind localizes to nuclear foci of aberrant RNA in myotonic dystrophy types 1 and 2. Hum Mol Genet. 2001;10(19):2165–70.
6. Steinbach P, Gläser D, Vogel W, Wolf M, Schwemmle S. The DMPK gene of severely affected myotonic dystrophy patients is hypermethylated proximal to the largely expanded CTG repeat. Am J Hum Genet. 1998;62(2):278–85.
7. Kamsteeg E-J, Kress W, Catalli C, Hertz JM, Witsch-Baumgartner M, Buckley MF, et al. Best practice guidelines and recommendations on the molecular diagnosis of myotonic dystrophy types 1 and 2. Eur J Hum Genet. 2012;20(12):1203.
8. Nadaj-Pakleza A, Łusakowska A, Sułek-Piątkowska A, Krysa W, Rajkiewicz M, Kwieciński H, et al. Muscle pathology in myotonic dystrophy: light and electron microscopic investigation in eighteen patients. Folia Morphol (Warsz). 2011;70(2):121–9.
9. Ranum LP, Day JW. Myotonic dystrophy: clinical and molecular parallels between myotonic dystrophy type 1 and type 2. Curr Neurol Neurosci Rep. 2002;2(5):465–70.
10. Streib EW, Sun SF. Distribution of electrical myotonia in myotonic muscular dystrophy. Ann Neurol. 1983;14(1):80–2.
11. Maddison P. Neuromyotonia. Clin Neurophysiol. 2006;117(10):2118–27.
12. Logigian E, Martens W, Moxley RT, McDermott M, Dilek N, Wiegner A, et al. Mexiletine is an effective antimyotonia treatment in myotonic dystrophy type 1. Neurology. 2010;74(18):1441–8.
13. Roses AD, Butterfield DA, Appel SH, Chestnut DB. Phenytoin and membrane fluidity in myotonic dystrophy. Arch Neurol. 1975;32(8):535–8.

Guillain-Barré Syndrome

20

Rajeev Ojha and Gaurav Nepal

Case Scenario

A 65-year-old female presented with chief complaints of upper and lower limb weakness for 10 days. She was well 3 weeks ago, and when she woke up in the morning, she had difficulty lifting bilateral lower limbs from bed. But she was still able to walk without support that day. Next day, she found that mild weakness developed in her both upper limbs. She had difficulty in holding things in her hands and can feed and perform household activities by herself, but with difficulty. There was also numbness in all her distal limbs, severe in lower limbs. Symptoms were further progressive for about 4–5 days. She then needed support of family members for walking. There was no facial deviation, but patient had difficulty forcefully closing her both eyes. There was no swallowing or respiratory difficulty. She was afebrile, with no loss of consciousness, diplopia, or hoarseness of voice. Since the symptoms were persistent, patient was then taken to a nearby hospital. Patient was admitted there for 9 days, and her symptoms were static then. Patient was referred to our center for diagnosis and further treatment.

R. Ojha (✉)
Department of Neurology, Tribhuvan University Institute of Medicine, Kathmandu, Nepal

G. Nepal
Department of Internal Medicine, Tribhuvan University Institute of Medicine, Kathmandu, Nepal

Patient had few episodes of diarrhea with mild fever 10 days before the onset of her symptoms. Patient is a smoker with a smoking history since the age of 12, 1 pack per day. On examination, blood pressure was 140/80 mmHg, pulse was 80/min, respiratory rate was 18/min, and temperature was 98 °F. Her general condition was fair. Mental status was alert and oriented. Her extraocular muscles were normal. Her face was mildly deviated to right side when patient was asked to show her teeth. There is weakness in bilateral forceful eye closure, severe in left side. Gag reflex was normal, and tongue movements were normal. Bulk was normal in upper and lower limbs, and tones were reduced in all limbs. Motor power of upper limbs was 4/5 and lower limbs was 3/5. Reflexes were absent in all the limbs. No cerebellar signs were present. Sensations to light touch and temperature, vibration, and proprioception were intact. Bilateral planters were flexor responses. Complete blood count was normal. Random sugar level was 5.2 mmol/L, normal renal function test, HIV/HBsAg/HCV/VDRL was negative, chest X-ray was normal, ECG: sinus, regular. CSF findings showed total cells: 0 cell, protein: 65 mg/dL, sugar: 4.5 mmol/L. Nerve conduction study (NCS) of upper and lower limbs was suggestive of motor demyelinating neuropathy. Diagnosis of Guillain-Barré syndrome (GBS) with acute inflammatory demyelinating polyneuropathy (AIDP) variant was made. Patient was admitted for about 10 days, and her power gradually started improving from the second day of admission. Patient was further rehabilitated, and her power improved to 4+/5 in upper limbs and 4/5 in lower limbs. Her bilateral facial weakness was also improved during discharge. Patient was followed up in Neurology Outpatient Department in about 2 months, and both her facial and limb weakness were completely improved.

20.1 Introduction

Guillain-Barré syndrome (GBS) is an acute neuromuscular paralysis characterized by rapidly progressive, symmetric progressive weakness, ascending pattern, and areflexia. Cranial nerve involvement and need of respiratory support are other features of GBS. In about 50–70% of patients, prodromal gastrointestinal or respiratory illness was due to Epstein-Barr virus, cytomegalovirus, mycoplasma pneumonia, hepatitis, varicella, and other herpes viruses. GBS can be classified into different variants: acute inflammatory demyelinating polyneuropathy (AIDP), Miller Fisher Syndrome (MFS), acute motor axonal neuropathy (AMAN), and acute motor and sensory axonal neuropathy (AMSAN). Rare variants are paraparetic variant, acute dysautonomia, acute ataxic neuropathy, pharyngeal–cervical–brachial variant, multiple cranial neuropathy, and facial diplegia.

20.2 Epidemiology

The incidence of GBS varies worldwide, ranges from 0.4 to 4 per 100,000 people [1]. GBS can affect people of all ages, though males are predominant in most studies. Incidence has been found to be associated with bimodal peak among two age-groups: 15–24 years and 65–74 years [1]. About two-thirds of the patients were found to have antecedent events before disease onset: upper respiratory or gastrointestinal, surgical procedures, immunizations, or trauma [2].

Usually, 1–6 weeks is the duration of such antecedent events. Common pathogens found to be associated with GBS are *Campylobacter jejuni, Haemophilus influenzae, Mycoplasma pneumoniae*, Epstein-Barr virus, cytomegalovirus, human immunodeficiency virus, varicella zoster virus, and Zika virus [3]. A global pooled analysis reported a greater incidence in winter compared to summer, which holds true even on subgroup analysis based on various geographical locations. Same study found that there was greater seasonal variation with respiratory prodrome than diarrheal prodrome [4].

20.3 Pathology

In AIDP, multifocal demyelination is the predominant feature, along with endoneural perivascular mononuclear cell infiltration. Primary lesions could be found in ventral roots, proximal peripheral nerves, and cranial nerves, but could affect all levels of nerves. Macrophages, class II positive monocytes, and T lymphocytes are found to involve in demyelination process. In severe conditions, axonal involvement with profound weakness with delayed recovery has been found. Whereas in AMAN, macrophages were found in the periaxonal spaces of myelinated internodes. Features of demyelination like segmental demyelination and remyelination which are secondary to axonal damage could be seen in some cases [5].

20.4 Pathogenesis

Although previous studies have suggested GBS as an immune disorder associated with humoral and cell mediated responses, it is still incompletely understood. Peripheral nerve injury, primarily myelin, due to the immune responses has been explained as the characteristics of AIDP variant of GBS. An antecedent infection is a trigger factor for autoimmune response, and host attacks body's own peripheral nerve (i.e., GM1 and GD1a gangliosides), which resembles epitopes (i.e., gly-cans) of infectious agent [6]. This response has also been described as "molecule mimicry." Antibodies to peripheral nerves were found to be gradually reduced with clinical recovery in patients. Inflammatory infiltrates found were class II-positive monocytes, macrophages, and T lymphocytes. Since class II antigen is highly expressed in Schwann cells, these cells might have involved in presenting the antigen to autoreactive T cells causing demyelination [7].

20.5 Clinical Manifestation

AIDP is most commonly reported from North America and Europe, accounting for about 80–90%, whereas this variant is about 20–40% in countries like China, Japan, Mexico, and India. AMAN is the most common GBS variant in Asia and was first reported in 1986. Even studies in Europe and United States have reported sporadic cases of AMAN. Young people are found to be more commonly affected. Infection by *Campylobacter jejuni* has been associated with AMAN and AMSAN variants [8]. AMSAN is similar to AMAN except it has severe sensory findings. Since both sensory and motor axons are involved, it is thus regarded as a severe and fulminant form of AMAN with severe axonal degeneration and delayed recovery.

Clinical manifestations are monophasic, rapidly progressive limb weakness with symmetricity, absence or reduced reflexes, and cranial nerve involvement, with bilateral facial nerves being common. Severity of symptoms reaches a plateau within 4 weeks, commonly in about 2–3 weeks. Along with limb weakness, bulbar and respiratory involvements are seen in 30–40%, and about one-third to one-fourth will require support from mechanical ventilation [3].

Sensory symptoms like tingling, burning, or radiating pain are common manifestations and are often experienced by the patient before the weakness becomes prominent. Even after months and years of resolution of motor weakness, persistent sensory symptoms might be problematic for patients. Dysautonomia is another common manifestation seen in more than 50% of GBS patients [9]. Tachycardia and a rise in systolic blood pressure are the frequent manifestations; rare but life-threatening features are arrhythmias, severe hypertension and hypotension, urinary retention, and adynamic ileus.

20.6 Diagnosis

The diagnosis of GBS is confirmed by correlating clinical presentations and supportive investigations, and excluding its mimics. The clinical presentation is usually a progressive, symmetric limb weakness with absent or depressed deep tendon reflexes. Cranial nerve and respiratory muscle involvement are also seen in many patients.

Cerebrospinal fluid (CSF) albuminocytological dissociation is the typical finding in patients with GBS. But only 50% might show some slight increase in protein in the first week, and subsequently protein elevation is seen after the second week. In about 10% of patients, CSF protein may remain normal throughout the disease course. Disruption of the blood nerve barrier and leakage of protein in the CSF are reasons for the rise in protein levels. Protein level usually varies from 45 to 200 mg/dL in most patients [10].

Nerve conduction study (NCS) has an important role in the diagnosis and classification of GBS subtypes. It further helps in ruling out different mimics like myopathies, motor neuron diseases, myasthenia gravis, and lambert eaten syndrome. Involvement of sensory or motor nerves, demyelination or axonal pattern, presence of conduction block and temporal dispersion, status of the F-wave, conduction velocity, and amplitudes of motor and sensory action potentials are important factors to be evaluated during NCS. Abnormalities are usually seen after 1 week of the onset of illness. Even in 2 weeks of disease duration, only 64% of patients fulfill definite criteria of AIDP [11].

20.7 Differential Diagnosis

20.7.1 Chronic Inflammatory Demyelinating Polyneuropathy (CIDP)

CIDP is usually characterized by symmetric limb weakness with diminished or absent reflexes, which progresses or causes relapses for more than 8 weeks. Clinically, CIDP is difficult to distinguish from GBS in early presentation. "Onion bulb formation," which is the pathological finding of repeated demyelination and remyelination, is the typical feature. Further, persistent development of weakness beyond 4 weeks, fluctuation of weakness more than three times, no loss of independent ambulation, and absence of cranial nerve involvement are the factors that help to distinguish CIDP from GBS.

20.7.2 Myasthenia Gravis

Myasthenia gravis is an autoimmune disorder characterized by a fluctuating degree of weakness of the ocular, bulbar, and limbs and can even involve respiratory muscles. Weakness is due to the antibody-mediated attack in postsynaptic acetylcholine receptors. Edrophonium and icepack tests are the common bedside tests. Acetylcholine receptor antibody or muscle-specific tyrosine kinase antibody test could further support the diagnosis. Thymic abnormalities are found to be associated with myasthenia patients. Acetylcholinesterase, steroids, immunomodulators, and thymectomy are the treatments available.

20.8 Treatment

Patients diagnosed with GBS should be admitted for close monitoring. Intubation might be needed in some patients with features of hypoxia, progressive declining respiratory function, and a weak cough. Most patients benefit with conservative treatment. Regular physiotherapy, proper diet and exercises, nutritional supplements, and pharmacological treatment for any sensory manifestations are the usual treatment considerations. Progression of skeletal muscle weakness may continue till the patient reaches the nadir even after intravenous immunoglobulin (IVIg) infusion or plasma exchange has been done. During or before the plateau phase, patients are at higher risk of developing respiratory failure and needing mechanical ventilation support. Close monitoring of respiratory function by measuring vital capacity and negative inspiratory force (NIF) should be done.

Plasma exchange includes the removal of the patient's plasma, immune complexes, and autoantibodies and the reinfusion of plasma back into the patient along with albumin solution. It is usually given in four to six cycles over 8–10 days (45–50 mL/kg). It is found to be effective if started within 1 week, but still beneficial if given within 4 weeks. Complications like hematoma at the puncture site, septicemia, hemodynamic instability, and blood product transfusion-related transmission of infections could be seen. A randomized trial comparing PE and IVIg treatment in GBS showed that they are equally efficient for the treatment of GBS [3].

IVIg contains anti-idiotypic antibodies that are able to bind and neutralize the pathogenetic antibodies. Other suggested mechanisms are downregulation of antibody production, increase of antibody metabolism, interference with antibody-dependent cytotoxicity mediated by macrophages, inhibition of cell adhesion, and induction of apoptosis. IVIg has been found to have better compliance and fewer blood product-related side effects. IVIg is given at a dose of 0.4 g/kg/day for 5 days. Side effects are rashes, aseptic meningitis, acute renal failure, hyperviscosity leading to stroke, and anaphylaxis in IgA deficiency patients. Combination treatments with IVIg and PE weren't found to be effective. Repeated course of IVIg has been suggested in the case of severe unresponsive GBS [12].

20.9 Prognosis

Prognostic factors for GBS recovery are older age, severe limb weakness during admission, rapid onset of symptoms, need for mechanical ventilation, and severe axonal neuropathy as detected by a nerve conduction study. GBS is a life-threatening disease, with mortality rates between 3 and 7% in Europe and North America. In the acute phase, patients have a likelihood of dying, most likely due to hypoventilation, pulmonary complications, or autonomic dysfunction, including arrhythmia [3]. One in four patients will require mechanical ventilation to prevent respiratory failure or protect the airway [13]. A systematic review regarding the association between Zika virus and GBS found that half of all cases were admitted to the ICU. This proportion was higher than expected based on the pathogen type. It may indicate that GBS following Zika infection is often severe, requiring intensive care. However, the percentage of mechanically ventilated patients (20%) was similar to other agents [14]. Patients who survive GBS often have residual discomfort and defects, including pain and fatigue, which can have a significant impact on the quality of life. Approximately 20% of GBS patients cannot be functionally independent 6 months after the onset [3].

Studies have shown that few chronic inflammatory demyelinating polyneuropathies (CIDP) are initially diagnosed as GBS, and relapses are seen in such patients.

References

1. Hughes RA, Rees JH. Clinical and epidemiologic features of Guillain-Barré syndrome. J Infect Dis. 1997;176(Suppl 2):S92–8.
2. Pritchard J. Guillain-Barré syndrome. Clin Med. 2010;10(4):399–401.
3. Willison HJ, Jacobs BC, van Doorn PA. Guillain-Barré syndrome. Lancet. 2016;388(10045):717–27.
4. Webb AJS, Brain SAE, Wood R, Rinaldi S, Turner MR. Seasonal variation in Guillain-Barré syndrome: a systematic review, meta-analysis and Oxfordshire cohort study. J Neurol Neurosurg Psychiatry. 2015;86(11):1196–201.
5. Nakano Y, Kanda T. Pathology of Guillain-Barre syndrome. Clin Exp Neuroimmunol. 2016;7:312–9.
6. Willison HJ, Yuki N. Peripheral neuropathies and anti-glycolipid antibodies. Brain. 2002;125(Pt 12):2591–625.
7. Allard DE, Wang Y, Li JJ, Conley B, Xu EW, Sailer D, et al. Schwann cell-derived periostin promotes autoimmune peripheral polyneuropathy via macrophage recruitment. J Clin Invest. 2018;128(10):4727–41.
8. Dimachkie MM, Barohn RJ. Guillain-Barré syndrome and variants. Neurol Clin. 2013;31(2):491–510.
9. Kondziella D. Autonomic dysfunction in Guillain-Barré syndrome puts patients at risk. Neurocrit Care. 2020;32(1):86–7. https://doi.org/10.1007/s12028-019-00793-6.
10. Illes Z, Blaabjerg M. Cerebrospinal fluid findings in Guillain-Barré syndrome and chronic inflammatory demyelinating polyneuropathies. Handb Clin Neurol. 2017;146:125–38.
11. Yadegari S, Nafissi S, Kazemi N. Comparison of electrophysiological findings in axonal and demyelinating Guillain-Barre syndrome. Iran J Neurol. 2014;13(3):138–43.
12. van Doorn PA, Kuitwaard K, Walgaard C, van Koningsveld R, Ruts L, Jacobs BC. IVIG treatment and prognosis in Guillain-Barré syndrome. J Clin Immunol. 2010;30(Suppl 1):S74–8.
13. Harms M. Inpatient management of Guillain-Barré syndrome. Neurohospitalist. 2011;1(2):78–84.
14. Leonhard SE, Bresani-Salvi CC, Lyra Batista JD, Cunha S, Jacobs BC, Ferreira MLB, et al. Guillain-Barré syndrome related to Zika virus infection: a systematic review and meta-analysis of the clinical and electrophysiological phenotype. PLoS Negl Trop Dis. 2020;14(4):1–24.

Inflammatory Muscle Diseases

21

Saraswati Nashi, Kiran Polavarapu, Seena Vengalil,
Veeramani Preethish-Kumar,
and Atchayaram Nalini

Case Scenario

A 32-year-old gentleman presented with limb weakness of 4 weeks of duration. The symptoms started with diffuse pain in arms and thighs followed by progressive proximal upper and lower limb weakness. He developed dark brownish discoloration of skin over forehead for 2 weeks and head drop for 1 week prior to presentation.

Examination revealed hyperpigmented dark brownish macular rashes over forehead and nose. There was muscle tenderness in the right arm. He had weakness of neck extensors, shoulder abductors and flexors, hip flexors and extensors, and waddling gait. Serum creatine kinase was elevated at 2529 IU/L. Urine for myoglobinuria was negative. ENMG showed myopathic pattern in right biceps and deltoid. Myositis profile for Anti-Mi-2β antibody was strongly positive and Anti-SRP was borderline positive. Paraneoplastic and vasculitis profiles were negative. Whole-body PET-MRI showed T2 stir hyperintense signal changes in muscles with myofascial oedema with no evidence of internal malignancy. Pulmonary function test revealed restrictive pattern of moderate severity.

He was treated with 5 g of IV methylprednisolone over 5 days during the hospital stay; subsequently he was maintained on 2 g/month of IV MP and 1.7 g of cyclophosphamide over 3 days/month for the next 6 months. After 4 months of treatment, he had recovered by 40% and was independent for all activities of daily living. He was also able to ride bike; however mild proximal upper limb weakness was persisting. This case vignette summarizes the clinical features, cardinal symptoms and signs, autoantibody profile and imaging features of a classical inflammatory myopathy. The subtyping is discussed below in this chapter.

21.1 Introduction

Inflammatory muscle diseases are a group of treatable myopathies which present in both adults and children. They are rare diseases which affect muscle and multiple other organs often causing impairment of the quality of life [1, 2]. They are traditionally divided into five main types based on the clinical and pathological features: dermatomyositis (DM), polymyositis (PM), necrotizing myopathy (NM), overlap myositis (OM) and inclusion body myositis (IBM).

The common symptoms are rapidly progressive proximal muscle weakness of the extremities at the onset, followed by distal muscle weakness, which occurs late, except in inclusion body myo-

S. Nashi (✉) · S. Vengalil · A. Nalini
Department of Neurology, National Institute of
Mental Health and Neurosciences, Bangalore, India

K. Polavarapu · V. Preethish-Kumar
Department of Clinical Neurosciences, National
Institute of Mental Health and Neurosciences,
Bangalore, India

© Springer Nature Singapore Pte Ltd. 2024
K. K. Oli et al. (eds.), *Case-based Approach to Common Neurological Disorders*,
https://doi.org/10.1007/978-981-99-8676-7_21

sitis, where it is seen early in the course of illness. Facial, neck and pharyngeal muscles can be involved but usually spare ocular muscles. Respiratory involvement may be seen in advanced disease. Muscle pains and tenderness are seen but are not a frequent finding. In long-standing cases, muscle atrophy sets in; however, atrophy is an early feature of inclusion body myositis.

Systemic manifestations in the form of fever, joint pains, cardiac arrhythmias, dyspnoea on exertion, interstitial lung disease (ILD) and internal malignancies are known. The treatment of IIMs is now rapidly expanding with newer immunosuppressive agents and biologics being tried successfully. Ongoing research in this area has led to further classification based on the numerous antibodies which are associated with the disease pathogenesis and clinical features [2*].

21.2 Incidence

The incidence rate is 4.27–7.89 cases per 1,00,000 individuals per year. DM has a prevalence of about 1–6 patients per 100,000 persons in the USA alone [3]. Overlap myositis forms the largest subgroup followed by dermatomyositis. The prevalence of polymyositis is controversial.

Also, with changing diagnostic criteria, the epidemiological data are changing. In general, the prevalence of myositis is higher in females than males, except for inclusion body myositis. There is significant morbidity and mortality associated with these diseases in view of the muscular and prominent extramuscular manifestations. A study done by Schiopu et al. observed a 10-year survival rate of 62% [1, 3].

21.3 Dermatomyositis (DM)

As the name implies, the classical manifestations are muscle weakness with skin changes. The weakness is generally proximal and symmetrical. The typical patient presents with a history of difficulty climbing stairs, rising from the floor, walking and lifting heavy objects, which is subacute or chronic in onset with or without myalgias. Further, diagnosis is supported by laboratory, pathology and neuroimaging findings (Figs. 21.1, 21.2, 21.3, 21.4 and 21.5).

The skin manifestations have a characteristic distribution—the shawl sign on the anterior upper chest or the posterior neck; Gottron papules (erythematous lesions) on the dorsum of hands; periungual erythema; telangiectasias;

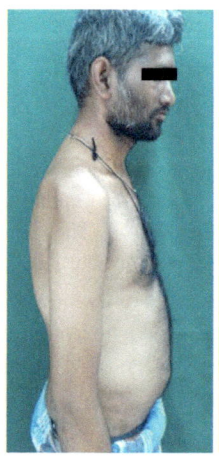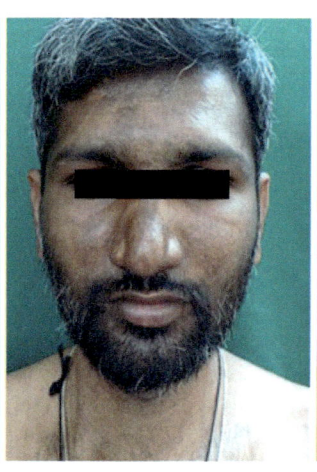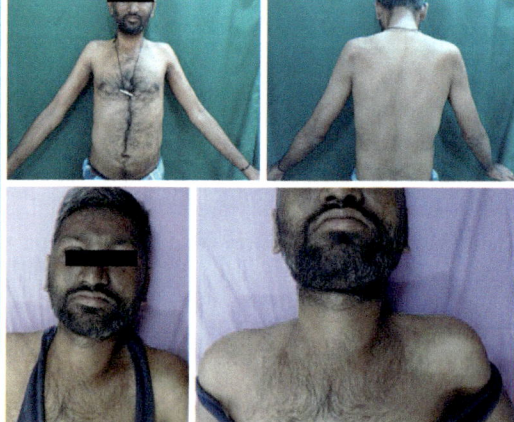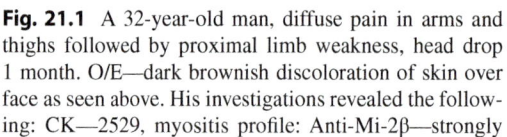

Fig. 21.1 A 32-year-old man, diffuse pain in arms and thighs followed by proximal limb weakness, head drop 1 month. O/E—dark brownish discoloration of skin over face as seen above. His investigations revealed the following: CK—2529, myositis profile: Anti-Mi-2β—strongly +ve; Anti-SRP—borderline +ve. Paraneoplastic and vasculitis profiles were negative; PET MR—myoedema; pulmonary function test (PFT)—restrictive pattern of moderate severity

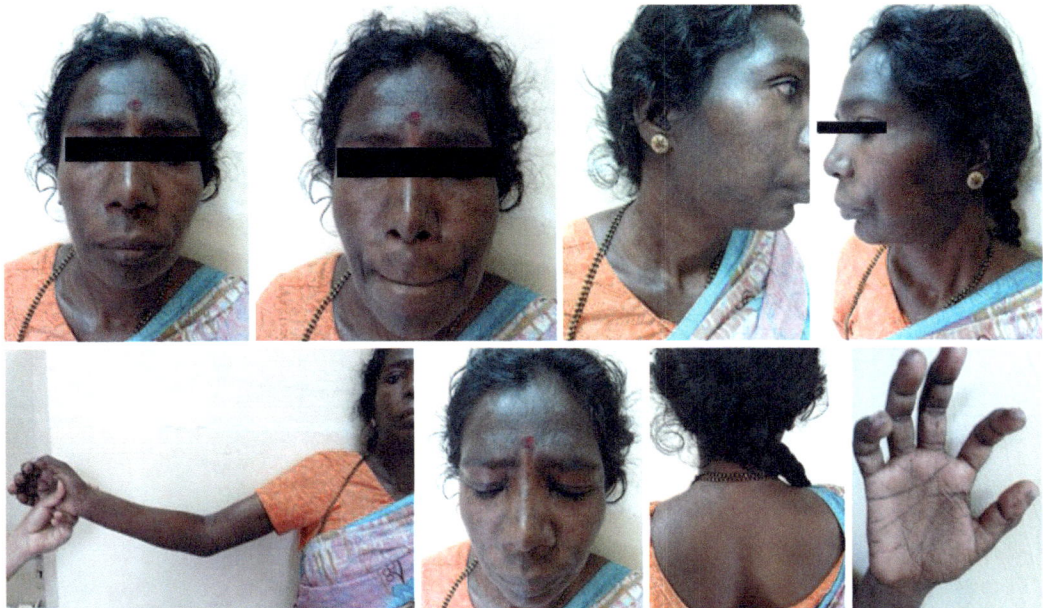

Fig. 21.2 A 43-year-old lady, fasciculations and muscle cramps of 2 years, proximal, truncal, neck, bulbar weakness with hyperpigmentation—1½ years. Her investigation reports are as follows: ESR: 29; CK: 2420; ANA profile, Paraneoplastic profile: negative; myositis profile: Mi-2B positive. Muscle biopsy: dermatomyositis; PFT: severe restrictive abnormality; PET-MRI: negative for malignancy

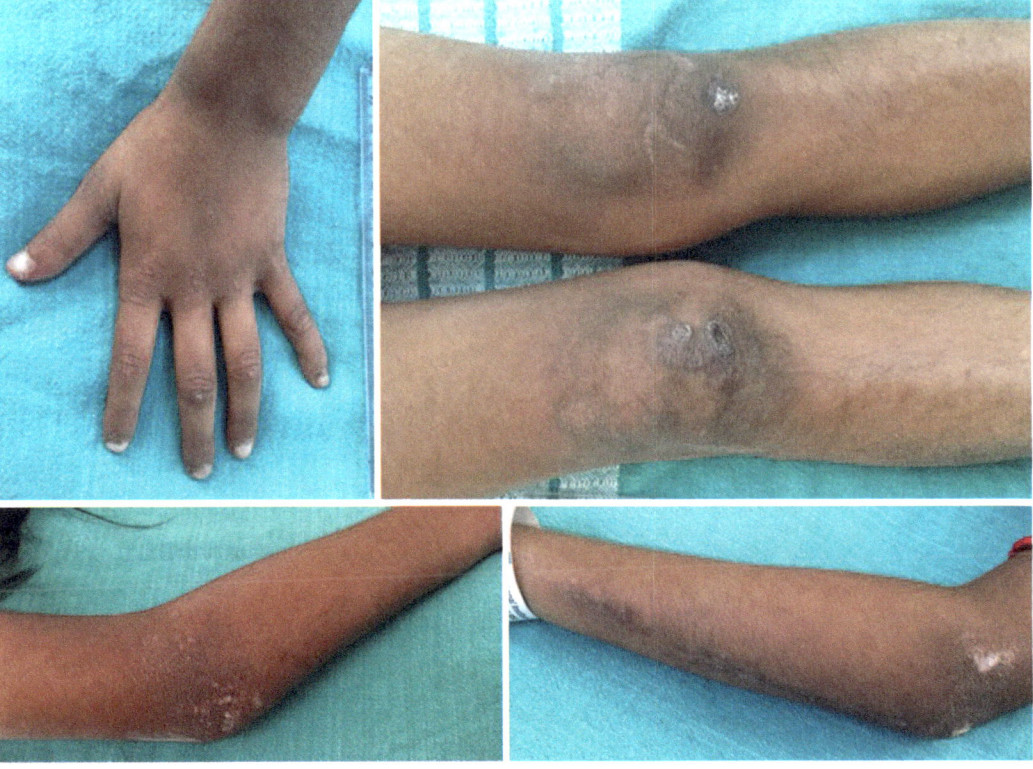

Fig. 21.3 A 7-year-old girl, rashes around eyes and cheeks followed by proximal weakness: 5 months. Heliotrope rash was present, Gottron's papules are seen above. Her investigations showed as follows: CK, 2207; myositis profile—Mi-2B: strongly positive; ANA: positive, speckled pattern; ANA profile: negative; CT thorax: no evidence of ILD

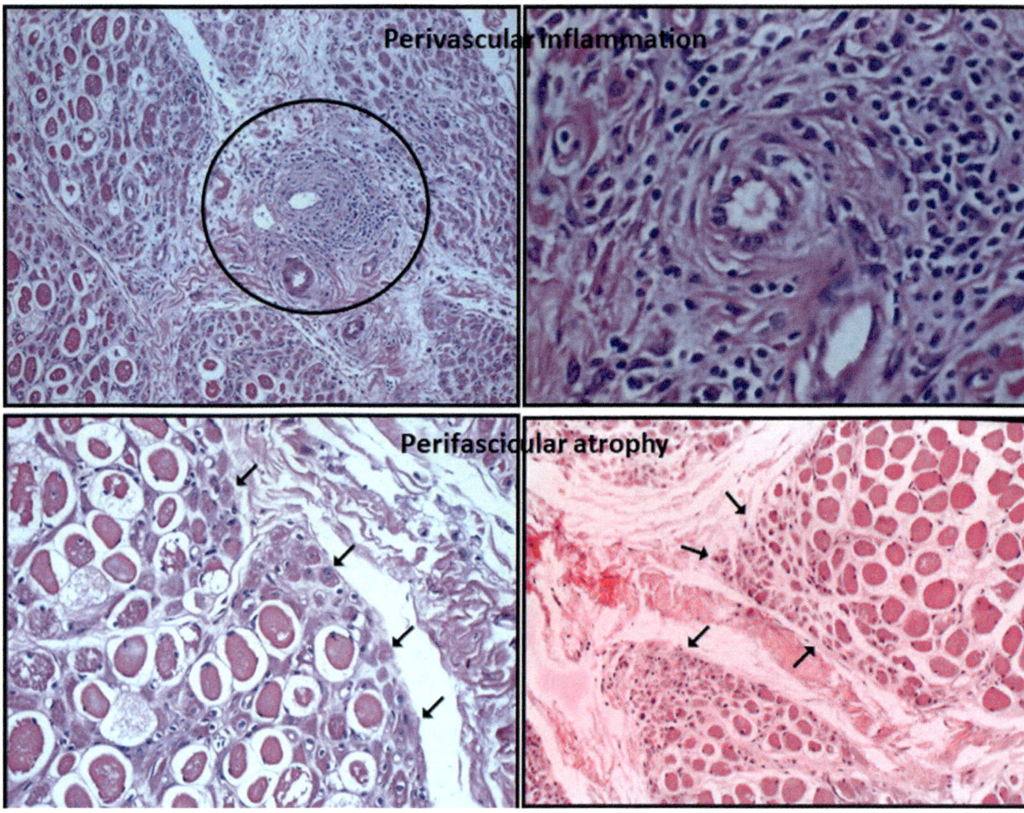

Fig. 21.4 Muscle biopsy in a case of dermatomyositis showing perifascicular inflammation and atrophy

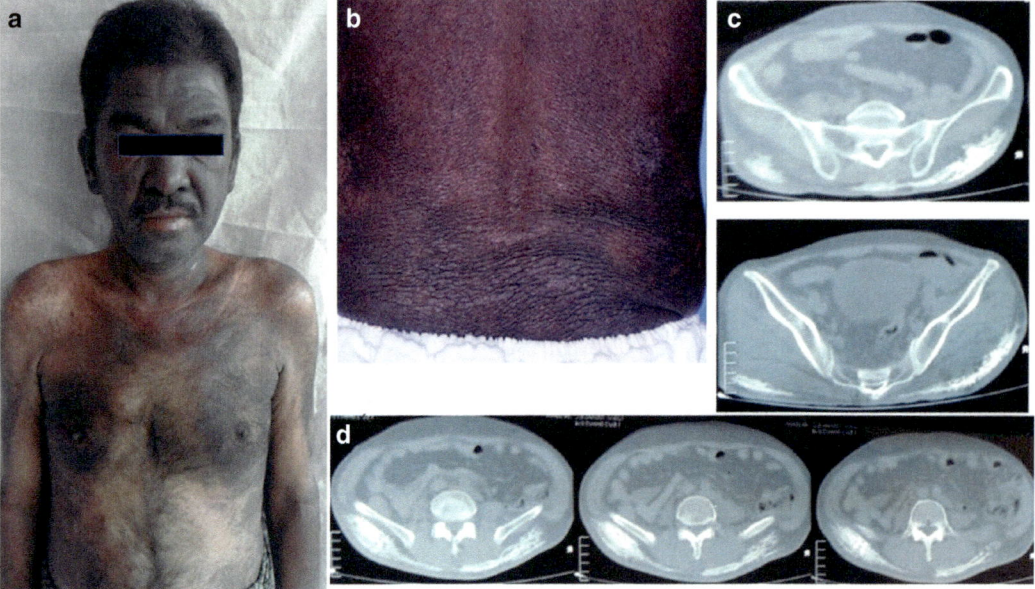

Fig. 21.5 (**a**) Hyperpigmentation of skin. (**b**) Hyperpigmented and indurated skin over the back. (**c, d**) Subcutaneous calcification seen on computed tomography images

cracked skin of the fingers and hands, also called mechanic's hands; heliotrope rashes over the eyelids and erythema of the face. Some of them may present without muscle weakness when they are called amyopathic dermatomyositis (20% of cases) and those without skin rashes are termed dermatomyositis sine dermatitis. There is increased incidence of interstitial lung disease (ILD) in amyopathic DM. Notable in this disease is the development of malignancy. The western literature reports an incidence of 15% within 3–5 years of diagnosis. They include colorectal, ovarian, lung, pancreatic and stomach cancers, and hence it is mandatory to investigate for these cancers.

Laboratory work-up reveals a creatine kinase elevation of 10–50 times the normal limit. The autoantibodies associated with this disease include the following:

1. Anti-Mi2 (component of nucleosome remodelling deacetylase chromatin remodelling complex) antibodies—in about 20% cases and present with classical clinical features.
2. Anti-NXP2 (nuclear matrix protein)—have both proximal and distal weakness, subcutaneous oedema, calcinosis and dysphagia; increased risk of malignancy. They are seen in juvenile dermatomyositis.
3. Anti-TIF-1 (transcriptional intermediary factor) (alpha/beta/gamma)—seen in one-third of cases; increased risk of malignancy, also seen in juvenile cases.

4. Anti-MDA5 (melanoma differentiation-associated gene-5)—in 10–30% of cases. They have severe skin involvement and are known to develop ulcers on the flexor surfaces of digits and palms: interstitial lung disease.
5. Anti-SAE (small ubiquitin-like modifier-activating enzyme)—classical form.
6. Antibody-negative dermatomyositis.

Routinely, line blot assay and enzyme-linked immunosorbent assay are used to detect autoantibodies, but immunoprecipitation is the standard test [4*] (Table 21.1).

Pathological features include
(a) Perifascicular atrophy (specificity >90%, sensitivity 25–50%, detected by routine histochemistry)
(b) Perimysial inflammation
(c) Perifascicular expression of MHC class I, binding of complement to capillaries and the surface of sarcolemma (less sensitive and specific)
(d) Perifascicular human myxovirus resistance protein 1 and retinoic acid-inducible gene 1 expression (sensitivity—71% and 50% respectively, detected by immunohistochemistry, i.e. IHC)
(e) Cellular infiltrates of dendritic cells, B-cells, CD4 T-cells and macrophages
(f) Microtubular inclusions in intramuscular capillaries (electron microscopy) and capillary drop-out [4*]

Table 21.1 Clinical features of different autoantibodies in dermatomyositis

Sl.	Antibody	Function of antigen	Adult/juvenile onset	CK	Muscle	Skin	Lung	Joint	Cancer
1	Anti-Mi2	Regulate gene transcription	Adult	Very high	Moderate severity	Moderate severity	Less common	Less common	Less common
2	Anti-TIF-1	Cell growth/differentiation, carcinogenesis	Adult/juvenile	High	Mild	Mild severity	Less common	Less common	High risk
3	Anti-NXP2	Regulate gene transcription	Adult/juvenile	Normal-high	Moderate severity	Mild severity	Less common	Less common	High risk
4	Anti-MDA5	Antiviral innate immunity		Normal-mild ↑	Mild/nil	Severe	High risk	Common	Unlikely
5	Anti-SAE	Post-translational modification	Adult	Normal-mild ↑	Mild	Moderate	Less common	Less common	Less common
6	Antibody –ve DM	–	Adult	High	Mild	Moderate	Unknown	Unknown	Unknown

See Refs. [4, 5]

21.4 Polymyositis (PM)

It is the most controversial form of myositis which accounts for about 5% of cases [6]. Many patients who have been diagnosed with polymyositis have either necrotizing autoimmune myositis, inclusion-body myositis or inflammatory dystrophy. It is diagnosed based on the exclusion of other types of myositis and is best defined as a subacute proximal myopathy in adults without rash, a family history of neuromuscular disease, a history of exposure to myotoxic drugs like penicillamine, statins and zidovudine and involvement of facial and extraocular muscles.

21.4.1 Muscle Pathology

Histopathologically, invasion of muscle fibres with endomysial cytotoxic CD8+ T-cells and upregulation of MHC class I is a characteristic feature seen [4*], but this histological feature is not just unique for PM, but even more common in IBM and also present in cases with DM or anti-synthetase syndrome (ASS).

21.5 Necrotizing Myopathy (NM)

It is a rapidly progressive and severe form of myositis. It clinically presents with limb weakness and swallowing difficulties. The creatine kinase values are very high, elevated 20–50-fold. They may be associated with anti-SRP, anti-HMGCR in two-thirds of cases or may be antibody-negative. Extramuscular manifestations are generally rare.

1. Anti-SRP antibody—they tend to have more severe muscle weakness and are refractory to treatment.
2. Anti-HMGCR antibody—they are usually associated with statin exposure. They have a higher risk of malignancy and a lesser risk of interstitial lung disease and cardiac involvement as compared to anti-SRP myopathy [4, 5].

21.5.1 Muscle Pathology

Pathologically, there are scattered necrotic fibres with focal upregulation of MHC class I, binding of complement to the sarcolemma and surface of capillaries, and membrane attack complex deposition on non-necrotic fibres. Histopathology findings in NM do not show primary inflammatory lesions as well as there are no tubuloreticular inclusions found in the endothelial cells [7]. However, some cases with anti-SRP or anti-HMGCR antibodies may have lymphocytic infiltrates.

21.6 Overlap Myositis (OM)

Patients with OM show profound elevation of CK which may rise up to 10–50 times the normal limit. OM is also associated various connective tissue disorders like Sjogren syndrome, systemic sclerosis, rheumatoid arthritis and systemic lupus erythematosus (SLE). The most common condition is the anti-synthetase syndrome, which includes myositis, Raynaud's phenomenon, arthritis, mechanic's hands and interstitial lung disease. The common antibodies associated are anti-Jo1, PL7, PL12, EJ, OJ, KS and anti-HA antibodies [4, 8]. Some of these present with predominant interstitial lung disease and only minimal myopathy. There are five other antibodies which are associated with both OM and connective tissue disorders; they are anti-PM/Scl, anti-U-snRNP, anti-Ku, anti-SS-A/Ro52/Ro60 and anti-SS-B-La [8].

21.6.1 Muscle Pathology

Perifascicular necrosis and perifascicular binding of MHC class 1 and class 2 antibodies and complement binding to sarcolemma are the histological findings in OM. Compared to dermatomyositis, the amount of necrosis is more in anti-synthetase syndrome biopsies. Nuclear actin aggregation is another feature of electron microscopy which is specific to this group.

21.7 Inclusion Body Myositis (IBM)

The clinical presentation of IBM varies from other variants. Males are affected more commonly than females. The disease progression is slower compared to other forms of myositis. Patients with IBM have an asymmetric onset of the disease, which may start with unilateral affection of a leg or an arm. In IBM, the affected muscles show profound muscle atrophy. In the early stages, long finger flexors, the quadriceps, and the tibialis anterior are weak. Dysphagia may be an initial symptom and leads to aspiration pneumonia; if not adequately addressed, it leads to a higher mortality rate.

cN1A (cytosolic 5′ nucleotidase 1A) is the antibody which is related to IBM; however, it is also seen in a small group of other inflammatory myopathies. The sensitivity and specificity are both poor for this antibody. cNIA is often associated with dysphagia, severe disease and mortality. However, myositis-specific antibodies are absent [9].

21.7.1 Muscle Pathology

Histologically, IBM is characterized by invasion of muscle fibres by endomysial cytotoxic CD8+ T-cells, upregulation of MHC class 1, amyloid deposition, tubulofilament inclusions in EM, signs of mitochondrial damage and paracrystalline inclusions (Table 21.2).

The initial criteria of IBM were based on histological criteria. IBM has been revisited by an ENMC workshop—the patients should be above 45 years and should have CK of less than a 15-fold increase, with the pattern of weakness being finger flexors weaker than shoulder abductors, quadriceps weaker than hip flexors.

The combination of the below three parameters of new ENMC criteria are ideal in diagnos-

Table 21.2 Classification criteria: Bohan and Peter criteria for polymyositis and dermatomyositis

First rule out all other forms of myopathy
(A) Symmetrical weakness, usually progressive, of the limb-girdle muscles
(B) Elevation of serum levels of muscle-associated enzymes CK, aldolase, LD, transaminases (ALT/SGPT and AST/SGOT)
(C) Electromyographic triad of myopathy (a) Short, small, low-amplitude polyphasic motor unit potentials (b) Fibrillation potentials, even at rest (c) Bizarre high-frequency repetitive discharges
(D) Muscle biopsy evidence of myositis—necrosis of type I and type II muscle fibres, phagocytosis, degeneration and regeneration of myofibres with variation in myofibre size, endomysial, perimysial, perivascular or interstitial mononuclear cells
(E) Characteristic rashes of dermatomyositis

See Ref. [10]

ing IBM at 90% sensitivity and 90% specificity—finger flexor weakness or quadriceps weakness, endomysial inflammation and invasion of non-necrotic muscle fibres or rimmed vacuoles as the characteristic features [11] (Table 21.3).

21.7.2 Pathogenesis

Dermatomyositis is a humoral-mediated disorder while polymyositis is cell mediated. In DM, complement-mediated microangiopathy and type-I interferon-initiated cascade play a major role. Muscle fibres secrete pro-inflammatory milieu, and there is local activation of the immune cells which in turn attack muscle fibres. Mediators of innate immune system are identified in myositis, and the expression of toll like receptors is present on sarcolemma of muscle fibres.

The exact pathomechanism of various antibodies is not yet clear. Anti-SRP and anti-HMGCR antibodies are shown to increase reactive oxygen species, TNF and IL-6 while

Table 21.3 Classification criteria for idiopathic inflammatory myopathies (except IBM) approved by the Myositis Study Group and the 119th European Neuromuscular Centre workshop

1	Clinical criteria
	  –Inclusion criteria
	    (a) Onset usually over 18 years (postpuberty), onset may be in childhood in DM and nonspecific myositis
	    (b) Subacute or insidious onset
	    (c) Pattern of weakness: symmetrical; Proximal > distal, neck flexor > neck extensor
	    (d) Rash typical of DM: heliotrope (purple) periorbital oedema; violaceous papules (Gottron's papules) or macules (Gottron's sign), scaly if chronic, at metacarpophalangeal and interphalangeal joints and other bony prominences; erythema of chest and neck (V sign) and upper back (shawl sign)
	  –Exclusion criteria
	    (a) Clinical features of IBM—asymmetrical weakness, wrist/finger flexors same or worse than deltoids; knee extensors and/or ankle dorsiflexors same or worse than hip flexors)
	    (b) Ocular weakness, isolated dysarthria, neck extensor > neck flexor weakness
	    (c) Toxic myopathy (e.g. recent exposure to myotoxic drugs), active endocrinopathy (hyper- or hypothyroid, hyperparathyroid), amyloidosis, family history of muscular dystrophy or proximal motor neuropathies (e.g. SMA)

2	Elevated serum creatine kinase level

3	Other laboratory criteria
	  (a) Electromyography
	    –Inclusion criteria
	      • Increased insertional and spontaneous activity in the form of fibrillation potentials, positive sharp waves or complex repetitive discharges
	      • Morphometric analysis reveals the presence of short duration, small amplitude, polyphasic MUAPs.
	    –Exclusion criteria
	      • Myotonic discharges that would suggest proximal myotonic dystrophy or other channelopathy
	      • Morphometric analysis reveals predominantly long-duration, large-amplitude MUAPs
	      • Decreased recruitment pattern of MUAPs
	  (b) MRI: diffuse or patchy increased signal (oedema) within muscle tissue on STIR images
	  (c) Myositis-specific antibodies detected in serum

4	Muscle biopsy inclusion and exclusion criteria
	  (a) Endomysial inflammatory cell infiltrate (T cells) surrounding and invading non-necrotic muscle fibres
	  (b) Endomysial CD8+ T-cells surrounding but not definitely invading non-necrotic muscle fibres, or ubiquitous MHC-1 expression
	  (c) Perifascicular atrophy
	  (d) MAC depositions on small blood vessels, reduced capillary density, tubuloreticular inclusions in endothelial cells on EM or MHC-1 expression of perifascicular fibres
	  (e) Perivascular, perimysial inflammatory cell infiltrate
	  (f) Scattered endomysial CD8+ T-cell infiltrate that does not clearly surround or invade muscle fibres
	  (g) Many necrotic muscle fibres as the predominant abnormal histological feature. Inflammatory cells are sparse or only slightly perivascular; perimysial infiltrate is not evident. MAC deposition on small blood vessels or pipestem capillaries on EM may be seen, but tubuloreticular inclusions in endothelial cells are uncommon or not evident.
	  (h) Rimmed vacuoles, ragged red fibres, cytochrome C oxidase-negative fibres that would suggest IBM
	  (i) MAC deposition on the sarcolemma of non-necrotic fibres and other indications of muscular dystrophies with immunopathology

DM dermatomyositis, *EM* electromyography, *IBM* inclusion body myositis, *MAC* membrane attack complex, *MHC* major histocompatibility complex, *MRI* magnetic resonance imaging, *MUAP* motor unit action potential, *SMA* spinal muscular atrophy, *STIR* short-tau inversion recovery. See ref. [11]

reducing IL4 and IL13 in cultured muscle cells, resulting in impaired myoblast fusion and muscle atrophy. Non-immune mechanisms are also present in myositis, including ER stress, NFkB activation and free radicals such as NO. The cell stress mechanisms weaken the skeletal muscles, leading to a chain of events. In IBM, many evidences suggest that there is a distinct interaction between inflammatory mediators, vacuolar transformations and the accumulation of amyloid.

It is suggested for two decades that myositis is associated with environmental factors like exposure to UV radiation [12*] and infections [13]. Environmental factors, in the presence or absence of genetic predisposition, can alter immune mechanisms that either reduce inhibitory factors or increase stimulatory effects thus triggering or aggravating an autoinflammatory cascade.

21.8   Laboratory Investigations

1. Creatine kinase, AST, ALT, LDH, rarely aldolase
2. Routine pathology and biochemical tests
3. Serum myositis-specific and myositis-associated autoantibodies
4. Muscle biopsy and enzyme histochemistry
5. Immunohistochemistry, electron microscopy if available
6. Electrophysiology—NCS and EMG
7. MRI of muscle
8. Pulmonary function test
9. High-resolution CT thorax
10. Electrocardiogram and echocardiogram
11. Video-fluoroscopy for dysphagia
12. Whole-body PET-MRI

(*AST* aspartate transaminase, *ALT* alanine transaminase, *LDH* lactate dehydrogenase, *NCS* nerve conduction study, *EMG* electromyography, *MRI* magnetic resonance imaging, *CT* computed tomography) [12] (Table 21.4).

Table 21.4 Autoantibodies in idiopathic inflammatory myopathies

Myositis-specific autoantibodies	Myositis-associated autoantibodies
Anti-aminoacyl-tRNA synthetases	
Anti-Jo-1	Anti-SSA/Ro
Anti-PL-12, 7	Anti-Ro52
Anti-EJ	Anti-Ro60
Anti-OJ	Anti-La
Anti-KS	Anti-PM-Scl 75
Anti-Zo	Anti-PM-Scl 100
Anti-YRS	Anti-Ku
Anti-Mi-2	Anti-U1RNP
Anti-SRP	Anti-cN-1A
Anti-TIF1-gamma	
Anti-NXP-2	
Anti-MDA5	
Anti-SAE	
Anti-HMGCR	
Anti-FHL1	

21.9   MRI Findings in Inflammatory Muscle Diseases

The inflammation is usually symmetrical and involves the proximal muscle groups in polymyositis and dermatomyositis, but the muscle involvement can be patchy and asymmetric. STIR can be used to differentiate between involved and uninvolved muscles. STIR and fat-saturated gadolinium-enhanced T1-weighted images often show high signal intensity in the active phase. In other times inflammation may extend only along individual muscles and muscle groups along the myofascial distribution. In chronic phase, fatty atrophy of the musculature is seen on T1-weighted images.

In dermatomyositis, the subcutaneous connective tissue septa and the muscle fasciae are also involved. Juvenile dermatomyositis generally takes a more severe clinical course, which is shown by the extent and intensity of cutaneous, subcutaneous and muscular signal abnormalities on MRI (Figs. 21.6 and 21.7). In immune-

Muscle MRI (Dermatomyositis)

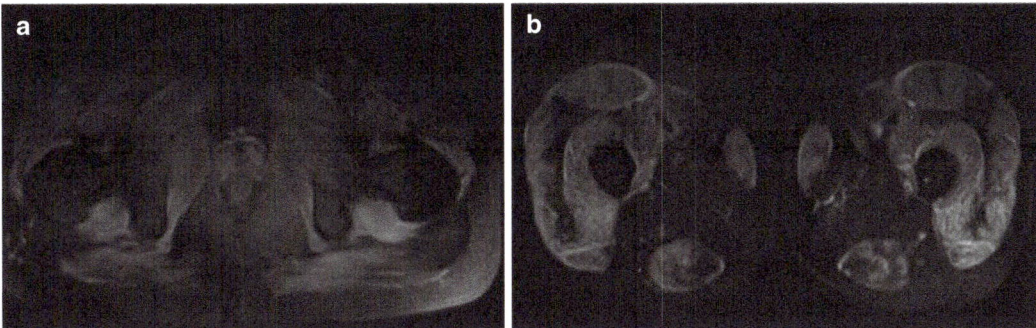

Fig. 21.6 T2-W FS axial images showing (**a**) hyperintensity involving bilateral obturator internus, pectineus, quadratus femoris, gluteus maximus muscles. (**b**) T2-W FS axial image showing hyperintensity involving bilateral vastus lateralis, intermedius and medialis muscles, bilateral rectus femoris, bilateral gracilis and bilateral semitendinosus muscles. Case of dermatomyositis with myofascial oedema noted in Fig. 21.2

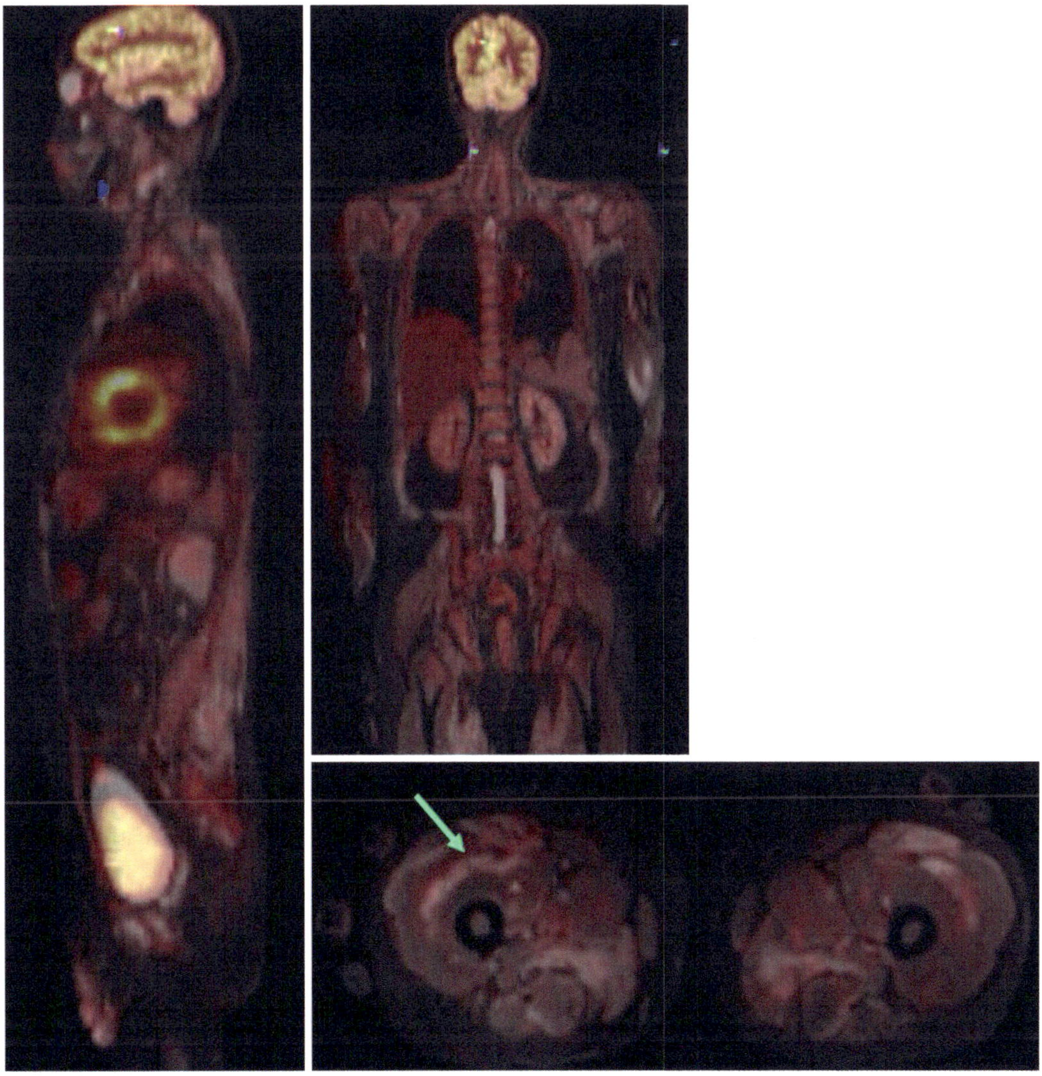

Fig. 21.7 FDG-PET MRI shows increased uptake in the oedematic muscles (metabolic activity) (arrow). No evidence of primary malignancy/secondaries (c/o dermatomyositis)

mediated necrotizing myopathy, MRI shows more widespread muscle oedema, atrophy and fatty replacement as compared to DM, PM and IBM. In inclusion body myositis, focal increased signal is seen on STIR and fat-saturated gadolinium-enhanced T1-weighted images, more in the anterior thigh compartment [14].

21.9.1 Course of Illness

The inflammatory myopathies respond well to immunomodulation. However, the response may not be adequate in some patients, especially when the treatment is delayed as the muscle tissue gets fibrosed or undergoes fatty changes. Some patients may worsen even on treatment. The course of the disease with regard to patient symptoms and respective treatment has been discussed below.

21.9.2 Risk of Malignancy and Extramuscular Manifestations in Myositis

There is an increased risk of malignancy by two- to sevenfold in variants of myositis except inclusion body myositis [15]. The risk of malignancy in myositis is associated with anti-TIF-1 or anti-NXP2 antibodies in DM cases and NM cases with anti-HMGCR antibodies. However, in some cases malignancy may occur even without these antibodies in NM. Patients are at risk of malignancy 1 year from the occurrence of myositis, and risk is elevated in the timeframe of next 3 years. Various associations with cancer are seen, the commonest being lung cancer, ovarian cancer, breast cancer and lymphoma. It would be ideal for patients to undergo CT scan or PET scan in cases of high suspicion as well as tumour markers. Tumour screening should be done at least once in a year and repeated for the next 3 years.

Extramuscular association is also seen in organs like lungs, kidneys, heart, joints and skin [4]. Their frequency depends upon the type of myositis. Pulmonary hypertension, serositis and ILD are common in specific types. Weakness of diaphragm and other muscles aiding breathing may lead to problems in ventilation. The anti-U-snRNP, anti-Ku, anti-MDA5, anti-PM/Scl and anti-SRP are the antibodies associated in patients with ILD in myositis [16]. Mortality rates significantly increase with the increase in the severity of ILD. Reticulation, linear and ground-glass opacity, traction bronchiectasis, peribronchovascular thickening and cystic spaces with thickened walls are the findings in patients with interstitial lung disease.

Cardiomyopathy, serositis or pericarditis, and conduction problems lead to increased mortality. ECG to detect arrhythmias, 2-D echocardiography and MRI of the heart are helpful. Along with symptomatic treatment for the heart, an intensified immunosuppression therapy is also undertaken. GIT and liver can also be affected. Renal involvement may lead to oedema of the legs, proteinuria and haematuria [12].

21.9.3 Treatment

The usual immunomodulation to start with is glucocorticoids [1], except in the case of inclusion body myositis. This is accepted universally and given at a dose of 1 mg/kg/day. For severe cases, intravenous glucocorticoids are initiated and later switched over to oral medication. The duration of treatment is guided by the clinical response and generally lasts up to 12 weeks followed by a slow taper initially by 10 mg every 1 or 2 weeks followed by 5 mg every week. Patients may require long-term maintenance treatment and hence have to be monitored for adverse effects like diabetes, hypertension, osteoporosis, cataracts, weight gain, mood swings, infections etc. [12]. They can be given calcium supplements.

Steroid-sparing immunomodulation has to be started in most cases. They include azathioprine, mycophenolate and methotrexate, which are commonly used. Other less commonly used immunosuppressants include cyclophosphamide, cyclosporin, IVIg and rituximab. In some trials, intravenous immune globulin has appeared to be effective in the treatment of polymyositis and necrotizing autoimmune myositis [12, 17]. Subcutaneous immune globulin has also been tried to sustain remission, and sometimes re-evaluation of patients is required if the disease is not responding to glucocorticoids and IVIg [17]. Patients with dermatomyositis have to be explained regarding skin manifestations, and they include the use of sunscreens, avoiding UV exposure and topical glucocorticoids. Azathioprine should be used only in patients with normal thiopurine methyltransferase activity. Methotrexate should be avoided in patients with interstitial lung disease. Calcineurin inhibitors are known to cause renal toxicity.

Creatine kinase levels do not correlate with the severity of disease or response to treatment. Anti-complement C3 drugs like eculizumab, effective in complement-mediated diseases, can be used to treat dermatomyositis and necrotizing autoimmune myositis.

Extramuscular manifestations require multispecialty care: dermatology, pulmonology, rheumatology, oncology referrals in case of manifestations are mandated. All patients should benefit from a structured rehabilitation programme and physiotherapy [12].

21.10 Management of Inclusion Body Myositis

Even though IBM has been extensively studied, currently no effective treatment plan is available. However, alemtuzumab provided transient improvement in a study. In another study, downmodulation of inflammatory markers was seen, without any change in the degenerative molecules [4]. Three placebo-controlled clinical trials assessed IVIg in IBM in 3–6 months: however, there was only a small increase in some of the outcomes, including *MRC* scale and swallowing function [17].

Nearly two-thirds of the patients suffer from impaired swallowing due to functional stenosis of the upper oesophageal sphincter, which is detected by video-fluoroscopy or real-time MRI. Certain local treatments include cricopharyngeal myotomy, pharyngoesophageal balloon dilatation and botulinum toxin to temporarily inactivate the muscle by injecting into the upper oesophageal sphincter. Cricopharyngeal myotomy is an effective technique, but it is irreversible; hence patients may later present with reflux or other swallowing difficulties [18, 19]. Percutaneous feeding tube can be advised.

Trials targeting muscle-inhibiting TGF-β molecules or muscle growth factors are being done. Resistance exercises with occupational and rehabilitation therapies are known to improve ambulation and balance and also avoid disuse atrophy and prevent joint contractures [20].

References

1. *Carstens PO, Schmidt J. Diagnosis, pathogenesis and treatment of myositis: recent advances. Clin Exp Immunol. 2014;175(3):349–58.
2. *Dalakas MC. Inflammatory muscle diseases. N Engl J Med. 2015;372(18):1734–47.
3. Furst DE, Amato AA, Iorga SR, Gajria K, Fernan-des AW. Epidemiology of adult idiopathic inflammatory myopathies in a U.S. managed care plan. Muscle Nerve. 2012;45(5):676–83.
4. *Selva-O'Callaghan A, Pinal-Fernandez I, Trallero-Araguás E, Milisenda JC, Grau-Junyent JM, Mammen AL. Classification and management of adult inflammatory myopathies. Lancet Neurol. 2018;17:816–28.
5. Uruha A, Suzuki S, Nishino I. Diagnosis of dermatomyositis: autoantibody profile and muscle pathology. Clin Exp Neuroimmunol. 2017;8(4):302–12.
6. *Uruha A, Suzuki S, Nishino I. Diagnosis of dermatomyositis: autoantibody profile and muscle pathology. Clin Exp Neuroimmunol. 2017;8(4):302–12.
7. Allenbach Y, Benveniste O, Goebel HH, Stenzel W. Integrated classification of inflammatory myopathies. Neuropathol Appl Neurobiol. 2017;43(1):62–81.
8. Lega JC, Fabien N, Reynaud Q, Durieu I, Durupt S, Dutertre M, et al. The clinical phenotype associated with myositis-specific and associated autoantibodies: a meta-analysis revisiting the so-called antisynthetase syndrome. Autoimmun Rev. 2014;13(9):883–91.
9. Schmidt K, Schmidt J. Inclusion body myositis. Advancements in diagnosis, pathomechanisms, and treatment. Curr Opin Rheumatol. 2017;29(6):632–8.
10. Bohan A, Peter JB. Polymyositis and dermatomyositis (parts 1 and 2). N Engl J Med. 1975;292:344–7.
11. Hoogendijk JE, Amato AA, Lecky BR, Choy EH, Lundberg IE, Rose MR, et al. 119th ENMC international workshop: trial design in adult idiopathic inflammatory myopathies, with the exception of

inclusion body myositis, 10–12 October 2003, Naarden, The Netherlands. Neuromuscul Disord. 2004;14:337–45.

12. *Schmidt J. Current classification and management of inflammatory myopathies. J Neuromuscul Disord. 2018;5(2):109–29.

13. Uruha A, Noguchi S, Hayashi YK, Tsuburaya RS, Yonekawa T, Nonaka I, et al. Hepatitis C virus infection in inclusion body myositis: a case-control study. Neurology. 2016;86(3):211–7.

14. Ukichi T, Yoshida K, Matsushima S, et al. MRI of skeletal muscles in patients with idiopathic inflammatory myopathies: characteristic findings and diagnostic performance in dermatomyositis. RMD Open. 2019;5:e000850.

15. Selva-O'Callaghan A, Trallero-Araguas E, Grau-Junyent JM, Labrador-Horrillo M. Malignancy and myositis: novel autoantibodies and new insights. Curr Opin Rheumatol. 2010;22(6):627–32.

16. Lega JC, Reynaud Q, Belot A, Fabien N, Durieu I, Cottin V. Idiopathic inflammatory myopathies and the lung. Eur Respir Rev. 2015;24(136):216–38.

17. Hoa SAT, Hudson M. Critical review of the role of intravenous immunoglobulins in idiopathic inflammatory myopathies. Semin Arthritis Rheum. 2017;46(4):488–508.

18. Olthoff A, Carstens PO, Zhang S, von Fintel E, Friede T, Lotz J, et al. Evaluation of dysphagia by novel real-time MRI. Neurology. 2016;87(20):2132–8.

19. Price MA, Barghout V, Benveniste O, Christopher-Stine L, Corbett A, de Visser M, et al. Mortality and causes of death in patients with sporadic inclusion body myositis: survey study based on the clinical experience of specialists in Australia, Europe and the USA. J Neuromuscul Dis. 2016;3(1):67–75.

20. Alexanderson H. Exercise in inflammatory myopathies, including inclusion body myositis. Curr Rheumatol Rep. 2012;14:244–51.

Part V

Neuroimmunology

Optic Neuritis

22

Sanjeeta Sitaula

Case Scenario

A 21-year-old male presented to the emergency department with the history of rapidly progressive diminution of vision in his right eye associated with headache and pain with eye movement for 5 days. It was not associated with double vision, tingling, numbness, or weakness of his body parts. He did not give any history of preceding fever, rashes, joint pain, oral ulcers, or recent immunization. His bowel and bladder habits were normal. However, he gave a history of similar problem occurring in his left eye 2 years back. His vision had improved after he was treated elsewhere with intravenous medications.

On ocular examination, his best corrected visual acuity in the right eye (RE) was 6/60 and in the left eye (LE) was 6/6, as measured by the Snellen chart. His extraocular motility was full in both eyes, but there was mild pain in abduction in the right eye. The pupillary assessment showed relative afferent pupillary defect (RAPD) in the RE. The rest of the anterior segment examination findings were normal. On dilated fundus examination, both the optic disks appeared normal with pink color and sharp margins. Macula was healthy with good foveal reflex. The vessels were of normal course and caliber, and the periphery was normal. Color vision (Farnsworth D-15

Dichotomous Color Blindness Test) showed normal results in both eyes; however, contrast sensitivity (Pelli-Robson chart) was decreased in RE (RE—1.20 log units and LE—1.90 log units). Goldman visual fields showed generalized constriction with enlarged blind spot in RE while it was normal in LE. Visual evoked potential (VEP) was suggestive of a bilateral conduction defect with decreased RE amplitudes for higher frequencies.

Magnetic resonance imaging (MRI) of the orbit and brain showed enlargement of the right optic nerve with high T2 signal intensity within right optic nerve (Fig. 22.1). Mild T2 high signal intensity was also noted in the left optic nerve. Multiple discrete T2 and FLAIR high signal intensity foci in the bilateral peri-ventricular region were oriented perpendicular to the ventricle and in the bilateral centrum semiovale, which was suggestive of multiple sclerosis (Fig. 22.2).

Patient was admitted with the diagnosis of right optic neuritis, and intravenous methylprednisolone 1 g was given once a day for 3 days. Lumbar puncture was done. CSF analysis showed raised IgG levels—61.30 mg/L (normal: 0.0–34 mg/L) and increased oligoclonal bands. The diagnosis was confirmed as right eye optic neuritis with multiple sclerosis.

S. Sitaula (✉)
Department of Ophthalmology, BP Koirala Lions Centre for Ophthalmic Studies, Tribhuvan University, Institute of Medicine, Kathmandu, Nepal

© Springer Nature Singapore Pte Ltd. 2024
K. K. Oli et al. (eds.), *Case-based Approach to Common Neurological Disorders*,
https://doi.org/10.1007/978-981-99-8676-7_22

Fig. 22.1 MRI orbit T2 FLAIR (**a**) and brain T2 fat-suppressed coronal section (**b**) showing hyperintense signal in right optic nerve

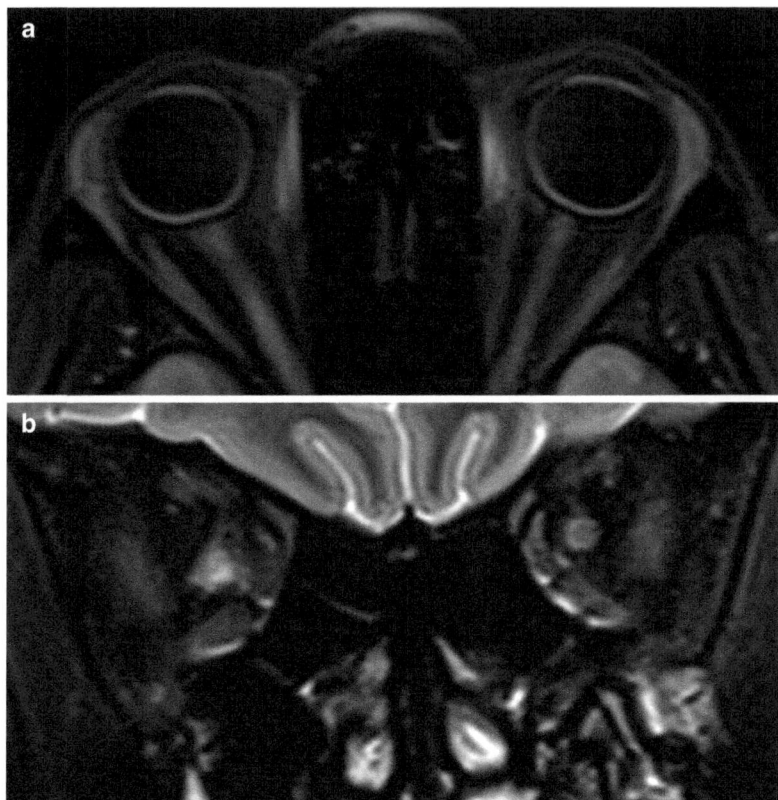

Fig. 22.2 MRI brain showing multiple discrete T2 and FLAIR high-signal-intensity foci in bilateral peri-ventricular region, oriented perpendicular to the ventricle, and in the bilateral centrum semiovale

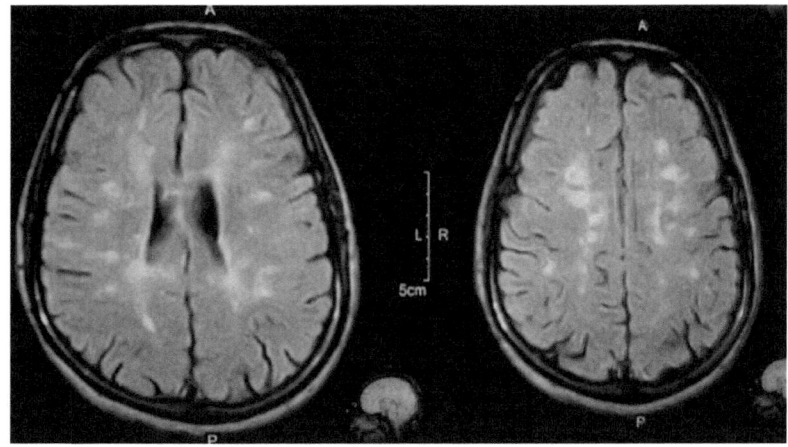

22.1 Introduction

Optic neuritis (ON) is the demyelinating inflammation of the optic nerve characterized by decreased vision and other features of optic nerve dysfunction, like decreased color and contrast vision, a visual field defect and the presence of a RAPD. It is often accompanied by periocular pain worse on eye movement.

It may be idiopathic but is often associated with multiple sclerosis (MS). Other demyelinating diseases like neuromyelitis optica (NMO), Schilder's disease, and encephalitis periaxialis concentrica are also associated with optic neuritis. Sometimes optic neuritis may occur following infections, post-vaccination, following inflammatory diseases like sarcoidosis, vasculitis (polyarteritis nodosa) or connective tissue disorders like systemic lupus erythematosus (SLE).

22.2 Anatomy

The optic nerve is a 50-mm-long, heavily myelinated tract extending from the eye to the optic chiasma. It consists of about 1.2 million axons derived from the retinal ganglion cells. These axons pass through the lamina cribrosa, a fenestrated sheet of connective tissue, forming the optic nerve.

It consists of four portions:

- Intraocular portion (the optic disk or the optic nerve head (ONH)—1 mm)
- Intraorbital portion (25 mm long)
- Intracanalicular portion (within the optic canal—9 mm long)
- Intracranial portion (about 16 mm long)

Topographically optic disk can be divided into four regions: superficial nerve fiber layer, prelaminar region, region of lamina cribrosa, and retrolaminar part. The ONH is a transition zone where the nerve fibers make a 90° turn as they enter the lamina cribrosa. Here the nerve fibers also pass from an area of relatively high intraocular pressure to the lower-pressure zone of the retro-orbital segment of the optic nerve. It receives the blood supply from the central retinal artery, branches of the posterior ciliary, and ophthalmic arteries. Myelination of optic nerve starts just behind the lamina cribrosa. Patients with a small cup-to-disk ratio (crowded disk) are at a risk to develop nonarteritic anterior ischemic optic neuropathy.

Orbital segment of the optic nerve is lax, and this redundancy helps to protect the optic nerve from damage by stretch even up to 9 mm of proptosis. The intraorbital segment of the optic nerve is enclosed by dural sheath which is continuous with that of the CNS. The superior rectus and the medial rectus muscles are closely attached to the dural sheath of the optic nerve, which accounts for the ocular pain in cases of retrobulbar neuritis during elevation and adduction of the globe. The intracanalicular (intraosseous) segment of the optic nerve exits the orbit through the optic foramen into the optic canal. The intracanalicular optic nerve is tightly fixed within the optic canal. Thus, even small lesions arising within the optic canal or force directed into the optic canal during indirect optic neuropathy may compress and damage the optic nerve. Intracranial segment of the optic nerve extends posteriorly, superiorly, and medially to join the optic chiasma.

Optic nerve receives most of its blood supply from the branches of the ophthalmic artery. The ophthalmic artery passes below the optic nerve in the optic canal. Inside the orbit, ophthalmic artery gives rise to two or three posterior ciliary arteries and central retinal artery, which pierces the optic nerve and travels along the optic nerve. Venous drainage of the ONH occurs via the central retinal vein.

22.3 Epidemiology

A typical case of optic neuritis is a young person (20–45 years old) with female preponderance (F:M = 3:2). The incidence of ON is higher among people living at higher latitudes compared with those living closer to the equator, which correlates with the prevalence of multiple sclerosis, one of the most common causes of optic neuritis [1, 2]. The annual incidence rate of optic neuritis in Japan is 1.62 per 100,000 person-years and Taiwan is 0.33 per 1000 person-years, while in the United States, it is 5.1 per 100,000 person-years [3]. The Asian Collaborative Longitudinal Optic Neuritis Epidemiology (ACLONE) was an observational cohort study done among an Asian population of 12–61-year-old patients in Singapore, Malaysia, Taiwan, and South Korea presenting with the first episode of ON [4]. The study revealed that Asian patients had a male-predominant bilateral optic neuritis with severe visual loss at presentation [4].

22.4 Pathophysiology

The pathology in optic neuritis is inflammatory demyelination of the optic nerve and myelin breakdown with perivascular edema in the myelinated nerve sheaths. It is believed that the optic neuritis is an immune-mediated demyelination disorder, but the specific mechanism and target antigens are unknown. Systemic T-cell activation occurs at the onset of symptoms, which leads to the release of cytokines and other inflammatory agents. B-cell activation against myelin basic protein also has a role in the pathogenesis of optic neuritis. Genetic susceptibility for optic neuritis is also suspected.

22.5 Symptoms and Signs

The diagnosis of optic neuritis is based on history and examination findings. Most of our current knowledge of this disease comes from the findings of Optic Neuritis Treatment Trial (ONTT) [5, 6], which was a multicentric randomized controlled trial conducted in 1990s. It included about 457 patients with acute unilateral optic neuritis and age ranging from 18 to 46 years.

Common clinical features of optic neuritis are acute vision loss progressing over a period of hours to days with a peak at around 1 or 2 weeks. It is usually monocular, but in approximately 10% of cases, it may have bilateral involvement, either in rapid succession or simultaneously. In younger children and in Asian patients, bilateral optic neuritis is frequently seen.

Ocular discomfort or pain especially with eye movement was present in 92% patients in ONTT. Other symptoms are phosphines (flashes of lights), "washed out" color vision, and loss of central vision or part of the peripheral vision. Uhthoff's phenomenon can be observed, which is the emerging of visual symptoms such as blurring of vision while exercising or bathing in hot water particularly when associated with MS.

The signs include decreased visual acuity (range from 6/6 to no light perception), abnormal color vision (abnormal in 94% cases in ONTT identified by Farnsworth–Munsell 100-Hue test),

relative afferent pupillary defect, diminished contrast sensitivity, and visual field defects (cecocentral, arcuate, altitudinal, and rarely hemianopic field defect). Based on ophthalmoscopic appearance, it is described as papillitis (anterior optic neuritis) when there is optic disk edema (seen in 35% cases in ONTT) and retrobulbar optic neuritis when the optic disk appears normal. Papillitis is frequently seen in children less than 14 years and in certain geographic regions like South Africa and Southeast Asia [7, 8].

22.6 Investigations and Laboratory Workup

1. Visual evoked response (VER): A slowed conduction in the optic nerve due to axonal demyelination leads to a delay in the P100 latency of the VER.
2. Imaging studies: It is done to rule out other optic nerve disorders and to evaluate the risk of progression to MS. MRI is superior to CT scan and is the imaging of choice for optic nerve and brain lesions. In acute optic neuritis, gadolinium-enhanced MRI of the brain and orbit shows enhancement of the optic nerve. MRI of the brain with FLAIR sequences can detect brain lesions >3 mm in size. "Dawson's Fingers" which are peri-ventricular white matter lesions involving the corpus callosum on FLAIR sequences are highly predictive of MS. Typical lesions in a brain MRI characteristic of MS are white matter abnormalities which are ovoid, peri-ventricular, and usually larger than 3 mm. In a 15-year follow-up data from the ONTT, mono-symptomatic patients with no white matter lesion had a 25% risk of MS, while those with one or more lesion had a 72% risk of MS. MRI of the spine is indicated, where there is a high suspicion of NMO.
3. Optical coherence tomography (OCT): OCT provides a non-invasive and a high-resolution imaging and is based on the principle of reflection of low-coherence radiation from tissues. The use of OCT is evolving to objectively monitor axonal loss and quantify and

detect optic atrophy at early stages. A number of studies have estimated that OCT may have a role in disease diagnosis and monitoring as it was noted that neuromyelitis optica (NMO) had a greater severity of optic nerve injury compared to optic neuritis associated with MS [9].

4. Lumbar puncture: It is not routinely done in all cases of optic neuritis. It is done for atypical optic neuritis (e.g., those with bilateral optic neuritis, pediatric ON, or symptoms suggesting infection) [10]. However, it may play an important role in confirming the diagnosis of MS and to rule out other conditions.

5. Antibodies: Serum NMO antibodies and MOG antibodies are done especially in unexplained bilateral simultaneous or sequential optic neuritis or ON with poor visual recovery. It is also considered if the MRI brain is normal apart for the findings in optic nerves/chiasma, in atypical ON, or in patients with transverse myelitis.

6. Others: Other investigations like serum angiotensin-converting enzyme, treponema pallidum hemagglutination assay, and antinuclear antibody tests are done in atypical ON to rule out sarcoidosis, syphilis, and SLE or other connective tissue disease respectively.

22.7 Differential Diagnosis

22.7.1 Anterior Ischemic Optic Neuropathy (AION)

AION results from ischemic damage to the anterior portion of the optic nerve, which is primarily supplied by the posterior ciliary artery. Arteritic AION (AAION) results from ischemia secondary to vasculitis, most commonly from giant cell arteritis (GCA). Visual loss from GCA is an ophthalmic emergency, and a high dose of intravenous steroids must be instituted immediately, which may provide some improvement in the visual acuity of the involved eye in addition to provide better protection for the fellow eye. Nonarteritic anterior ischemic optic neuropathy

(NAION) is the most common acute optic neuropathy occurring in individuals above 50 years. In contrast to ON, NAION is usually associated with systemic vascular risk factors, like diabetes mellitus, hypertension, hyperlipidemia, and ischemic heart diseases, and also other factors like nocturnal hypotension, anemia, and structural abnormalities of the optic nerve head like a crowded optic disk.

22.7.2 Compressive and Infiltrative Optic Neuropathy

Compressive and infiltrative optic neuropathies may present with progressive visual loss with a RAPD, headache, proptosis, signs of orbital congestion, and limitation of ocular motility. A variety of lesions like thyroid eye disease, mucocele, orbital pseudotumor, orbital hemorrhage, and neoplasias like meningioma (optic nerve sheath, sphenoid wing), pituitary tumor, intraorbital tumor (hemangioma, lymphangioma, metastasis), and craniopharyngioma can cause compression of the optic nerve. Infiltration of the optic nerve can occur in sarcoidosis and other neoplasias like optic nerve glioma (pilocytic astrocytoma), metastatic carcinoma, sinonasal tumors, lymphoma, leukemia and meningeal carcinomatosis.

22.7.3 Infectious Optic Neuropathy

Optic neuropathy has been reported in association with a wide variety of infectious agents, like viruses, bacteria, fungi, and parasites. The common causes of infectious optic neuropathy are bacteria like tuberculosis, Cat-scratch disease, Lyme disease, and syphilis; viruses like Herpes and HIV, and parasites like toxoplasma. Common presentations are neuroretinitis, papillitis, retrobulbar optic neuritis, and optic disk edema, along with neurological manifestations such as encephalopathy, cranial neuropathy, and focal neurological deficits, and systematic manifestations such as fever, headache, vomiting, myalgia, and rashes.

22.7.4 Hereditary Optic Neuropathy

The hereditary optic neuropathies are a group of optic nerve disorders which are inherited. They are diagnosed based on familial expression or genetic analysis. Based on the pattern of inheritance they can be autosomal dominant, autosomal recessive, and maternal (mitochondrial). The diagnosis of hereditary optic neuropathy should be considered in any patient with unexplained, sequential or bilateral, painless, central visual loss.

22.8 Management

From the results of ONTT, the recommended treatment for acute optic neuritis is high-dose intravenous methylprednisolone (IVMP), 1 g/day for 3 days followed by oral prednisone, 1 mg/kg daily for 11 days, followed by a 4-day taper. However, high-dose steroids hasten the rate of recovery and not the ultimate visual outcome, so it is important to take into consideration the risk, benefits, and side effects based on patient preference and underlying medical illness. The ONTT showed that treatment with IVMP followed by oral prednisone decreased the rate of MS development for the first 2 years; however, this protective effect was not seen at 3 years. Another striking finding in the ONTT study was that low-dose oral steroids alone increased the rate of recurrent optic neuritis in cases of acute optic neuritis, especially in patients with MS in the ONTT study. The recurrence rate was 30% at 2 years in oral prednisone group compared to 16% in placebo group and 13% in the IVMP group.

If MRI features are suggestive of demyelinating disease, the patient can be started on disease-modifying drugs like interferons or glatiramer acetate, weighing the risk-benefit ratio. Several studies like the Controlled High-Risk Subjects Avonex Multiple Sclerosis Prevention Study (CHAMPS) [11] in North America, Early Treatment of MS Study (ETOMS) [12] in Europe, and the Betaseron in Newly Emerging MS for Initial Treatment (BENEFIT) [13] in Canada and Europe, which were multi-center, randomized, and placebo-controlled trials conducted to assess the effects of interferon-β in the disease course of MS in patients with clinically isolated syndrome. These studies found that treatment with interferon is beneficial by delaying a second relapse and reducing the cumulative probability of clinically definite MS.

Atypical optic neuritis may benefit from early intravenous steroids by both decreasing the severity of the attack and speeding the recovery. Therapeutic plasmapheresis and intravenous immunoglobulins may be tried in steroid-unresponsive cases. Chronic immunosuppressive therapy with agents like azathioprine, rituximab, and mycophenolate mofetil may be required, especially after recurrent attacks with incomplete recovery.

22.9 Prognosis

Visual prognosis is excellent for typical optic neuritis, with 94% achieving 20/40 or better vision at 5 years and only 3% having a vision <20/200 at 5 years in ONTT. The visual recovery starts by 1 month and completes by 3 months but sometimes may even require about a year.

References

1. Shams P, Plant G. Optic neuritis: a review. Int MS J. 2009;16(3):82–9.
2. Pau D, Al Zubidi N, Yalamanchili S, Plant G, Lee AG. Optic neuritis. Eye. 2011;25(7):833.
3. Woung L-C, Chung H-C, Jou J-R, Wang K-C, Peng P-H. A comparison of optic neuritis in Asian and in Western countries. Neuro-ophthalmology. 2011;35(2):65–72.
4. Seah B, Tow S, Ong OK, Yang C, Tsai C, Lee K, et al. The natural history of optic neuritis in Asian patients: an observational cohort study. Neurol Asia. 2017;22(4):341–8.
5. Beck RW. The optic neuritis treatment trial. Arch Ophthalmol. 1988;106(8):1051–3.
6. Optic Neuritis Study Group. The clinical profile of optic neuritis: experience of the optic neuritis treatment trial. Arch Ophthalmol. 1991;109:1673–8.
7. Wakakura M, Minei-Higa R, Oono S, Matsui Y, Tabuchi A, Kani K, et al. Baseline features of idiopathic optic neuritis as determined by a multi-

center treatment trial in Japan. Jpn J Ophthalmol. 1999;43(2):127–32.

8. Wang JC, Tow S, Aung T, Lim SA, Cullen JF. The presentation, aetiology, management and outcome of optic neuritis in an Asian population. Clin Exp Ophthalmol. 2001;29(5):312–5.

9. Ratchford J, Quigg M, Conger A, Frohman T, Frohman E, Balcer L, et al. Optical coherence tomography helps differentiate neuromyelitis optica and MS optic neuropathies. Neurology. 2009;73(4):302–8.

10. Beck RW, Trobe JD, Optic Neuritis Study Group. What we have learned from the optic neuritis treatment trial. Ophthalmology. 1995;102(10):1504–8.

11. O'Connor P. The effects of intramuscular interferon beta-Ia in patients at high risk for development of multiple sclerosis: a post hoc analysis of data from CHAMPS. Clin Ther. 2003;25(11):2865–74.

12. Comi G, Filippi M, Barkhof F, Durelli L, Edan G, Fernández O, et al. Effect of early interferon treatment on conversion to definite multiple sclerosis: a randomised study. Lancet. 2001;357(9268):1576–82.

13. Kappos L, Polman C, Freedman M, Edan G, Hartung H, Miller D, et al. Treatment with interferon beta-1b delays conversion to clinically definite and McDonald MS in patients with clinically isolated syndromes. Neurology. 2006;67(7):1242–9.

Autoimmune Encephalitis

23

M. Netravathi

Case Scenario

A 12-year-old girl presented with behavioural disturbances (decreased interaction, decline in scholastic performance, abusive behaviour and abnormal involuntary movements of the right hand with generalised seizures for 6 weeks). After 1–2 weeks, she progressively developed involuntary perioral movements, refractory status epilepticus and mutism. There was no fever, headache, myoclonic jerks, visual complaints, weight loss or any systemic complaints. At the time of admission, she had intermittent respiratory disturbances, was in altered sensorium with status epilepticus, and had perioral dyskinesias and right upper limb dystonic posturing with the presence of pyramidal signs. She was then intubated and kept in mechanical ventilation. Routine lab investigations including anti-TPO antibody level were within normal limits. MRI brain and CSF studies showed no abnormalities. Electroencephalography showed generalised theta-delta range slowing with "delta brush" and focal epileptiform discharges as well (Fig. 23.1). CSF anti-NMDA receptor antibody was positive. She was treated with a course of intravenous methylprednisolone followed by intravenous immunoglobulins (IVIg) but showed no signs of improvement. She was then started on large-volume plasmapheresis along with oral steroids. She made mild-to-moderate improvement. She was extubated, weaned off the ventilator, and shifted to the ward where she continued to have mutism and mild Parkinsonism with stereotypy movements of the hand. She improved significantly, and presently she is on low dosage of steroids.

M. Netravathi (✉)
Department of Neurology, National Institute of
Mental Health and Neurosciences (NIMHANS),
Bangalore, India

© Springer Nature Singapore Pte Ltd. 2024
K. K. Oli et al. (eds.), *Case-based Approach to Common Neurological Disorders*,
https://doi.org/10.1007/978-981-99-8676-7_23

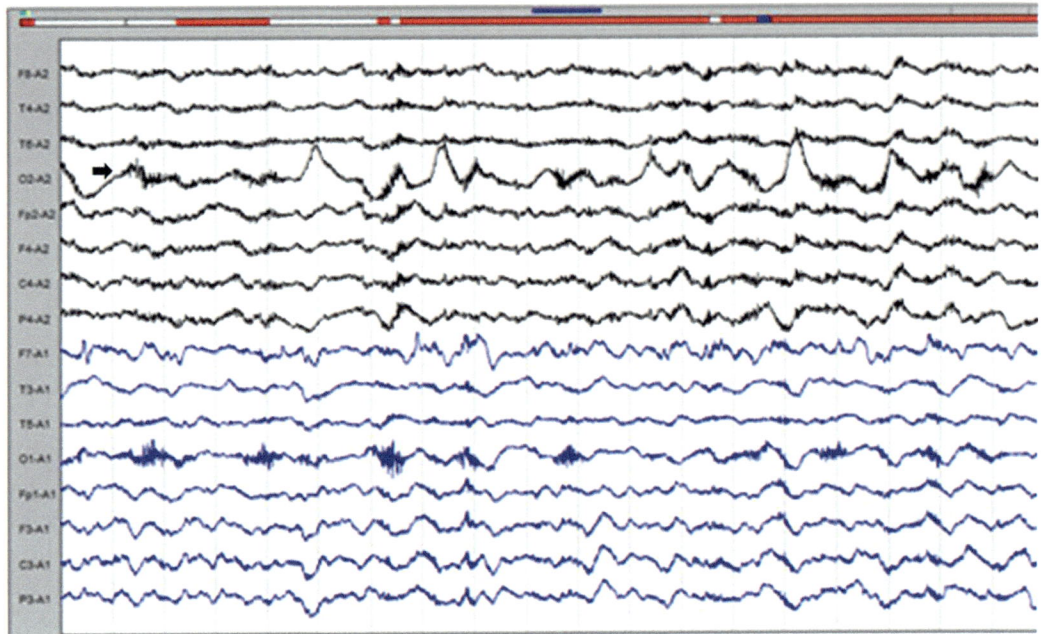

Fig. 23.1 EEG showing mild diffuse background slowing of 4–6 Hz with intermittent delta brush pattern (arrow) in the occipital leads

23.1 Introduction

Von economo's Encephalitis lethargica was described in 1916–1927, wherein patients presented with features of headache, malaise, ophthalmoplegia, Parkinsonism, and sleep changes [1]. Aetiological basis of this disorder was largely unknown and was presumed to be triggered by influenza virus. Many such disorders have been described in recent times with associated autoantibodies and have been termed as autoimmune encephalitis (AIE). Autoimmune encephalitis is a group of autoantibody-mediated inflammatory, non-infectious encephalitis being increasingly recognised in clinical practice [2]. It encompasses a group of clinical syndromes which are immune mediated, maybe associated with anti-bodies, and responds well to immunotherapy if initiated in the early stages. AIE has diverse clinical manifestations, such as cognitive dysfunction, behavioural and personality changes, seizures, movement disorders, autonomic disturbances and decreased level of sensorium. Some of them may have an underlying neoplasm. The initial diagnostic criteria were mostly reliant on antibody reports and response to various immunomodulation therapies [3]. But these criteria may not always be practical, as antibody results may come negative in a few cases and immunotherapy responsiveness may not occur, especially when treatment is initiated late in the course of illness [3]. A consensus statement proposed a practical approach to the diagnosis of AIE, which is enumerated in Table 23.1.

Table 23.1 Diagnostic criteria for autoimmune encephalitis (AIE)

Definitive diagnosis is made when all four of the following criteria have been met:
1.	Subacute onset (rapid progression of less than 3 months) of working memory deficits, seizures or psychiatric symptoms
2.	MRI brain showing abnormalities on T2-weighted fluid-attenuated inversion Recovery images involving the medial temporal lobes (or FDG-PET showing similar changes)
3.	At least one of the following: 1. CSF pleocytosis (white blood cell count >5 cells per mm³) 2. EEG with epileptic or slow-wave activity involving the temporal lobes
4.	Exclusion of alternative causes
Possible diagnosis is made when all three of the following criteria have been met:
1.	Subacute onset (rapid progression of less than 3 months) of working memory deficits (short-term memory loss), altered mental status (altered sensorium, lethargy, personality change) or psychiatric symptoms
2.	At least one of the following: 1. New focal CNS findings 2. Seizures not explained by a previously known seizure disorder 3. CSF pleocytosis (white blood cell count >5 cells/mm³)
3.	MRI features suggestive of encephalitis
4.	Reasonable exclusion of alternative causes

23.2 Epidemiology

The annual incidence of all forms of encephalitis is 5–8/100,000 persons/year. The California Encephalitis Project reported higher incidence of NMDAR encephalitis than viral encephalitis. Increased recognition of the disorder with increased availability of antibody testing has resulted in accurate diagnosis and management of AIE. A prospective multicentre study found AIE to be the third most common form of encephalitis after viral and post-infectious acute demyelinating encephalomyelitis [4, 5]. Exact incidence and prevalence cannot be ascertained in India in view of limited case reports and case series.

23.3 Pathophysiology

The most common triggers for AIE are tumours and viral encephalitis, followed by cryptogenic causes. HLA association has been noticed in anti-LGI1 encephalitis in two independent cohorts from Dutch [6] and Korea [7] suggesting genetic basis. The implicated HLA genes are HLA-DRB1*07 (DR7), HLA-DRB4 in a Dutch population and DRB1*07:01–DQB1*02:02 in a Korean population. Few viruses like herpes simplex virus (HSV) [8] and Japanese encephalitis (JE) virus [9] have been implicated in triggering the NMDAR antibodies.

In recent years, the reporting of antibodies associated with AIE has increased. These are divided into three major categories [10, 11] (Table 23.2):

1. **Intraneuronal antigens (INAab):** They are also known as onconeural antibodies, are not directly pathogenic and result from an epiphenomenon of T-cell-mediated immune response. They are more often paraneoplastic, seen in elderly patients and have a poor response to immunotherapy. The antibodies to these antigens serve as diagnostic markers.
2. **Cell-surface antigens (CSAab):** The antibodies target molecules involved in neurotransmission leading to neuronal dysfunction. They are usually seen in younger adults, less often paraneoplastic and respond well to immunotherapy in early treatment.
3. **Extracellular location of antigens against synaptic antigens (SyAab):** It results in the alteration of neurotransmitter release.

Some patients may have more than one type of antibody as well, and CSAab and SyAab have been reported together with anti-INAab, especially in paraneoplastic AIE.

Table 23.2 Antibodies implicated in autoimmune encephalitis (AIE)

Antigen	Clinical features	Diagnostic assay	Frequency of malignancy	Types of malignancy
Intracellular antigens				
AGNA (SOX1)	Limbic encephalitis, LEMS, neuropathy			Small-cell lung cancer (SCLC)
Amphiphysin	Stiff-person syndrome, cerebellar degeneration, limbic encephalitis, encephalomyelitis, myelopathy, peripheral neuropathy, opsoclonus myoclonus		~85%	Breast, small-cell lung cancer
ANNA-1 (anti-Hu)	Sensory neuronopathy, limbic encephalitis, cranial neuropathies, cerebellar degeneration, encephalomyelitis, partial epilepsy, status epilepticus, autonomic dysfunction-intestinal pseudo-obstruction, opsoclonus myoclonus	Western blot	~80%	Small-cell lung cancer, neuroblastoma, prostate cancer
ANNA-2 (anti-Ri)	Opsoclonus myoclonus, brainstem encephalitis, cerebellar degeneration		~60%	Breast, gynaecologic, lung, bladder cancer
ANNA-3	Cerebellar degeneration, encephalomyelitis, sensory neuronopathy		~60%	Lung cancer
BRSK2				Small-cell lung cancer
CRMP-5 (anti-CV2)	Cerebellar degeneration, limbic encephalitis, optic neuritis, retinopathy, uveitis, chorea, encephalomyelitis, sensorimotor neuropathy		~75%	Small-cell lung cancer, thymoma
EFA6A				Ovarian
GAD-65	Encephalitis, stiff-person syndrome, cerebellar ataxia, seizures, opsoclonus myoclonus, encephalomyelitis, PERM, palatal myoclonus, hyperekplexia	Radioimmunoassay	~10%	Lung cancer, neuroendocrine tumour, thymoma, breast cancer
GFAP	Encephalitis, myelitis, meningoencephalitis, encephalomyelitis, neuropathy, meningitis, ataxia		34%	Ovarian teratoma
Anti-Ma1, Ma2 (Ta)	Ma1 and Ma2: cerebellar and brainstem dysfunction Ma2 (only): limbic encephalitis, hypothalamic dysfunction, brainstem encephalitis	Western blot	>~90%	Ma1 and Ma2—breast, colon, parotid, non-small-cell lung cancer; Ma2 (only)—germ cell testicular seminoma
PCA-1 (anti-Yo)	Paraneoplastic cerebellar syndrome, peripheral neuropathy		~90%	Breast, gynaecologic, lung cancer
PCA-2 (MAP1B)	Encephalomyelitis, cerebellar degeneration, LEMS		~90%	Lung cancer
Striational	Myasthenia gravis; common with muscle AChR antibodies		~30%	Thymoma

Table 23.2 (continued)

Antigen	Clinical features	Diagnostic assay	Frequency of malignancy	Types of malignancy
ZIC	Encephalomyelitis, cerebellar degeneration, opsoclonus			Small-cell lung cancer
Cell-surface antigens				
AChR (muscle and ganglionic)	Muscle: myasthenia gravis when paraneoplastic Ganglionic: autonomic dysfunction, encephalopathy, seizures, peripheral neuropathy		Muscle: ~10% Ganglionic: ~30%	Muscle: thymoma Ganglionic: breast, prostate, lung, gastrointestinal cancer
AMPAR	Limbic encephalitis, nystagmus, epilepsy, ataxia, insomnia	Cell-based assay	~70%	Lung, breast, thymoma
AQP4	NMOSD	Cell-based assay	~5–20%	Breast, lung, thymic, carcinoid, B cell lymphoma
CASPR2	Encephalitis, Morvan's syndrome, neuromyotonia	Cell-based assay	~0–40%	Thymoma
D2 (dopamine) receptor	Basal ganglia encephalitis	Cell-based assay	0%	–
DPPX	Diarrhoea and profound weight loss common Encephalitis with CNS hyperexcitability: confusion, psychiatric manifestations, tremor, myoclonus, nystagmus, hyperekplexia, PERM-like symptoms, ataxia	Cell-based assay	<10%	Rare B-cell neoplasms
GABA$_A$R	Refractory seizures, status epilepticus, epilepsia partialis continua, stiff-person syndrome, opsoclonus	Cell-based assay	<5%	Thymoma
GABA$_B$R	Stiff-person syndrome, PERM, limbic encephalitis, cerebellar degeneration, or optic neuritis, abnormal orolingual movements, fluent aphasia, epilepsy, sleep disturbances, agrypnia	Cell-based assay	50%	Small-cell lung cancer
GlyαR	Stiff-person syndrome, PERM, limbic encephalitis, cerebellar degeneration, optic neuritis, hyperekplexia			Infrequent
GQ1b	Bickerstaff's brainstem encephalitis	ELISA	0%	
IgLON5	Abnormal sleep movements and behaviours, obstructive sleep apnoea, stridor, dysarthria, dysphagia, ataxia, chorea			None reported
mGluR1	Cerebellar degeneration, ataxia intention tremor			Hodgkin's lymphoma; may occur without tumour
mGluR5	Ophelia syndrome: limbic encephalitis, myoclonus	Cell-based assay	70%	Hodgkin's lymphoma; may occur without tumour

(continued)

Table 23.2 (continued)

Antigen	Clinical features	Diagnostic assay	Frequency of malignancy	Types of malignancy
MOG	NMOSD-like phenotype, optic neuritis and/or longitudinally extensive transverse myelitis; ADEM, especially in children	Cell-based assay	0%	Infrequent
Neurexin-3α	Fever, headache or gastrointestinal symptoms, followed by confusion, seizures and decreased level of consciousness, seizures			None
NMDAR (GluN1)	Behavioural and psychiatric manifestations, insomnia, reduced verbal output, seizures, amnesia, movement disorders, catatonia, dyskinesia, stereotypy, catatonia, hypoventilation, autonomic instability, coma	Cell-based assay	~10–45%	Ovarian teratomas, rarely carcinomas
PCA-Tr (anti-DNER)	Cerebellar degeneration, limbic encephalitis		~90%	Hodgkin's lymphoma
VGCC (P/Q, N-type)	P/Q and N: LEMS P/Q: cerebellar degeneration, seizures N: variable; includes encephalopathy, seizures		LEMS: ~50%	Small-cell lung cancer
LGI-1 and CASPR2 double negative VGKC complex	Variable, including dementia and pain syndromes	Cell-based assay		Variable
Extracellular location of antigens				
LGI-1	Limbic encephalitis, faciobrachial dystonic seizures, REM sleep behaviour disorder, myoclonus, hyponatremia	Cell-based assay	<~10%	Small-cell lung cancer, thymoma

Adapted from: Bradshaw MJ, 2018
AChR acetylcholine receptors, *ADEM* acute disseminated encephalomyelitis, *AGNA* antiglial nuclear antibody, *AMPAR* α-amino-3-hydroxy-5-methyl-4-isoxazolepropionic acid receptor, *ANNA* antineuronal nuclear antibody, *AQP4* aquaporin-4, *CASPR2* contactin-associated protein-like-2, *CNS* central nervous system, *CRMP-5* collapsing response mediator protein-5, *DNER* delta/notch-like epidermal growth factor-related receptor, *DPPX* dipeptidyl-peptidase-like protein-6, *EEG* electroencephalography, *GAB_AR* gamma-amino-butyric acid receptor, *GAD-65* glutamic acid decarboxylase, *GluN1* ionotropic NMDA glutamate receptor 1, *GlyαR* glycine α-receptor, *IgLON5* immunoglobulin-like family member 5, *LEMS* Lambert-Eaton myasthenic syndrome, *LGI-1* leucine-rich, glioma-inactivated 1, *mGluR* metabotropic glutamate receptor, *MOG* myelin oligodendrocyte glycoprotein spectrum disorder, *NMDAR* N-methyl-D-aspartic acid receptor, *NMOSD* neuromyelitis optica, *PCA* Purkinje cell cytoplasmic antibody, *PERM* progressive encephalomyelitis with rigidity and myoclonus, *REM* rapid eye movement, *VGCC* voltage-gated calcium channel, *VGKC* voltage-gated potassium channel complex, *SOX1* sex-determining region Y box 1 transcription factor, *ZIC* zinc finger protein

23.4 Clinical Manifestations

Approach to a patient with autoimmune encephalitis: A patient with rapidly progressive behavioural, cognitive disorder is suspected to have autoimmune encephalitis if the patient fulfils the criteria as mentioned in Table 23.1. Cognitive dysfunction refers to the inability to form new, long-term memory or executive dysfunction associated with psychiatric features and a depressed level of consciousness. If a patient has rapid progressive clinical symptoms with no evidence of positive antibodies or an MRI brain that is non-contributory, then the patient can be given a trial of immunomodulation therapy, as delayed diagnosis and treatment have poor long-term prognosis. Few of the salient features observed in various AIE (Table 23.2) are:

(a) **Anti-NMDAR encephalitis**: is one of the most common causes of AIE that predominantly affects children and young female patients. The clinical features can be divided into following stages:

1. Prodromal features associated with fever and headache.
2. Early stage: characterised by behavioural changes in the form of psychosis, confusion, amnesia and speech disturbances (mutism), seizures which may be focal, generalised or progress to status epilepticus.
3. Late stage: evolves over 1–2 weeks which is characterised by movement disorders (choreoathetosis, stereotypy, orofacial dyskinesias and dystonia), autonomic dysfunction, encephalopathy, catatonia, hyperhidrosis, hyperthermia, BP fluctuations, with hypoventilation. Some patients may develop mutism and catatonia.

There are underlying malignancies associated mainly in patients of age range 12–45 years; ovarian teratomas are the most common (94%), followed by extraovarian teratomas (2%) and other malignancies (4%): Hodgkin's lymphoma, small-cell lung, pancreatic, and breast cancer [12]. Apart from these, few viruses (herpes simplex virus-1 encephalitis—HSV; Japanese encephalitis—JE) are known to trigger anti-NMDAR encephalitis.

The MRI brain of an AIE is usually normal. Abnormal findings may be seen in nearly 30% of the patients, which involve the temporal lobe, cortical, subcortical and basal ganglia regions. CSF may show mild-to-moderate lymphocytic pleocytosis. The diagnosis of anti-NMDAR is established by the detection of serum and CSF antibodies against the GluN1 subunit of NMDAR. Serum may be falsely negative in around 14% of patients. EEG may show background slowing. Few patients may show extreme delta brush pattern (Fig. 23.1), which consists of superimposed beta fast activity on delta waves [13].

(b) **Anti-LGI1 and anti-CASPR2 encephalitis—Formerly these formed the VGKC-Complex antibodies**-*mediated encephalitis*: Initial description of anti-VGKC antibodies was described in patients with neuromyotonia, limbic encephalitis etc. Eventually, the anti-VGKC antibodies have been found to be directed against proteins that form a complex with leucine-rich glioma-inactivated 1 (LGI1) and contactin-associated protein-like 2 (CASPR-2). Each of these antibody subtypes presents with specific clinical syndrome [10]. Patients with LGI1 encephalitis present with seizures, limbic encephalitis, faciobrachial dystonic seizures, hyponatremia (60%) and rapid eye movement behavioural abnormalities. These symptoms are most common in elderly males; paraneoplastic aetiology is found in very few patients, and most common tumour is small-cell lung carcinoma. MRI brain shows abnormalities in 40% of patients with changes involving the medial temporal lobe. Relapse occurs in 20% of subjects.

Anti-CASPR2 encephalitis presents with peripheral and central nerve hyperexcitability with symptoms of fasciculations, myokymia, insomnia, autonomic dysfunction, behavioural changes, anxiety, panic attacks and neuropathic pain. This disorder is most common in males, and nearly 30% of them can have malignancy affecting the thymus, lung or endometrium [10].

(c) **Anti-AMPAR encephalitis**: This is common in elderly females; they present with features of limbic encephalitis with prominent psychiatric disturbances. Few may also have clinical features of extrapyramidal and sleep disturbances. Paraneoplastic aetiology affecting the thymus, lung, ovary or breast is common in 65–70%.

(d) **Anti-GABA-A receptor encephalitis**: Refractory seizures, or status epilepticus, along with mild encephalopathy, are the usual presentation of this encephalitis. Less than 27% of them are associated with malignancy.

(e) *Anti-GABA-B receptor encephalitis*: This presents with limbic encephalitis, seizures, ataxia and myoclonus. Nearly 50% of them are paraneoplastic affecting the lungs.

(f) *Anti-GAD (GAD65 & GAD67)*: They can occur alone or in association with other antibodies such as $GABA_AR$ and Glycine receptor (GlyR). They have been associated with various autoimmune disorders which include insulin-dependent diabetes mellitus, thyroiditis and other systemic autoimmune disorders. Stiff-person syndrome, cerebellar ataxia, epilepsy and limbic encephalitis are the main neurological syndromes associated with anti-GAD antibodies. There are rarely paraneoplastic.

(g) *Anti-GlyR encephalitis*: Glycine receptors are chloride channels that facilitate inhibitory neurotransmission in the central nervous system. They have been associated with patients with progressive encephalomyelitis with rigidity and myoclonus (PERM), stiff-person syndrome, cerebellar ataxia, muscle stiffness, hyperactive startle responses and limb spasms. They have been detected in few patients of optic neuritis and multiple sclerosis; however, their clinical significance remains unclear. These antibodies are usually not associated with tumours.

(h) *Anti-DPPX encephalitis*: Dipeptidyl peptidase-like protein 6 (DPPX) is a subunit of Kv4.2 potassium channels expressed in the brain (hippocampus, cerebellum, striatum) and gut (myenteric plexus). Patients usually present with severe diarrhoea, followed by neuropsychiatric manifestations (confusion and agitation), seizures, myoclonic jerks, tremor, startle response and stiff-person syndrome. In addition, features of dysautonomia such as arrhythmias, thermodysregulation, diaphoresis, urinary symptoms and sleep disorders can be associated.

(i) *Encephalopathy associated with anti-IgLON5 antibodies*: The IgLON family member 5 (IgLON5) is a neuronal cell adhesion molecule of the immunoglobulin superfamily. Common presentations are sleep disorders like non-REM (rapid eye movement) and REM parasomnia, obstructive sleep apnoea, stridor, and episodic central hypoventilation, cognitive impairment, limb ataxia, chorea, dysarthria, dysphagia, dysautonomia and supranuclear gaze palsy. They have a similar clinical presentation as tauopathies such as progressive supranuclear palsy and frontotemporal dementia. They are also found to be associated with alleles HLA-DQB1*0501 and HLA-DRB1*1001, suggesting a genetic susceptibility. Investigations such as MRI brain, EEG, and CSF studies and electromyography are usually normal. Clinical deterioration is usually rapid, and response to immunotherapy is still in debate. Death usually occurs due to dysautonomia.

(j) *Anti-mGluR1 and anti-mGluR5 encephalitis*: Metabotropic glutamate receptor 1 (mGluR1) and metabotropic glutamate receptor 5 (mGluR5) are both G-protein-coupled receptors that are involved in modulating synaptic functions including long-term depression. Anti-mGluR1 antibodies are found in association with ataxia, diplopia, dysgeusia, paranoia and cognitive deficits. Haematologic malignancies and prostate adenocarcinoma are common tumours associated. Response to immunomodulation therapy is variable. Patients with anti-mGluR5-abs encephalitis may present with memory loss and psychosis in association with Hodgkin's lymphoma, which is called "Ophelia syndrome".

(k) *Hashimoto's encephalopathy:* It is a steroid-responsive encephalopathy characterised by fluctuating or progressive encephalopathy, myoclonus, seizures and stroke. Patients have elevated antibodies, such as antithyroid peroxidase antibodies (antithyroid microsomal antibodies) and antithyroglobulin antibodies.

23.5 Diagnosis

23.5.1 Electroencephalography (EEG)

Abnormalities on EEG are usually non-specific. It helps in the diagnosis of subclinical seizures or status epilepticus. Few of the EEG changes observed are:

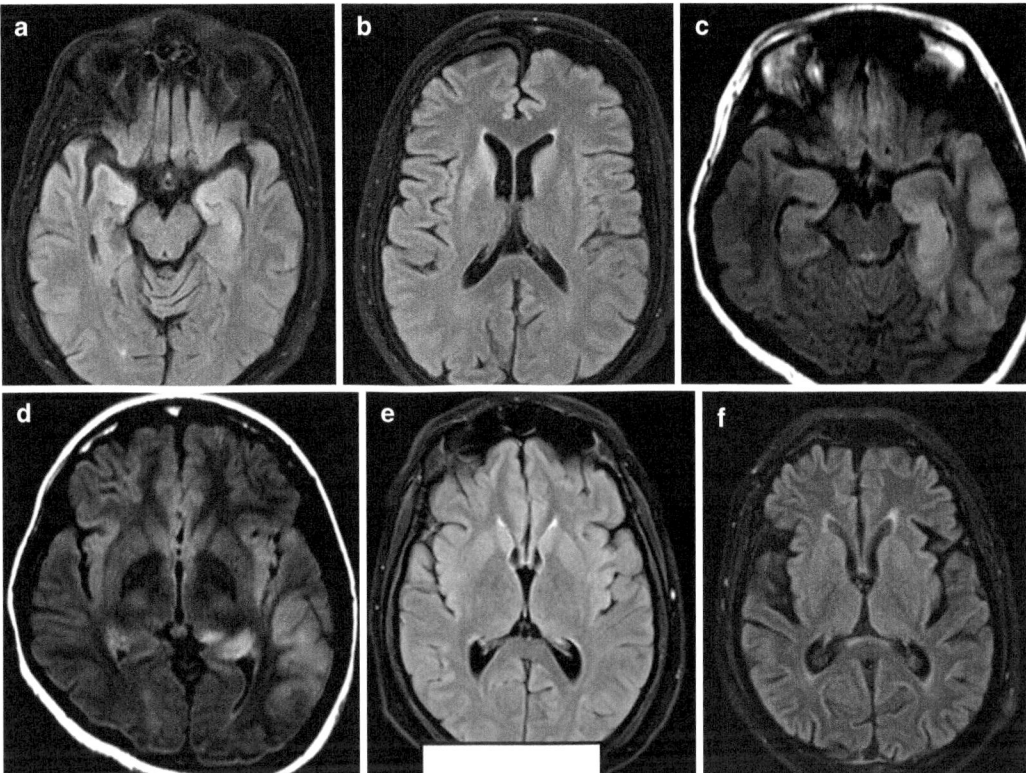

Fig. 23.2 MRI brain showing (**a**) flair sequence showing medial temporal hyperintensities in patient with anti-VGKC antibodies. (**b**) Flair sequence showing bilateral caudate (Rt > Lt) and right putamen hyperintensities in a patient with anti-VGKC antibodies. (**c**) Flair hyperintensities in bilateral (Lt > Rt) medial and lateral temporal lobes in a patient with anti-NMDA antibodies which were triggered by HSV. (**d**) Flair hyperintensities involving left temporal cortex, left thalamus and bilateral insular regions in a patient with anti-NMDA antibodies. (**e**) Normal MRI brain in a patient with anti-GAD antibody. (**f**) Mild diffuse cerebral atrophy in a patient with Hashimoto's encephalopathy

1. Normal.
2. Diffuse or focal background slowing.
3. Delta brush pattern of 1–3 Hz delta activity with superimposed 20–30 Hz beta fast activity observed in 33% of NMDAR encephalitis (Fig. 23.1).
4. Electrodecremental slowing or slow frontal activity prior to the onset of faciobrachial dystonic seizures in LG1–1 encephalitis.
5. Focal or interictal epileptiform discharges.
6. Triphasic waves, especially in Hashimoto's encephalopathy.

23.5.2 Imaging

MRI brain (Fig. 23.2) can detect abnormalities such as mesial temporal T2 flair hyperintensities in few cases or can be normal. With delayed treatment, mesial temporal sclerosis or diffuse cerebral atrophy may be observed. PET MRI has been found to be more informative, showing abnormalities in 85% cases, while MRI brain shows abnormalities in 40% cases [5] (Fig. 23.2).

23.5.3 Cerebrospinal Fluid (CSF) Analysis

CSF analysis can show pleocytosis with increased protein and normal sugars. CSF studies can be normal, depending on when the CSF analysis is done. It has been found to show abnormalities in the initial peak period and return to normalcy with the progression of the disease. CSF IgG

Fig. 23.3 NMDA positivity: transfected cell showing granular cytoplasmic fluorescence

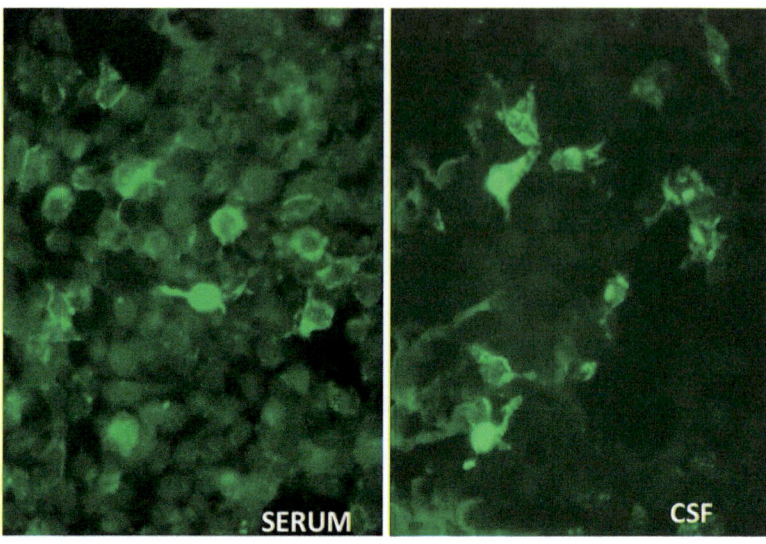

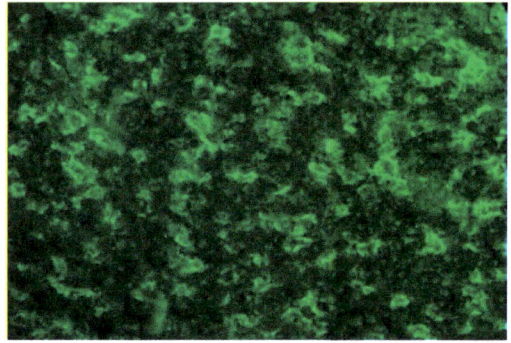

Fig. 23.4 GAD positivity: cerebellum section showing characteristic "leopard skin like" immunofluorescence of the granular layer with the patient's serum

index may be elevated, and there may be the presence of oligoclonal bands.

23.5.4 Autoantibody Test

Antibody testing can be performed based on the clinical suspicion, especially in resource-poor settings. It is preferable to test both serum and CSF for both autoimmune and paraneoplastic antibodies. Various antibody testing (Figs. 23.3 and 23.4) methods available include indirect tissue immunofluorescence, radiolabelled immunoprecipitation, immunoblotting, cell-based assays and flow cytometry assays. Positive antibody reports need to be interpreted cautiously, especially with low titres or multiple positive antibodies. The clinical syndrome, age, gender and positive antibody have to be taken into picture prior to further evaluation and treatment.

23.5.5 Investigating for Malignancy

Malignancy search should be guided based on the patient's age, gender, personal history, tobacco usage, personal/family history of malignancy and neural antibody. Combined PET/CT has a higher specificity in detecting malignancy, except in thymus, ovarian, testicular and few gastrointestinal malignancies during which ultrasound, MRI or duodenoscopy or colonoscopy assist in cancer detection.

23.6 Differential Diagnosis

Rapidly progressive neurological disorder such as those due to HIV, infections, syphilis, Creutzfeldt–Jakob disease and human herpes virus-6-associated encephalitis should be ruled out. The other differential diagnosis includes Hashimoto's and other steroid-responsive encephalopathies, acute disseminated encephalomyelitis, neuromyelitis optica spectrum disorders, vasculitis, lupus, angiocentric lymphoma and Rasmussen's encephalitis [10].

23.7 Treatment and Prognosis

Treatment should be initiated as soon as possible without any delay. Early immunotherapy and prevention of complications may result in complete reversibility of the neurological disorder. In the initial acute period patients need to be treated with intravenous methylprednisolone with or without plasmapheresis or IV immunoglobulin. The combination of steroids with plasmapheresis has been found to be more beneficial. Following these patients can be continued on oral steroids. Second immunomodulation will be required in the case of non-responders. The second immunotherapy includes azathioprine, mycophenolate, rituximab or cyclophosphamide. If the aetiological factor is an associated malignancy, then tumour resection or chemotherapy will be required. Good prognostic factors include early immunotherapy, non-requirement of intensive care and non-paraneoplastic aetiology.

References

1. Dale RC, Church AJ, Surtees RAJ, et al. Encephalitis lethargica syndrome: 20 new cases and evidence of basal ganglia autoimmunity. Brain. 2004;127(1):21–33.
2. Ramanathan S, Mohammad SS, Brilot F, Dale RC. Autoimmune encephalitis: recent updates and emerging challenges. J Clin Neurosci. 2014;21:722–30.
3. Graus F, Titulaer MJ, Balu R, Benseler S, Bien CG, Cellucci T, et al. A clinical approach to diagnosis of autoimmune encephalitis. Lancet Neurol. 2016;15(4):391–404.
4. Granerod J, Ambrose HE, Davies NW, et al. Causes of encephalitis and differences in their clinical presentations in England: a multicentre, population-based prospective study. Lancet Infect Dis. 2010;10:835–44.
5. Probasco JC, Solnes L, Nalluri A, et al. Abnormal brain metabolism on FDG-PET/CT is a common early finding in autoimmune encephalitis. Neurol Neuroimmunol Neuroinflamm. 2017;4(04):e352.
6. van Sonderen A, Roelen DL, Stoop JA, et al. Anti-LGI1 encephalitis is strongly associated with HLA-DR7 and HLA-DRB4. Ann Neurol. 2017;81:193–8.
7. Kim TJ, Lee ST, Moon J, et al. Anti-LGI1 encephalitis is associated with unique HLA subtypes. Ann Neurol. 2017;81:183–92.
8. Armangue T, Moris G, Cantarín-Extremera V, et al. Autoimmune post-herpes simplex encephalitis of adults and teenagers. Neurology. 2015;85:1736–43.
9. Shaik RS, Netravathi M, Nitish LK, Mani RS, Shah P, Damodar T, Anita M, Pal PK. A rare case of Japanese encephalitis-induced anti-N-methyl-D-aspartate receptor encephalitis. Neurol India. 2018;66(5):1495–6.
10. Dutra LA, Abrantes F, Toso FF, Pedroso JL, Barsottini OGP, Hoftberger R. Autoimmune encephalitis: a review of diagnosis and treatment. Arq Neuropsiquiatr. 2018;76(1):41–9.
11. Bradshaw MJ, Linnoila JJ. An overview of autoimmune and paraneoplastic encephalitides. Semin Neurol. 2018;38:330–43.
12. Khadilkar S, Soni G, Patil S, Huchche A, Faldu H. Autoimmune encephalitis: an update. J Assoc Physicians India. 2017;65(2):62–9.
13. Kamble N, Netravathi M, Saini J, Mahadevan A, Yadav R, Nalini A, Pal PK, Satishchandra P. Clinical and imaging characteristics of 16 patients with autoimmune neuronal synaptic encephalitis. Neurol India. 2015;63(5):687–96.

Part VI

Movement Disorders

Shweta Prasad and Pramod Kumar Pal

Case Discussion

A 60-year-old man presented with a 2-year history of progressive difficulty in walking, with occasional unprovoked falls, especially in the backward direction which occurred while walking, sitting without support and getting up from a chair. Family members reported a constant staring expression, reduced volume and output of speech, and change in behaviour—disinterest in routine activities and occasional inappropriate laughing or crying. There was no history of tremor. There was also a history of occasional difficulty swallowing liquids, choking, and spillage of food while eating. There was no family history of Parkinsonism. Though the patient was started on dopaminergic medications, there was no significant improvement.

On examination the patient had a staring expression with reduced blink rate. Speech was hypophonic and dysarthric. There was supranuclear vertical gaze palsy (both upward and downward) with a slowing of vertical and horizontal saccades. Rigidity was symmetrical, and the axial rigidity was disproportionate greater than limb rigidity. Bradykinesia was moderate and bilaterally symmetrical. There was no apraxia or myoclonus. Motor perseveration was observed. Frontal release signs, i.e., the palmomental reflex and rooting, were present, and deep tendon reflexes were brisk. Upon being asked to stand, the patient stood up rapidly from the chair and displayed significant imbalance. The patient walked with a broad-based lurching gait, and the pull test was positive.

Magnetic resonance imaging of the brain revealed significant midbrain atrophy, and the "humming bird" and "morning glory" signs were observed.

24.1 Introduction

Progressive supranuclear palsy (PSP) or Steele–Richardson–Olszewski syndrome, first described in 1964 [1], is an atypical Parkinsonian disorder and the second most common form of neurodegenerative Parkinsonism. It is the most common primary tauopathy and belongs to the family of 4R tauopathies [2]. At present, there are 10 clinical phenotypes [3] of PSP, and the classical variant of PSP, i.e., PSP-Richardson syndrome (PSP-RS), has a prevalence of 5–7 per 100,000 [4]. The mean age of onset of PSP is usually

S. Prasad
Department of Neuroimaging and Interventional Radiology, National Institute of Mental Health and Neurosciences (NIMHANS), Bangalore, Karnataka, India

Department of Neurology, National Institute of Mental Health and Neurosciences (NIMHANS), Bangalore, Karnataka, India

P. K. Pal (✉)
Department of Neurology, National Institute of Mental Health and Neurosciences (NIMHANS), Bangalore, Karnataka, India

© Springer Nature Singapore Pte Ltd. 2024
K. K. Oli et al. (eds.), *Case-based Approach to Common Neurological Disorders*,
https://doi.org/10.1007/978-981-99-8676-7_24

66.4 ± 12 years, with an average life span of 7 ± 3.7 years after the onset of symptoms [5]. The clinical phenotypes of PSP-Parkinsonism (PSP-P) and PSP-pure akinesia with gait freezing (PSP-PAGF) have relatively benign courses with a survival period of more than a decade [6]. Patients with PSP-RS typically present with progressive postural instability with falls, supranuclear vertical gaze palsy, pseudobulbar palsy, levodopa-unresponsive Parkinsonism and frontal cognitive disturbances [1, 7]. Until recently, the clinical criteria from the National Institute of Neurological Disorders and Stroke and the society for PSP (NINDS-SPSP) were the most widely used diagnostic criteria [7]. The International Parkinson and Movement Disorder Society (MDS) PSP study group published the MDS-PSP criteria in 2017 to include the wide spectrum of clinical phenotypes observed in PSP [8].

24.2 Aetiopathogenesis

24.2.1 Aetiology

The exact aetiology of PSP is uncertain, and several genetic factors, environmental factors and mitochondrial dysfunction have been implicated.

24.2.1.1 Genetics

Genome-wide association studies (GWAS) have reported several genes associated with PSP. The most common risk allele for PSP is the H1 haplotype of the MAPT gene, which encodes for tau [8]. This haplotype was observed in over 90% of patients with PSP. Three additional genes which were found to be associated with a risk of developing PSP are EIF2AK3 (eukaryotic translation factor 2-α kinase 3), STX6 (syntaxin-6) and MOBP (myelin-associated oligodendrocyte basic protein) [8].

24.2.1.2 Environmental Factors and Mitochondrial Dysfunction

A possible role of complex I inhibition in the aetiology of PSP was suggested based on the consumption of a tropical fruit containing annon-acin (a complex I inhibitor) and a higher prevalence of PSP [9]. Chronic administration of rotenone, a natural complex I inhibitor, to rats produced a neurodegeneration pattern similar to PSP [10]. Hence, experimental and clinical data suggest that complex I inhibition may play a role in the pathogenesis of PSP.

24.2.2 Neuropathology

PSP is the most common primary tauopathy and belongs to the family of 4R tauopathies, implying the accumulation of the tau isoform with four repeats in the microtubule binding domain [2]. The pathology is characterised by neuronal loss, gliosis and tau accumulation in the basal ganglia and brainstem. The tau accumulations are best observed with Gallyas silver stain or tau immunohistochemistry. Globose neurofibrillary tangles (NFTs) are observed in the nucleus basalis of Meynert and brainstem nuclei, whereas flame-shaped nuclei are observed in other regions. The characteristic neuropathological lesions in PSP are tufted astrocytes, which are densely packed tau-positive fibres located close to the centre of an astrocyte [11]. The pathological diagnostic criteria require the presence of NFTs and neuropil threads in the pallidum, subthalamic nucleus, substantia nigra, pons (at least three locations) and low-to-high density of neuropil threads or NFTs in other locations [11].

24.3 Clinical Features

PSP has a wide phenotypic spectrum, and the classical PSP phenotype, i.e., PSP-RS, is characterised by symmetric axial Parkinsonism, postural instability with early falls, vertical supranuclear gaze palsy and a frontal-subcortical dementia. The initial signs in PSP are often vague and non-specific. Patients may complain of clumsiness, unsteadiness, difficulty walking, unprovoked falls or visual symptoms. Family members may report softening of speech, depression, irritability, apathy or introversion. A correct diagnosis of PSP may often be delayed to 3–4 years after symptom onset [12, 13]. The symptoms described below are commonly observed in the PSP-RS phenotype. The clinical features of other PSP phenotypes are briefly described in Table 24.1.

Table 24.1 Key features of the clinical phenotypes of progressive supranuclear palsy [3]

Phenotype	Key clinical feature
PSP-Richardson's syndrome	Early-onset postural instability and falls
	Vertical ocular motor dysfunction
PSP-Parkinsonism	Initially resembles Parkinson's disease and progresses to develop symptoms of PSP-RS
	Levodopa responsive in the early stages
PSP-pure akinesia with gait freezing	Present as an isolated gait disorder with start (PSP-progressive gait freezing) hesitation and progressive freezing of gait
PSP-corticobasal syndrome	Progressive asymmetric limb dysfunction—limb apraxia, parietal sensory impairment, dystonia, myoclonus, levodopa-unresponsive rigidity, bradykinesia and occasionally alien limb phenomenon
	Postural instability and supranuclear downward gaze palsy
PSP-progressive non-fluent aphasia (PSP-speech/language disorder)	Progressive apraxia of speech, non-fluent/agrammatic primary progressive aphasia
PSP-behavioural variant of FTD (PSP-frontal)	Frontal cognitive or behavioural presentation
PSP-postural instability	Predominant postural instability
PSP-with predominant cerebellar ataxia (PSP-cerebellar ataxia)	Patients present with cerebellar ataxia as the initial and predominant symptom
PSP-postural instability	Predominant postural instability
PSP-ocular motor	Predominant ocular motor dysfunction

FTD fronto-temporal dementia, *PSP* progressive supranuclear palsy

24.3.1 Motor Symptoms

24.3.1.1 Postural Instability and Falls

Postural instability manifesting as falls within the first year of symptom onset is the most frequent symptom at presentation in PSP [12, 14]. In the NINDS study, 96% of patients with PSP had a history of postural instability and falls at the first visit to a specialised neurology clinic [14]. Patients walk with a broad-based lurching gait, resembling that of a drunken sailor or a dancing bear, and often tend to pivot on one foot when turning, which further compromises balance. Although backward falls are common in PSP, they may occur in any direction. As the disease progresses, gait ignition failure and freezing are commonly observed. Axial rigidity, oculomotor abnormalities and motor recklessness secondary to frontal lobe dysfunction contribute to falls [15].

24.3.1.2 Extrapyramidal Signs

Bradykinesia and rigidity are often absent in the early stages of the PSP-RS phenotype and develop as the disease progresses [1]. In the NINDS study, at the first visit to a specialised neurology clinic, 63% had axial (neck) rigidity and 88% had bilateral bradykinesia. Patients with PSP exhibit axial rigidity which is disproportionate to limb rigidity. This often leads to an upright extended posture, and occasionally retrocollis may be observed. Patients may report difficulty and clumsiness in fine finger movements. Repetitive finger tapping although hypokinetic does not show a decrement [16]. Handwriting is small and untidy, and "fast micrographia" may be observed in the PSP-PAGF subtype [16, 17].

24.3.2 Ocular Motor Abnormalities

The classical supranuclear gaze palsy associated with PSP-RS develops over the course of the disease, and the early ophthalmologic features are non-specific. The eye movement abnormalities observed in PSP vary based on the stage of the disease. Patients may complain of blurred vision, diplopia, dry eyes, photophobia, and difficulty focusing during the early stages. Occasionally, observant patients may report difficulty ascending or descending stairs or looking down at a plate of food while eating. As the disease progresses patients tend to lose the ability to read due to abnormalities in generating saccades.

24.3.2.1 Early Stage

1. Hypometric and slow saccades: Prior to a reduction in the range of vertical gaze, slowing of the vertical saccades are observed in PSP. Slowing of downward saccade is highly suggestive of PSP [18]. Additionally, the trajectory of vertical saccades may be curved or oblique ("round the houses" sign) [19].
2. Abnormal downward optokinetic nystagmus.
3. Square-wave jerks.
4. Impaired convergence, accommodation reflex and slowing of the quick phase of optokinetic or caloric-induced nystagmus [20].

24.3.2.2 Middle Stage

1. Supranuclear vertical gaze palsy.
2. Reduced blink rate with lid retraction (Collier's sign).
3. Apraxia of eyelid opening or closing.
4. Impairment of anti-saccade task [21].

24.3.2.3 Late Stage

1. The reduction of vertical and horizontal eye movements eventually leading to complete ophthalmoplegia.
2. Blepharospasm.
3. Loss of oculocephalic reflex.
4. Dysconjugate gaze.

The combination of a markedly reduced blink rate, ophthalmoplegia and focal dystonia of the procerus (procerus sign) leads to the characteristic astonished and worried facial expression observed in PSP.

24.3.3 Behavioural and Cognitive Features

Frontal lobe abnormalities are consistently observed in PSP and manifest early in course of the disease. Apathy, behavioural changes and difficulty planning routine activities may be early features. Disinhibition with emotional lability—inappropriate, uncontrollable laughter or crying, and anger outbursts—is frequently observed. Patients with PSP demonstrate a subcortical-type dementia with slowing of information processing, motor execution and executive dysfunction. Executive dysfunction observed in PSP comprises difficulties in motor sequencing, problem-solving, abstract thinking, shifting mental sets and sorting [22].

Frontal release signs such as rooting, sucking, grasping and palmomental reflexes can be elicited. Echolalia, echopraxia, reduced verbal fluency and motor perseveration ("applause sign") are often present [23]. Patients frequently demonstrate motor recklessness and tend to rapidly rise out of chairs ("rocket sign") without paying heed to the presence of balance impairment [23].

24.3.4 Speech, Swallowing and Other Neurological Signs

Patients with PSP classically have hypokinetic-spastic dysarthria. Although hypophonia may be prominent early in the disease, a slow slurred growling speech is commonly observed [24]. Swallowing disturbances and severe sialorrhoea occur early in the course of the disease. Drooling of saliva and down gaze palsy often lead to patients dropping food while eating and produces the "dirty tie" sign.

Brisk reflexes with a positive Babinski sign may be observed in one-fifth of patients with PD [5]. Although orthostatic hypotension is not observed in PSP, urinary disturbances, constipation and erectile dysfunction are commonly observed as the disease progresses. In comparison to Parkinson's disease, patients with PSP report a higher prevalence of non-motor symptoms in the domains of mood, attention, gastrointestinal and urinary disturbances [25]. Patients with PSP also have significant sleep abnormalities, including lower sleep efficiency, rapid eye movement (REM) sleep behaviour disorder and REM sleep without atonia [26].

24.4 Diagnostic Criteria

There are two main diagnostic criteria for the diagnosis of PSP—NINDS-SPSP criteria and the MDS-PSP criteria. The NINDS-SPSP criteria are the most widely used diagnostic criteria for PSP [7] (Table 24.2). Based on this, patients may be classified into clinically "possible" and clinically "probable" PSP. A diagnosis of definitive PSP

Table 24.2 NINDS-SPSP diagnostic criteria for PSP [7]

Clinically "possible" PSP
1. Gradually progressive illness
2. Age at onset: 40 years or older
3. No evidence of other disease that could explain the observed features
4. Vertical gaze palsy **OR** slowing of vertical saccades with postural instability and falls within the first year of illness
Clinically "probable" PSP
1. Gradually progressive illness
2. Age at onset: 40 years or older
3. No evidence of other diseases that could explain the observed features
4. Vertical gaze palsy **AND** slowing of vertical saccades with postural instability and falls within the first year of illness
"Definitive" PSP
1. Clinically "possible"/"probable" PSP
2. Histopathological confirmation
Supportive criteria
1. Symmetric akinesia or proximal > distal rigidity
2. Retrocollis
3. Early dysphagia and dysarthria
4. Poor response to levodopa
5. Early cognitive impairment
6. At least one of the following signs: apathy, frontal signs, abstract thought alterations, language alterations, imitation or utilisation behaviour
Mandatory exclusion criteria
1. Recent history of encephalitis
2. Alien limb syndrome, cortical sensory deficits, focal frontal or temporoparietal atrophy
3. Hallucinations or delusions unrelated to dopaminergic therapy
4. Cortical dementia of Alzheimer type
5. Prominent, early cerebellar signs
6. Unexplained dysautonomia
7. Severe asymmetric Parkinsonian signs
8. Imaging evidence of relevant structural abnormality
9. Whipple's disease

requires histological confirmation. However, this criterion is limited to the diagnosis of PSP-RS and does not provide guidelines for the other phenotypic presentations.

The recently introduced MDS-PSP criteria provide guidelines for the diagnosis of the clinical phenotypes of PSP [8]. Application of the MDS-PSP criteria requires assessment of the core features of ocular motor dysfunction, postural instability within 3 years, akinesia and cognitive dysfunction. The criteria describe levels of certainty or a predictive value for each core feature and provide specific combinations of these core features based on the clinical phenotype and the level of certainty [3].

24.5 Differential Diagnosis

Arriving at a diagnosis of PSP is relatively easy in the later stages of illness; however, several differential diagnoses may be considered in the early stages, where symptoms tend to be vague.

PSP should be differentiated from other neurodegenerative disorders, especially Parkinson's disease and other atypical Parkinsonian disorders such as multiple system atrophy, corticobasal degeneration and dementia with Lewy bodies [27, 28]. Although neuroimaging of the brain may aid in differentiating these disorders, several key clinical differences exist between these disorders (Table 24.3).

Apart from neurodegenerative disorders, several genetic, infective, acquired or drug-induced, vascular, structural, paraneoplastic and autoimmune disorders may mimic PSP [28].

24.6 Investigations

Although PSP is predominantly a clinical diagnosis, several abnormalities in brain neuroimaging have been proposed to be specific to PSP [29]. The most clinically useful MRI abnormalities are signs of midbrain atrophy, superior cerebellar peduncle atrophy, and frontal and parietal atrophy [29, 30]. The "humming bird sign", often known as "penguin sign" or "sil-

Table 24.3 Clinical features of atypical Parkinsonian disorders [27]

Characteristics	PSP	MSA	CBS	DLB
Postural instability and falls	Initial	Early	Present	Early
Oculomotor abnormalities	Vertical gaze palsy Slow vertical saccades	Square-wave jerks Nystagmus	Impaired horizontal and vertical saccades	Variable
Parkinsonism	Symmetric Axial >> distal	Asymmetric Distal > axial	Asymmetric	Asymmetric
Levodopa response	Poor to absent Initial response in PSP-P	Moderate in MSA-P	Variable Initial response may be present	Variable
Cognitive disturbances	Early	Late	Lateralised sensory or visual neglect, apraxia, aphasia	Early
	Severe frontal	Mild frontal		Cortical
Myoclonus	Absent	Present	Present—stimulus sensitive	Present
Dystonia	Retrocollis	Antecollis	Asymmetric—limbs	Present
Pyramidal signs	Late, bilateral	Early, bilateral	Asymmetric	Late, bilateral

CBS corticobasal syndrome, *DLB* dementia with Lewy bodies, *MSA* multiple system atrophy, *MSA-P* multiple system atrophy with predominant Parkinsonian features, *PSP* progressive supranuclear palsy

Fig. 24.1 (a) The "hummingbird sign" in PSP. Midsagittal section of the brainstem shows a concave superior border of the midbrain that is disproportionately atrophied in comparison to the pons. (b) The "morning glory sign" in PSP. Axial section of the midbrain shows concave lateral margins of the midbrain tegmentum

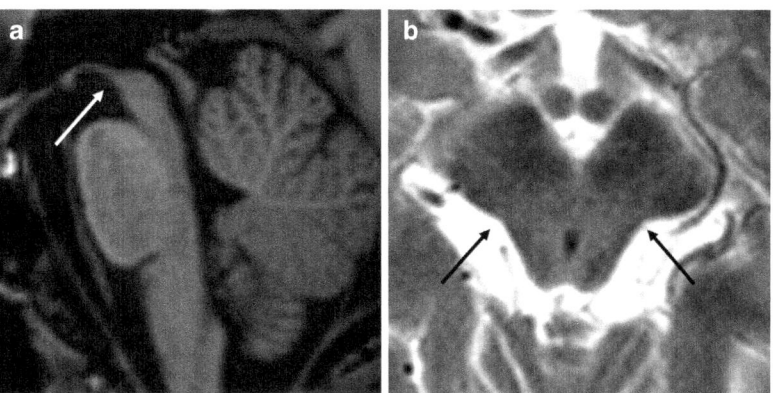

houette sign", and the "morning glory sign" are signs representing midbrain atrophy and are considered pathognomonic to PSP (Fig. 24.1) [31, 32]. Other structural imaging metrics such as the midbrain:pons ratio and magnetic resonance Parkinsonism index are also useful in differentiating PSP from other disorders [29].

The utility of functional imaging, dopamine transporter imaging, PET or SPECT in diagnosing PSP is debatable since all atypical Parkinsonian disorders tend to show abnormalities.

At present, apart from neuroimaging there are no specific diagnostic tools for PSP. Novel diagnostic approaches for PSP and biomarkers such as proteins in cerebrospinal fluid are still in the research phase [33].

24.7   Management

Currently there are no effective symptomatic or neuroprotective treatments for PSP [34]. The management of PSP with medication alone is unsatisfactory, and a multidisciplinary approach, involving speech therapy, physiotherapy and psychological counselling, is required to provide some benefit and improve the quality of life [27].

24.7.1 Medication

Dopaminergic Medication Levodopa provides negligible improvement in the Parkinsonism observed in PSP. Patients with the PSP-P variant are more likely to respond to levodopa, especially in the early stages of illness. Amantadine may be useful in improving gait and postural instability.

Antidepressants Selective serotonin receptor inhibitors and amitriptyline can be used in cases of apathy and depression and may help improve the pseudobulbar affect.

Others Benzodiazepines such as clonazepam may be given to improve the sleep disturbances commonly observed in PSP. Botulinum toxin injections are useful in patients with troublesome blepharospasm and retrocollis. There is emerging evidence of the utility of co-enzyme Q10 for neuroprotection in PSP.

24.7.2 Physical Therapy and Other Supportive Measures

Physiotherapy Gait and balance training exercises play a significant role in the management of PSP. Frequent falls add to the morbidity of the disease, and appropriate strategy training and gait aids may benefit patients.

Swallowing Evaluation Dysphagia is a major problem in PSP with significant weight loss and risk of aspiration as the disease progresses. Appropriate swallowing evaluation and interventions such as a feeding tube or gastrostomy should be considered to maintain adequate nutrition and avoid complications.

24.8   Conclusion

Progressive Supranuclear Palsy is an atypical parkinsonian disorder and a tauopathy which is characterised by symmetric parkinsonism, supranuclear palsy of vertical gaze, early postural instability with falls backwards, subcortical dementia, dysarthria, and dysphagia. There are no specific diagnostic tools or biomarkers and diagnosis requires good clinical acumen. Treatment is predominantly supportive and symptomatic with an aim to reduce morbidity and improve quality of life. However, all patients should receive a trial of dopaminergic medications.

References

1. Steele JC, Richardson JC, Olszewski J. Progressive supranuclear palsy. A heterogeneous degeneration involving the brain stem, basal ganglia and cerebellum with vertical gaze and pseudobulbar palsy, nuchal dystonia and dementia. Arch Neurol. 1964;10:333–59.
2. Dickson DW, Ahmed Z, Algom AA, Tsuboi Y, Josephs KA. Neuropathology of variants of progressive supranuclear palsy. Curr Opin Neurol. 2010;23(4):394–400.
3. Armstrong MJ. Progressive supranuclear palsy: an update. Curr Neurol Neurosci Rep. 2018;18(3):12.
4. Coyle-Gilchrist IT, Dick KM, Patterson K, et al. Prevalence, characteristics, and survival of frontotemporal lobar degeneration syndromes. Neurology. 2016;86(18):1736–43.
5. Williams DR, de Silva R, Paviour DC, et al. Characteristics of two distinct clinical phenotypes in pathologically proven progressive supranuclear palsy: Richardson's syndrome and PSP-Parkinsonism. Brain. 2005;128(Pt 6):1247–58.
6. Williams DR, Lees AJ. Progressive supranuclear palsy: clinicopathological concepts and diagnostic challenges. Lancet Neurol. 2009;8(3):270–9.
7. Litvan I, Agid Y, Calne D, et al. Clinical research criteria for the diagnosis of progressive supranuclear palsy (Steele–Richardson–Olszewski syndrome): report of the NINDS-SPSP international workshop. Neurology. 1996;47(1):1–9.
8. Hoglinger GU, Melhem NM, Dickson DW, et al. Identification of common variants influencing risk of the tauopathy progressive supranuclear palsy. Nat Genet. 2011;43(7):699–705.
9. Lannuzel A, Michel PP, Caparros-Lefebvre D, et al. Toxicity of Annonaceae for dopaminergic neurons: potential role in atypical Parkinsonism in Guadeloupe. Mov Disord. 2002;17(1):84–90.
10. Hoglinger GU, Lannuzel A, Khondiker ME, et al. The mitochondrial complex I inhibitor rotenone triggers a cerebral tauopathy. J Neurochem. 2005;95(4):930–9.
11. Litvan I, Hauw JJ, Bartko JJ, et al. Validity and reliability of the preliminary NINDS neuropathologic criteria for progressive supranuclear palsy and related disorders. J Neuropathol Exp Neurol. 1996;55(1):97–105.
12. Maher ER, Lees AJ. The clinical features and natural history of the Steele–Richardson–Olszewski syndrome (progressive supranuclear palsy). Neurology. 1986;36(7):1005–8.
13. Golbe LI, Davis PH, Schoenberg BS, Duvoisin RC. Prevalence and natural history of progressive supranuclear palsy. Neurology. 1988;38(7):1031–4.
14. Litvan I, Mangone CA, McKee A, et al. Natural history of progressive supranuclear palsy (Steele–Richardson–Olszewski syndrome) and clinical predictors of survival: a clinicopathological study. J Neurol Neurosurg Psychiatry. 1996;60(6):615–20.
15. Ling H. Clinical approach to progressive supranuclear palsy. J Mov Disord. 2016;9(1):3–13.
16. Ling H, Massey LA, Lees AJ, Brown P, Day BL. Hypokinesia without decrement distinguishes progressive supranuclear palsy from Parkinson's disease. Brain. 2012;135(Pt 4):1141–53.
17. Niall Q, Mikko K. Fast micrographia and pallidal pathology. Mov Disord. 2003;18(9):1067–9.
18. Rivaud-Pechoux S, Vidailhet M, Gallouedec G, et al. Longitudinal ocular motor study in corticobasal degeneration and progressive supranuclear palsy. Neurology. 2000;54(5):1029–32.
19. Quinn N. The "round the houses" sign in progressive supranuclear palsy. Ann Neurol. 1996;40(6):951.
20. Troost BT, Daroff RB. The ocular motor defects in progressive supranuclear palsy. Ann Neurol. 1977;2(5):397–403.
21. Rafal RD, Posner MI, Friedman JH, Inhoff AW, Bernstein E. Orienting of visual attention in progressive supranuclear palsy. Brain. 1988;111(Pt 2):267–80.
22. Gerstenecker A, Mast B, Duff K, et al. Executive dysfunction is the primary cognitive impairment in progressive supranuclear palsy. Arch Clin Neuropsychol. 2013;28(2):104–13.
23. Litvan I. Cognitive disturbances in progressive supranuclear palsy. J Neural Transm Suppl. 1994;42:69–78.
24. Nath U, Ben-Shlomo Y, Thomson RG, Lees AJ, Burn DJ. Clinical features and natural history of progressive supranuclear palsy: a clinical cohort study. Neurology. 2003;60(6):910–6.
25. Radicati FG, Martinez Martin P, Fossati C, et al. Non motor symptoms in progressive supranuclear palsy: prevalence and severity. NPJ Parkinsons Dis. 2017;3:35.
26. Sixel-Doring F, Schweitzer M, Mollenhauer B, Trenkwalder C. Polysomnographic findings, video-based sleep analysis and sleep perception in progressive supranuclear palsy. Sleep Med. 2009;10(4):407–15.

27. Stamelou M, Bhatia KP. Atypical Parkinsonism: diagnosis and treatment. Neurol Clin. 2015;33(1):39–56.
28. Stamelou M, Quinn NP, Bhatia KP. "Atypical" atypical Parkinsonism: new genetic conditions presenting with features of progressive supranuclear palsy, corticobasal degeneration, or multiple system atrophy—a diagnostic guide. Mov Disord. 2013;28(9):1184–99.
29. Stezin A, Lenka A, Jhunjhunwala K, Saini J, Pal PK. Advanced structural neuroimaging in progressive supranuclear palsy: where do we stand? Parkinsonism Relat Disord. 2017;36:19–32.
30. Longoni G, Agosta F, Kostic VS, et al. MRI measurements of brainstem structures in patients with Richardson's syndrome, progressive supranuclear palsy-Parkinsonism, and Parkinson's disease. Mov Disord. 2011;26(2):247–55.
31. Kato N, Arai K, Hattori T. Study of the rostral midbrain atrophy in progressive supranuclear palsy. J Neurol Sci. 2003;210(1–2):57–60.
32. Adachi M, Kawanami T, Ohshima H, Sugai Y, Hosoya T. Morning glory sign: a particular MR finding in progressive supranuclear palsy. Magn Reson Med Sci. 2004;3(3):125–32.
33. Boxer AL, Yu JT, Golbe LI, et al. Advances in progressive supranuclear palsy: new diagnostic criteria, biomarkers, and therapeutic approaches. Lancet Neurol. 2017;16(7):552–63.
34. Stamelou M, de Silva R, Arias-Carrion O, et al. Rational therapeutic approaches to progressive supranuclear palsy. Brain. 2010;133(Pt 6):1578–90.

Multiple System Atrophy

25

Malligurki Raghurama Rukmani,
Talakad N. Sathyaprabha, and Ravi Yadav

Case Scenario A 59-year-old female was admitted in the neurology ward with complaints of difficulty in walking, recurrent falls, stiffness of whole body, slowness of activities of daily living, tremors of left lower limb, urge incontinence, postural giddiness, speech disturbance, constipation, and sleep disturbances for the past 2.5 years. She had become wheelchair bound within 2 years of disease onset. She had a history of difficulty initiating sleep, intermittent awakenings, violent dreams, and dream-enacting behavior such as speaking, shouting, laughing, sudden limb movements, and occasionally hitting the bed partner. She did not have any other significant medical or surgical history. She was born out of non-consanguineous marriage with a negative family history of similar illness. Her past treatment history revealed that she was initially diagnosed as having Parkinson's disease (PD) and was on 500 mg levodopa per day. She reported only 10–15% symptomatic improvement with levodopa.

On examination, she was alert, conscious, and oriented. Her MMSE score was 28/30. She had hypomimia. Her speech was slow and hypophonic. Examination of her cranial nerves was normal. Her pupils were bilaterally equal and reactive to light. She had gaze-evoked nystagmus at an eye position of more than 45°, slow saccades, jerky pursuit, and saccadic hypometria. She had slight and intermittent rest tremor of left lower limb, and postural and action tremor of bilateral upper limbs. Rigidity was present at rest in bilateral upper limbs, lower limbs, and neck. Severe bradykinesia was noted in bilateral upper limbs during finger taps, handgrips, hand pronation, and supination, and bilateral lower limbs during foot taps. She was unable to arise from chair without help. Her deep tendon reflexes were normal. She was able to walk with one person support with severely stooped posture, reduced gait speed, and reduced arm swing on both sides. There was no incoordination during the finger-nose test or knee-heel-shin test. Her bilateral plantar responses were flexor. Her bulk, tone, and power were normal in bilateral limbs. Her superficial sensation, joint and position sensation, and vibration sensation were normal. Her pulse was 80 beats/min. Her supine BP was 170/110 mmHg. Within 3 min of standing, there was 30/20 mmHg drop in BP. She was negative for HIV/HbsAg/HCV/VDRL. Her complete hemogram, liver function test, renal function test, and thyroid function tests were normal. Her paraneoplastic

M. R. Rukmani · T. N. Sathyaprabha
Department of Neurophysiology, National Institute of Mental Health and Neuro Sciences (NIMHANS), Bangalore, India

R. Yadav (✉)
Department of Neurology, National Institute of Mental Health and Neuro Sciences (NIMHANS), Bangalore, India

© Springer Nature Singapore Pte Ltd. 2024
K. K. Oli et al. (eds.), *Case-based Approach to Common Neurological Disorders*,
https://doi.org/10.1007/978-981-99-8676-7_25

panel was negative. The patient's MRI brain showed putaminal atrophy, diffuse pontocerebellar atrophy, and "hot cross bun sign" in pons. Tilt table test also showed orthostatic hypotension. Her ultrasound scanning of abdomen showed significant post-void residual volume of 90 mL. Levodopa off-state and on-state assessment did not show any significant improvement in UPDRS motor scores. A diagnosis of probable MSA-P was made. Levodopa drug dosage was adjusted. She was also advised clonazepam (0.5 mg at night) for RBD; tolterodine (2 mg o.i.d.) for urge incontinence; fludrocortisone (0.1 mg o.i.d.), increased fluid and salt intake, and elastic compression stockings for orthostatic hypotension; and increased insoluble fiber consumption for constipation. She was also referred to speech therapist, occupational therapist, physiotherapist, and psychiatric social worker.

25.1 Introduction

Multiple system atrophy (MSA) is an adult-onset, sporadic, and rapidly progressive neurodegenerative disorder. It manifests with a combination of symptoms such as parkinsonism, dysfunction of the autonomic system, impairment of the cerebellum, involvement of the pyramidal tract, and a poor response to medications targeting dopamine. The pathological features of MSA include the loss of cells, gliosis, and the presence of abnormal α-synuclein protein aggregates in oligodendroglia in various structures of the central nervous system. Clinically, MSA can be classified into two phenotypes based on the primary motor system affected: the parkinsonian variant (MSA-P) and the cerebellar variant (MSA-C) [1, 2].

The initial clinical observation of multiple system atrophy (MSA) was documented by Dejerine and Thomas in 1900. They provided a detailed account of two patients who exhibited sporadic ataxia in adulthood, along with extrapyramidal, urinary, and postural symptoms. Pathological examination indicated a potential condition known as "olivopontocerebellar atrophy." Later, in 1960, Shy and Drager identified a clinical syndrome characterized by autonomic failure, severe parkinsonism, and ataxic features, which became known as "Shy-Drager syndrome." In 1961, Adams et al. coined the term "striatonigral degeneration" to represent similar clinical picture. In 1969, Graham and Oppenheimer proposed to use the term "Multiple System Atrophy" to include the overlapping progressive pre-senile multisystem degenerations (olivopontocerebellar atrophy, Shy-Drager syndrome, and striatonigral degeneration) [1, 3, 4]. Research by Papp et al. led to the identification of glial cytoplasmic inclusion (Papp-Lantos bodies) in MSA, which was later confirmed by Spillantini et al. to contain α-synuclein protein. This evidence provided a pathological link between Parkinson's disease, dementia with Lewy bodies (DLB), and MSA, and the term α-synucleinopathies was coined [5, 6].

25.2 Epidemiology

MSA is a rare neurological disorder. The prevalence rate of MSA ranges between 1.9 and 4.9 per 100,000 [4]. Distribution of phenotypes suggest a predominance of MSA-P in Europe [7], North America [8, 9], and Korea [10], whereas MSA-C is more common in Japan [11, 12]. MSA affects both men and women equally. It generally starts in the sixth decade of life. Even environmental factor hasn't been known to impact the risk of MSA [7–12].

25.3 Pathology

From a pathological perspective, MSA is distinguished by the specific susceptibility of the striatonigral and olivopontocerebellar systems, as well as the autonomic nervous system.

25.3.1 Macroscopy

Upon visual examination, the brain affected by MSA may exhibit notable atrophy of the cerebellum, middle cerebellar peduncle, and pontine base. Additionally, mild diffuse cortical atrophy in the frontal lobes may be observed, while the overall weight of the brain typically remains unchanged. In individuals with MSA-P, significant atrophy and a darkened appearance of the putamen can be observed, with the most severe effects occurring posteriorly. Conversely, individuals with MSA-C tend to display pronounced cerebellar atrophy [4, 13, 14].

25.3.2 Histopathology

The key characteristics of MSA involve the selective neuronal loss and degeneration of axons. This is accompanied by distinctive cellular pathology characterized by the presence of α-synuclein immunoreactive inclusions. These inclusions primarily manifest as cytoplasmic inclusions in oligodendroglial cells, with less frequent occurrences in glial nuclei, neuronal cytoplasm, and neuronal nuclei. Additionally, astroglial cells exhibit similar cytoplasmic inclusions. Furthermore, observable effects include a reduction in myelin content, referred to as myelin pallor, accompanied by gliosis, which signifies the proliferation of glial cells [4, 13–16]. The degree of neuronal loss and cellular inclusions in different regions of the brain is related to MSA phenotype. The presence of argyrophilic, oligodendroglial cytoplasmic inclusions (OGCIs) is the histological hallmark of MSA. They are composed of α-synuclein and classical cytoskeletal antigens including ubiquitin, tau, and large number of multi-functional proteins [4, 13–17].

25.4   Pathogenesis

The specific process by which MSA develops is not fully understood. Recent research indicates that several factors may play a crucial role in the development of MSA, including increased production of α-synuclein in oligodendroglial cells, changes in the structure of proteins such as p25α that are specific to oligodendroglia, oxidative stress, malfunctioning mitochondria, excessive stimulation of neurons leading to cell damage (excitotoxicity), and neuroinflammation mediated by microglia [2, 4, 18]. The combined influence of various mechanisms can lead to the formation of abnormal clumps of α-synuclein in the brain of individuals with MSA. These aggregations of α-synuclein may then spread to other networks that are functionally connected, contributing to a distinct pattern of neurodegeneration specific to the affected system. However, the exact source of the abnormal α-synuclein in oligodendrocytes and the mechanisms through which it spreads are still not fully understood [2, 14, 18–20].

Despite being considered a non-heritable disorder, recent investigations into genetics have revealed that certain genetic factors might contribute to an elevated risk of developing MSA. Studies have identified that dysfunctional versions of the COQ2 gene are linked to a higher susceptibility for both familial and sporadic cases of MSA [21]. However, the genetic underpinnings of MSA remain largely elusive [4].

25.5   Clinical Manifestation

In clinical terms, MSA is distinguished by two primary motor manifestations: parkinsonism and cerebellar ataxia. These prominent motor symptoms are used to classify individuals with MSA into two subtypes: MSA-P (with predominant parkinsonism) and MSA-C (with predominant cerebellar ataxia). However, urogenital and cardiovascular dysautonomic symptoms, although less common, may occur initially in a small proportion of MSA patients (around 5–30%) [1, 2, 4, 7, 9].

Parkinsonism: Regardless of the phenotype, a significant majority of MSA patients (87–98%) will eventually develop parkinsonism over the course of the disease. Parkinsonism associated with MSA is typically characterized by symptoms such as akinesia, rigidity, and postural instability. In some MSA patients, the parkinsonism can exhibit varying degrees of asymmetry, similar to Parkinson's disease. Irregular and jerky postural tremors are commonly observed in MSA, while resting tremors are less common. Falls within the first year of the disease have been reported in approximately 20% of MSA cases.

MSA patients are generally considered unresponsive to levodopa, a common medication used in the treatment of Parkinson's disease. However, it is worth noting that up to 83% of MSA patients may initially show a positive response to dopaminergic medications. This initial benefit from dopaminergic treatment is transient and typically lasts for a short duration of less than 3 years.

Cerebellar Signs: A broad-based ataxic gait, limb kinetic ataxia, scanning dysarthria, intentional tremor, and cerebellar oculomotor abnormalities (gaze-evoked nystagmus, jerky pursuit, slow saccades, saccadic hypometria/hypermetria) are observed in MSA patients, predominantly in the MSA-C phenotype [1, 2, 4, 7, 9, 22].

Speech Impairment: Dysarthria is seen in early stages of both MSA phenotypes. MSA-C patients typically present with scanning dysarthria, while MSA-P patients present with hypophonic, high-pitched, quivery and croaky voice [1, 2, 4, 7, 9, 22].

25.6 Autonomic Dysfunction

- *Urogenital Dysfunction:* Erectile dysfunction, reduced genital sensitivity, increased urinary frequency, urgency, urge incontinence, and nocturia are the most common urogenital symptoms. Bladder disturbances may be the only dysautonomic complaint in 50% of the MSA patients [4, 22, 23].
- *Cardiovascular Autonomic Dysfunction:* MSA patients who experience orthostatic hypotension typically exhibit distinctive symptoms such as dizziness, blurred vision, weakness, palpitations, and recurrent episodes of fainting in response to sudden changes in posture or prolonged periods of standing. Additionally, MSA patients may also present with supine hypertension, nocturnal hypertension, and postprandial hypotension [1, 2, 4, 7, 9, 22–25].
- *Respiratory Dysfunction:* Respiratory dysfunction in MSA is characterized by various symptoms, including stridor (noisy breathing during inspiration), sleep-related breathing disorders, respiratory insufficiency of the pump failure type, and involuntary sighs. Inspiratory stridor, which is caused by vocal cord palsy, is considered a negative indicator of prognosis in MSA [4, 24, 26].
- *Gastrointestinal Dysfunction:* Chronic constipation is a major feature of lower gastrointestinal tract dysfunction and is observed in one-third of MSA cases. Anal sphincter denervation may lead to fecal incontinence in a small number of MSA patients [27]. Upper gastrointestinal tract dysfunction may cause mild-to-moderate dysphagia. Severe dysphagia is a poor prognostic predictor [28].
- *Dermatological Dysfunction:* Anhidrosis or hypohidrosis occurs frequently in MSA, possibly due to degeneration of the preganglionic sympathetic sweat fibers. Impaired vasomotor sympathetic skin response, skin temperature regulation, and heat tolerance are also observed in MSA. Cold hand sign, described as cold, dusky, violaceous hands with poor circulatory return after blanching, is also observed in MSA patients [24, 29].
- *Pupillomotor Dysfunction:* Pupillomotor abnormalities with accommodation difficulties and pupillary hypersensitivity to sympathomimetic agents may occur in MSA patients due to central noradrenergic failure [30].

25.6.1 Pyramidal Signs

Generalized hyperreflexia and a positive Babinski sign are documented in 30–50% of MSA patients, predominantly MSA-C cases. However, significant pyramidal weakness or overt spastic paraparetic gait does not support the diagnosis of MSA [4, 22].

25.6.2 Cognitive Dysfunction and Behavioral Disturbances

Overt dementia points against the diagnosis of MSA [24]. However, it does not imply that dementia does not occur in MSA. Overt dementia has been sporadically reported in pathologically proven MSA series [31]. Memory and attention deficits, visuospatial dysfunction, and executive dysfunction are the major cognitive domains affected in MSA [32, 33]. Emotional incontinence is reported in one-third of MSA patients [4, 22]. Depression and anxiety disorder are the most common psychiatric disorders in MSA [34].

25.6.3 Sleep Disturbances

Sleep quality is severely affected in individuals with MSA due to various disturbances, including REM behavior disorder (RBD), decreased and fragmented sleep, excessive daytime sleepiness, sleep-disordered breathing, and restless leg syndrome. RBD, in particular, has been observed in a high percentage of MSA cases, ranging from 90.5% to 100% [35, 36]. Other sleep-related symptoms include obstructive sleep apnea (40%), day time and nocturnal stridor (20–42%), and excessive daytime sleepiness (17–28%) [22, 37, 38].

25.6.4 Red Flags

The indicative symptoms or warning signs that suggest the presence of MSA include a rapid decline in clinical condition (referred to as the "wheelchair sign"), early onset of postural instability, stridor, involuntary deep sighs, bulbar dysfunction characterized by dysphonia, dysphagia, dysarthria, a phenomenon known as the "cold hand sign," and abnormal postures such as camptocormia, Pisa syndrome, disproportionate antecollis, and contractures of the hands and/or feet without evidence of arthritis-related deformities. The presence of these warning signs in a patient presenting with parkinsonism or ataxia can provide support for a diagnosis of MSA [4, 24].

25.7 Diagnosis

Diagnosing MSA poses significant challenges in neurology clinics. In the early stages, MSA-P can be difficult to differentiate from idiopathic Parkinson's disease (PD), while the clinical features of advanced MSA-P may overlap with those of progressive supranuclear palsy (PSP) or dementia with Lewy bodies (DLB). Similarly, the clinical presentation of MSA-C can resemble that of inherited ataxias or late-onset ataxia caused by acquired factors. The diagnosis of MSA primarily relies on a thorough medical history and a meticulous neurological examination.

25.7.1 Clinical Diagnostic Criteria

The second consensus statement of diagnosis of MSA is now considered the standard clinical diagnostic criteria. These criteria delineate clinical symptoms into definite, probable, and possible MSA [Tables 25.1 and 25.2]. They also provide a list of features supporting (red flags) and non-supporting the diagnosis of MSA [Table 25.3] [24].

Investigations are helpful to support the diagnosis of MSA, rule out the potential mimicking disorders, and design the treatment plan. These include structural and functional brain imaging, autonomic function tests, olfactory tests, and cognitive assessment [4, 24, 39].

25.7.2 Imaging

Imaging of the brain is included as supportive criteria and for ruling out other pathological conditions with similar presentation.

- *Magnetic Resonance Imaging:* MRI remains the gold standard imaging technique in MSA patients. MRI shows several abnormalities including atrophy of the putamen, middle cerebellar peduncles, cerebellum, medulla oblongata, pons and midbrain, as well as signal intensity alterations. Characteristic MRI signal intensity abnormalities in MSA brain include the "hot cross bun sign," a cruciform hypointensity in the pons [Fig. 25.1], and the "putaminal slit" sign, hyperintense signal in the dorsolateral margin of the putamen [Fig. 25.2]. Patients with early "hot cross bun sign" are more likely to develop severe cerebellar symptoms, while patients with early bilateral

Table 25.1 Second consensus criteria for the diagnosis of MSA (Reproduced from Gilman et al. 2008)

Criteria for the diagnosis of definite MSA

A sporadic, progressive, adult (>30 years) onset disease characterized by

- Neuropathologic findings of widespread and abundant CNS α-synuclein–positive glial cytoplasmic inclusions (Papp–Lantos inclusions) in association with neurodegenerative changes in striatonigral or olivopontocerebellar structures

Criteria for the diagnosis of probable MSA

A sporadic, progressive, adult (>30 years) onset disease characterized by

- Autonomic failure involving urinary incontinence (inability to control the release of urine from the bladder, with erectile dysfunction in males) or an orthostatic decrease of blood pressure within 3 min of standing by at least 30 mmHg systolic or 15 mmHg diastolic AND
- Poorly levodopa-responsive parkinsonism (bradykinesia with rigidity, tremor, or postural instability) OR
- A cerebellar syndrome (gait ataxia with cerebellar dysarthria, limb ataxia, or cerebellar oculomotor dysfunction)

Criteria for the diagnosis of possible MSA

A sporadic, progressive, adult (>30 years) onset disease characterized by

- Parkinsonism (bradykinesia with rigidity, tremor, or postural instability) OR
- A cerebellar syndrome (gait ataxia with cerebellar dysarthria, limb ataxia, or cerebellar oculomotor dysfunction) AND
- At least one feature suggesting autonomic dysfunction (otherwise unexplained urinary urgency, frequency, or incomplete bladder emptying, erectile dysfunction in males, or significant orthostatic blood pressure decline that does not meet the level required in probable MSA) AND
- At least one of the additional features specified in Table 25.2

9.9. 25.2 Additional features for possible MSA (Reproduced from Gilman et al. 2008)

Possible MSA-P or MSA-C

- Babinski sign with hyperreflexia
- Stridor

Possible MSA-P

- Rapidly progressive parkinsonism
- Poor response to levodopa
- Postural instability within 3 years of motor onset
- Gait ataxia, cerebellar dysarthria, limb ataxia, or cerebellar oculomotor dysfunction
- Dysphagia within 5 years of motor onset
- Atrophy on MRI of putamen, middle cerebellar peduncle, pons, or cerebellum
- Hypometabolism on FDG-PET (FDG: [18^F] fluorodeoxyglucose) in putamen, brainstem, or cerebellum

Possible MSA-C

- Parkinsonism (bradykinesia and rigidity)
- Atrophy on MRI of putamen, middle cerebellar peduncle, or pons
- Hypometabolism on FDG-PET (FDG: [18^F] fluorodeoxyglucose) in putamen
- Presynaptic nigrostriatal dopaminergic denervation in SPECT or PET

Table 25.3 Features supporting (red flags) and not supporting the diagnosis of MSA (Reproduced from Gilman et al. 2008)

Supporting features	Non-supporting features
- Orofacial dystonia	- Classic pill-rolling rest tremor
- Disproportionate antecollis	- Clinically significant neuropathy
- Camptocormia (severe anterior flexion of the spine) and/or Pisa syndrome (severe lateral flexion of the spine)	- Hallucinations not induced by drugs
	- Onset after the age of 75 years
- Contractures of hands or feet	- Family history of parkinsonism or ataxia
- Inspiratory sighs	- Dementia (on DSM-IV)
- Severe dysphonia	- White matter lesions suggesting multiple sclerosis
- Severe dysarthria	
- New or increased snoring	
- Cold hands and feet	
- Pathological laughter or crying	
- Jerky, myoclonic postural/action tremor	

putaminal rim sign are more likely to develop MSA-P. However, these signal changes can be seen in other conditions too. However, MRI has very low specificity to distinguish MSA from other atypical parkinsonian conditions [4, 24, 39]. Magnetic resonance volumetry may also be helpful in the differential diagnosis of MSA [39, 40]. These include the MR parkinsonism index [MRPI index = (pons/midbrain)*(middle cerebellar peduncle/superior cerebellar peduncle)], which seems to have high sensitivity and specificity to distinguish MSA-P from PD and PSP [41].

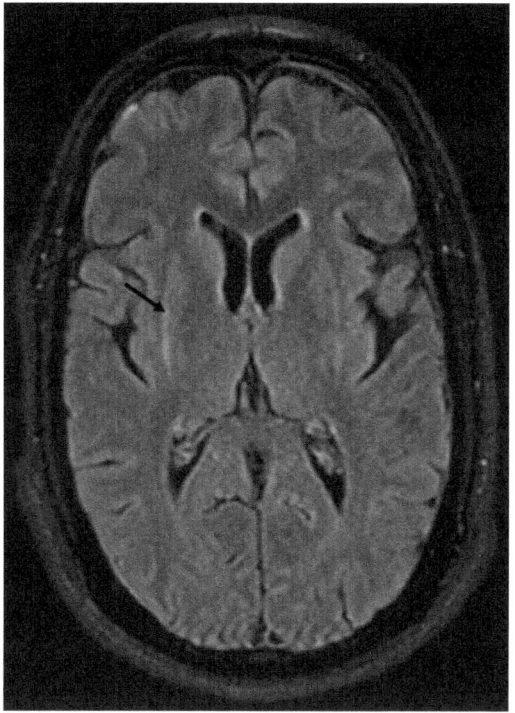

Fig. 25.1 T2 flair showing "putaminal slit" sign in MSA-P patient

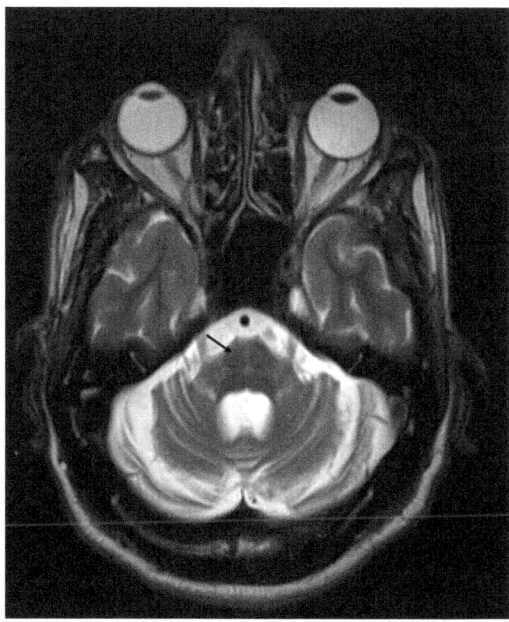

Fig. 25.2 T2 showing "hot cross bun" sign in MSA-C patient

- *Positron Emission Tomography:* ^{18}F-fluorodeoxyglucose positron emission tomography (FDG-PET) is being used to differentiate MSA from other mimicking conditions. FDG-PET has shown that glucose metabolic rates are decreased only in brainstem and cerebellum in sporadic cerebellar degeneration, while in MSA, there is reduced glucose metabolic rate in basal ganglia, thalamus, and cerebral cortex in addition to cerebellum and brainstem [42]. FDG-PET studies have shown that there is reduced striatal metabolism in MSA-P patients as compared to PD [43, 44]. It has a highly specific positive predictive value of 97% [45].

- *Single-Photon Emission Computed Tomography (SPECT):* Bosman et al. have reported that putaminal perfusion patterns are different in MSA as compared to PD using SPECT scan. However, the diagnostic accuracy is poor [46].

- *Dopaminergic Imaging:* Nuclear imaging techniques are being widely applied to assess presynaptic and postsynaptic dopaminergic neuronal function in parkinsonian disorders. ^{18}F-Dopa tracer is used to assess dopamine storage capacity, ^{11}C-dihydrotetrabenazine for vesicular monoamine transporter function, and ^{123}I-β-CIT and [123]IFPCIT for assessing dopamine transporter binding. Presynaptic dopaminergic metabolism may be useful to distinguish MSA-C from other adult-onset cerebellar ataxias. MSA patients also show a marked reduction in postsynaptic D2 receptor binding in the putamen as compared to PD. However, one has to be cautious in interpreting this because one-third of MSA patients show normal postsynaptic D2 receptor binding [4, 39, 47].

- *MIBG Scintigraphy:* ^{123}I-metaiodobenzylguanidine (MIBG) scintigraphy is employed to assess the cardiac sympathetic postganglionic innervation, which is modestly reduced in MSA and PSP. Neuroimaging evidence of intact cardiac sympathetic innervations almost certainly excludes PD, but neuroimaging evidence of cardiac sympathetic denervation does not exclude MSA [4, 39].

25.7.3 Cardiac Autonomic Function Tests

Orthostatic hypotension in MSA should be investigated first by recording supine blood pressure, followed by taking the BP after 3 min of standing in the neurology clinic. About 50% of MSA patients have delayed orthostatic hypotension, and tilt table test is advisable in most cases. Cardiac autonomic function tests including Ewing's protocol, heart rate variability, and tilt table testing have shown that cardiac autonomic dysfunction is more severe in MSA as compared to PD [4, 39]. The diagnostic gold standard to detect nocturnal hypertension in MSA patients is ambulatory 24-h BP monitoring (ABPM) [48].

25.7.4 Sudomotor Testing

Sudomotor function is assessed by thermoregulatory sweat test (TST) and the quantitative sudomotor axon reflex test. Thermoregulatory sweat test (TST) assesses the functional integrity of both preganglionic and postganglionic sudomotor pathways. Quantitative sudomotor axon reflex testing (QSART) evaluates the functional integrity of postganglionic sympathetic sudomotor axons. TST is abnormal in MSA patients, whereas QSART is normal in MSA as compared to PD [4]. However, recent studies have shown that QSART is also abnormal in 30% of MSA patients [49, 50]. Despite this, the exact diagnostic value of these tests needs further validation [4, 51].

25.7.5 Urological Evaluation

Ultrasound scanning with post-void residual volume assessment and routine urine analysis are advised in MSA [4]. Urodynamic studies are useful in determining the bladder abnormalities in MSA, such as detrusor underactivity, detrusor sphincter dyssynergia, and urethral hypertonia in the voiding phase, and inhibited external sphincter relaxation and bladder neck dysfunction in the filling phase [52]. To assess the functional capability of the external sphincter muscle, it is recommended to perform external sphincter electromyography (EMG), which involves measuring the electrical activity during both contraction and relaxation. In the majority of MSA patients, an abnormal sphincter EMG is detected [1]. However, abnormal sphincter EMG findings were not able to differentiate MSA from PD and other parkinsonian disorders [53].

25.7.6 Olfactory Tests

Substantial hyposmia is present in PD and pure autonomic failure, while mild hyposmia is present in only a small percentage of MSA patients [4, 39]. Olfactory function tests may be useful to differentiate MSA from other mimicking disorders [54].

25.7.7 Other Investigations

Neuropsychological assessment may be done to assess the cognitive impairment associated with MSA. Videopolysomnography in addition to sleep-related questionnaires might help in the assessment of sleep disturbances seen in MSA patients [4].

25.7.8 Unified MSA Rating Scale (UMSARS)

The unified MSA rating scale (UMSARS) is utilized to evaluate the extent of functional impairment in MSA patients. UMSARS consists of four components: a historical review of disease-related impairments (Part I, consisting of 12 items), a motor examination (Part II, consisting of 14 items), an autonomic examination (Part III), and a global disability scale (Part IV). Each item is assigned a score on a scale of 0 (indicating no impairment) to 4 (indicating severe impairment) [55].

25.8 Differential Diagnosis

Parkinson's disease (PD), progressive supranuclear palsy (PSP), and dementia with Lewy bodies (DLB) are major conditions that can resemble MSA-P, making diagnosis challenging. PD diagnosis is relatively easier when patients exhibit gradually progressing, asymmetrical parkinsonism, classic rest tremor resembling pill rolling, and an excellent response to levodopa. However, some PD patients may present with symmetrical parkinsonism, early autonomic dysfunction, and a moderate response to levodopa, resembling MSA-P. In such cases, the presence of red flags outlined in the second consensus criteria and the occurrence of cerebellar symptoms or sleep-disordered breathing should be considered, which would favor a diagnosis of MSA. Some MSA-P patients initially display asymmetrical parkinsonism with an initial positive response to levodopa, leading to a misdiagnosis of PD. Neuroimaging findings such as the "hot cross bun" sign and "putaminal rim" sign may support the diagnosis of MSA [4, 56].

In the early stages of PSP-P, patients have normal eye movements, poor levodopa responsiveness, prominent axial symptoms, and early postural instability, similar to MSA-P. If predominant autonomic dysfunction is observed, it may favor a diagnosis of MSA-P. However, it is important to note that some MSA patients develop autonomic disturbances 2–3 years after the onset of motor symptoms, further complicating the accurate diagnosis. PSP with prominent cerebellar ataxia (PSP-C) can resemble MSA-C. DLB patients typically have poor responsiveness to levodopa, exhibit rapid eye movement sleep behavior disorder (RBD), and experience autonomic dysfunction similar to MSA-P patients. The most distinctive distinguishing feature of DLB from MSA-P is the presence of dementia with fluctuating cognition and visual hallucinations, which are not characteristic of MSA. In rare cases, motor neuron disease can be misdiagnosed as MSA-P due to features such as pyramidal slowing and hyperreflexia [4, 56].

MSA-C can resemble sporadic adult-onset ataxia of unknown origin in the early stages before the onset of autonomic symptoms, making it difficult to differentiate between the two. The presence of mild parkinsonism can aid in diagnosing MSA-C. Genetic disorders such as spinocerebellar ataxias, autosomal recessive cerebellar ataxias, hereditary spastic paraplegia, and late-onset Huntington's disease can also mimic MSA. Factors that may help distinguish MSA from genetic disorders include a younger age of symptom onset, positive family history, pedigree analysis, observation of features typical for the genetic disorders but atypical for MSA, and a slower progression of the disease. Genetic testing may be recommended when feasible. MSA can be mistaken for vascular parkinsonism and normal-pressure hydrocephalus, and neuroimaging can aid in ruling out these conditions. Paraneoplastic cerebellar degeneration and autoimmune disorders can also resemble MSA-C, but they typically exhibit a more rapid deterioration. Testing for autoimmune and paraneoplastic panels, along with whole-body PET scanning, can aid in the differential diagnosis. Chronic alcoholism is a common cause of progressive cerebellar ataxia, and less commonly, phenytoin and lithium use can contribute to this condition. A thorough history can help rule out these toxin-related causes. However, distinguishing whether cerebellar ataxia is solely caused by toxins or is a result of a neurodegenerative disorder can be challenging. Accurate diagnosis of MSA is crucial, as misdiagnosis can lead to delays in treating potentially treatable conditions and incorrect predictions about the clinical course and prognosis [4, 56].

25.9 Treatment and Prognosis

Researchers around the globe are dedicated to developing therapeutic approaches that can modify the course of MSA. However, as of now, no definitive cure has been identified. The primary focus of MSA treatment involves managing and alleviating the symptoms associated with the disease. Symptomatic treatment targeting various clinical manifestations and providing palliative care during the advanced stages of MSA form the cornerstone of current treatment strategies.

25.9.1 Parkinsonism

If necessary and well tolerated, a trial of levodopa (combined with a decarboxylase inhibitor) up to a maximum dosage of 1000 mg per day may be administered. However, the dosage of levodopa may be limited due to potential side effects such as exacerbation of orthostatic hypotension, nausea, or excessive sleepiness. In cases where levodopa is not well tolerated, dopamine agonists are prescribed as a second-line treatment option. These include pramipexole ER (up to 3.15 mg per day if tolerated) and ropinirole ER (up to 24 mg per day if tolerated). As a third-line option, amantadine, a non-selective NMDA antagonist, may be given at a dosage of 100 mg up to three times daily. While anticholinergic medications like trihexyphenidyl are generally ineffective in treating parkinsonism in MSA, they may provide some degree of benefit if dystonia or sialorrhea (excessive drooling) is present. Non-pharmacological measures for managing parkinsonism in MSA include speech therapy with the provision of communication aids, physiotherapy involving lower-limb resistance training, balance and flexibility exercises, and occupational therapy focusing on environmental adaptations, providing walking aids, and wheelchair provision [1, 4, 22, 57].

25.9.2 Camptocormia

Levodopa therapy and botulinum toxin injection in rectus abdominis bilaterally might be given to improve camptocormia in MSA patients. Physiotherapy, wearing a back orthosis, and wearing a backpack weighing around 6 kg are the non-pharmacological measures for camptocormia [4].

25.9.3 Focal Dystonia

To address focal dystonia, such as blepharospasm (eye muscle spasms) and hand contractures, localized injections of botulinum toxin can be given with the aim of improving symptoms. There is a lack of empirical data regarding oral treatments for dystonia. Nevertheless, there have been reports of off-label use of anticholinergic medications like trihexyphenidyl (administered at a dosage of up to 10–12 mg per day) and baclofen, which have shown to provide symptomatic relief in some cases [1, 4, 22, 57].

25.9.4 Cerebellar Dysfunction

At present, there are no specific medications available for the treatment of cerebellar dysfunction in MSA. However, there have been reports suggesting that low doses of clonazepam (0.5–1 mg at bedtime) administered off-label can be effective in managing myoclonus or kinetic tremors associated with MSA [4]. Non-pharmacological approaches such as speech therapy, physiotherapy, and occupational therapy play a crucial role in managing cerebellar dysfunction in MSA. Speech therapy involves providing communication aids to enhance communication abilities. Physiotherapy focuses on lower-limb resistance training, as well as balance and flexibility exercises. Occupational therapy includes environmental adaptations, provision of walking aids, and supplying wheelchairs when necessary. Neurorehabilitation programs have shown effectiveness in both MSA-P and MSA-C patients, aiding in the prevention of falls, choking episodes, and improving communication abilities [1, 4, 22, 57].

25.9.5 Orthostatic Hypotension

Non-pharmacological approaches are the primary method for managing orthostatic symptoms in MSA. Patients should be educated to recognize pre-syncopal symptoms and employ counter-pressure maneuvers such as leg crossing, bending forward, or clenching the buttocks or fists to alleviate symptoms. They should also avoid sudden changes in posture, straining during urination or bowel movements, exposure to hot temperatures, and excessive physical exertion. Wearing elastic compression stockings and increasing fluid and salt intake may help improve orthostatic hypotension in MSA patients. However, it is important for neurologists to ensure that MSA patients do not have a history of heart failure, liver, or kidney dysfunction before recommending increased salt and fluid intake [58]. The use of dopaminergic medications may potentially worsen orthostatic symptoms. The risk-benefit ratio of increasing the dosage of dopaminergic medications should be continuously evaluated, considering the cardiovascular side effects in MSA patients. Additional pharmacological options for managing orthostatic hypotension include the use of plasma expanders and vasoconstrictive agents. Plasma expanders include medications such as fludrocortisone (administered at a dosage of 0.1–0.4 mg once daily) and desmopressin (available as a nasal spray at a dosage of 10–40 µg or as a tablet at a dosage of 100–400 µg). Vasoconstrictive agents consist of medications like midodrine (administered at a dosage of 2.5–10 mg three times daily), etilefrine (available as an extended-release tablet at a dosage of 25 mg once or twice daily), and droxidopa (administered at a dosage of 300 mg twice daily) [1, 4, 22, 57].

25.9.6 Supine Hypertension/ Nocturnal Hypertension

MSA patients experiencing nocturnal or supine hypertension may be recommended to have a light snack prior to bedtime and sleep in a head-up tilted position of approximately 30°. Pharmacological interventions for managing nocturnal hypertension include the use of short-acting calcium antagonists (such as nifedipine at a dosage of 30 mg taken at night), medications like losartan or clonidine to be administered 1 h before sleeping, and the application of a transdermal nitroglycerine patch specifically during nighttime (at a dosage of 0.1–0.2 mg per hour) [1, 4].

25.9.7 Postprandial Hypotension (PPH)

In MSA patients, consuming water rapidly during meals and having caffeine after meals may help alleviate postprandial hypotension (PPH) symptoms. It is important for patients to avoid excessive intake of alcohol and refined carbohydrates during a single meal. Octreotide, administered subcutaneously at a dosage of 25–50 µg before meals, may be considered as a treatment option for PPH. However, the use of octreotide is limited due to the need for parenteral administration and potential gastrointestinal side effects such as nausea and pain [1, 4].

25.9.8 Urological Dysfunction

The most common complication in MSA patients with bladder dysfunction is urinary tract infection (UTI). It is crucial to promptly assess and manage UTIs by using antibiotics tailored to the specific antibiogram. Anti-muscarinic agents are the preferred medications for relieving symptoms of urgency and urinary incontinence caused by overactive bladder. Examples of these medications include oxybutynin (administered at a dosage of 5 mg twice or three times daily), tolterodine (2 mg three times daily), solifenacin (5 mg once daily), darifenacin (dosage range of 7.5–15 mg once daily), and trospium chloride (60 mg extended-release once daily). However, it is important to note that these medications carry the risk of increasing post-void residual volume, as well as causing dry mouth (xerostomia), constipation, and blurred vision. In some cases, injecting botulinum toxin-A into the detrusor muscle has been reported to improve urinary continence in MSA patients. Sanitary pads and condom catheters are non-pharmacological measures for urinary incontinence. Bedtime desmopressin (10-40 µg/nasal spray or 100-400 µg/tablet) may alleviate nocturia and reduce sleep fragmentation. In MSA patients presenting with urinary retention, post-void residual volume of 100 mL or more is considered as a cut-off value to start intervention. In early stages of MSA when the patient is still ambulant, clean intermittent self-catheterization is advised. For long-term management of urinary retention in MSA, suprapubic indwelling catheterization is considered. Pharmacological approaches targeting the bladder for urinary retention involve the use of cholinergic agents such as distigmine chloride (at a dosage of 10–15 mg per day) or bethanechol chloride (at a dosage of 30–45 mg per day). However, a limitation of these agents is that they can worsen urinary incontinence in MSA patients who also have detrusor overactivity. Another pharmacological approach, targeting the urethra, is the administration of α-adrenergic receptor (α-AR) antagonists such as prazosin (1 mg three times daily) or tamsulosin (0.4 mg once daily). It is important to note that the main side effect associated with these medications is syncope (fainting) [1, 4, 22, 57].

25.9.9 Sexual Dysfunction

Apomorphine injection (2–4 mg subcutaneously), sildenafil (50–100 mg), or alprostadil (10-20 μg intracavernous injection) on demand are the available choices for the pharmacological management of erectile dysfunction in men. However, they have potential side effects, which need to be considered. There is no proven therapy for the management of sexual dysfunction in women [1, 4].

25.9.10 Respiratory Dysfunction

Administering botulinum toxin-A through unilateral injection into the thyroarytenoid muscle provides relief for both diurnal and nocturnal stridor in MSA patients. However, this treatment approach may worsen respiratory insufficiency, dysphagia, and dysphonia. The use of continuous positive airway pressure (CPAP) within the range of 6–8 cm H_2O or, in cases of resistance, biphasic positive airway pressure (BiPAP) may improve nocturnal stridor and address obstructive sleep apnea in MSA patients. CPAP and BiPAP can also enhance sleep quality and reduce daytime sleepiness. Laryngeal surgery options such as vocal cord lateralization, cordectomy, or laser arytenoidectomy can potentially increase the openness of the glottis and reduce stridor; however, these procedures may worsen dysarthria and increase the risk of aspiration pneumonia.

Tracheostomy eliminates both nocturnal and diurnal stridor as well as prevents respiratory crisis due to paroxysmal vocal cord abductor palsy. MSA patients with sleep-disordered breathing might be advised to sleep in a lateral position rather than supine to ameliorate nocturnal laryngeal patency. Speech therapy with provision of communication aids might help patients with dysarthria [1, 4, 22, 57].

25.9.11 Gastrointestinal Dysfunction

To manage sialorrhea (excessive drooling), botulinum toxin-A can be injected into the parotid and submandibular glands, and anticholinergic drugs may also be prescribed. To prevent aspiration pneumonia in dysphagic patients, strategies such as chin-down positioning during swallowing and adding thickeners (such as honey) to thin liquids may be recommended. In severe cases of dysphagia, MSA patients may require nasogastric tube or percutaneous endoscopic gastrostomy (PEG) feeding. To alleviate constipation, moderate exercise and an increase in water and insoluble fiber intake are important. In resistant cases, osmotic bulking agents like macrogol (administered at a dosage of 13–39 g per day) or calcium polycarbophil (0.5 mg three times daily) may be prescribed [1, 4, 22, 57].

25.9.12 REM Behavior Disorder

Clonazepam (0.5 mg–1 mg at bedtime) is effective in treating RBD. However, it should not be advised if the MSA patient has stridor or sleep apnea, for clonazepam worsens upper airway obstruction [1, 4, 22, 57]. Melatonin (0.5–1 mg at night) is the alternative for clonazepam [4].

25.9.13 Depression

Tricyclic anti-depressants worsen orthostatic hypotension. Hence, selective serotonin reuptake inhibitors (SSRI) such as paroxetine or fluoxetine are preferred for the management of depression in MSA patients [4].

25.10 Prognosis of MSA

MSA is a rapidly advancing neurodegenerative condition that currently lacks a cure. The prognosis of MSA is generally quite grim. Most individuals with MSA undergo a progressive deterioration in motor function, characterized by early postural instability and frequent falls within 3 years of the onset of the disease. Consequently, many patients require walking aids during this early phase to maintain mobility [1, 4, 7, 9]. Time from disease onset to "wheel chair sign" has been reported to last 3–6 years, while time to reach bed-ridden state has been reported to last 5–8 years from MSA onset [4, 57, 59]. Mean survival has been reported to be 6–10 years from the symptomatic onset of MSA. Major causes of death in MSA are sudden death, bronchopneumonia, and urinary tract infections [1, 4, 7, 9]. Patients who experience autonomic failure within 2.5 years from the onset of the disease face a significantly higher risk of sudden death, approximately seven times greater, compared to those who develop autonomic dysfunction at a later stage in the course of the disease [59]. Older age at disease onset, early and more severe autonomic failure, parkinsonian phenotype, and female gender are the negative prognostic factors in MSA [7, 9, 11, 28, 59]. Cerebellar phenotype and late-onset cardiovascular autonomic failure have been reported to be positive predictors for survival in MSA [60–62].

References

1. Wenning GK, Colosimo C, Geser F, Poewe W. Multiple system atrophy. Lancet Neurol. 2004;3(2):93–103.
2. Stefanova N, Bücke P, Duerr S, Wenning GK. Multiple system atrophy: an update. Lancet Neurol. 2009;8(12):1172–8.
3. Quinn N. Multiple system atrophy – the nature of the beast. J Neurol Neurosurg Psychiatry. 1989;S2(Suppl):78–89.
4. Wenning GK, Fanciulli A, editors. Multiple system atrophy. Wien: Springer-Verlag; 2014.
5. Papp MI, Kahn JE, Lantos PL. Glial cytoplasmic inclusions in the CNS of patients with multiple system atrophy (striatonigral degeneration, olivopontocerebellar atrophy and shy-Drager syndrome). J Neurol Sci. 1989;94(1–3):79–100.
6. Spillantini MG, Crowther RA, Jakes R, Cairns NJ, Lantos PL, Goedert M. Filamentous alpha-synuclein inclusions link multiple system atrophy with Parkinson's disease and dementia with Lewy bodies. Neurosci Lett. 1998;251(3):205–8.
7. Wenning GK, Geser F, Krismer F, Seppi K, Duerr S, Boesch S, Kollensperger M, Goebel G, Pfeiffer KP, Barone P, Pellecchia MT, Quinn NP, Koukouni V, Fowler CJ, Schrag A, Mathias CJ, Giladi N, Gurevich T, Dupont E, Ostergaard K, Nilsson CF, Widner H, Oertel W, Eggert KM, Albanese A, del Sorbo F, Tolosa E, Cardozo A, Deuschl G, Hellriegel H, Klockgether T, Dodel R, Sampaio C, Coelho M, Djaldetti R, Melamed E, Gasser T, Kamm C, Meco G, Colosimo C, Rascol O, Meissner WG, Tison F, Poewe W. The natural history of multiple system atrophy: a prospective European cohort study. Lancet Neurol. 2013;12:264–74.
8. May S, Gilman S, Sowell BB, Thomas RG, Stern MB, Colcher A, Tanner CM, Huang N, Novak P, Reich SG, Jankovic J, Ondo WG, Low PA, Sandroni P, Lipp A, Marshall FJ, Wooten F, Shults CW. Potential outcome measures and trial design issues for multiple system atrophy. Mov Disord. 2007;22:2371–7.
9. Low PA, Reich SG, Jankovic J, Shults CW, Stern MB, Novak P, et al. Natural history of multiple system atrophy in the USA: a prospective cohort study. Lancet Neurol. 2015;14(7):710–9. https://doi.org/10.1016/S1474-4422(15)00058-7.
10. Kim HJ, Jeon BS, Lee JY, Yun JY. Survival of Korean patients with multiple system atrophy. Mov Disord. 2011;26:909–12.
11. Watanabe H, Saito Y, Terao S, Ando T, Kachi T, Mukai E, Aiba I, Abe Y, Tamakoshi A, Doyu M, Hirayama M, Sobue. Progression and prognosis in multiple system atrophy: an analysis of 230 Japanese patients. Brain. 2002;125:1070–83.
12. Ozawa T, Tada M, Kakita A, Onodera O, Ishihara T, Morita T, Shimohata T, Wakabayashi K, Takahashi H, Nishizawa M. The phenotype spectrum of Japanese multiple system atrophy. J Neurol Neurosurg Psychiatry. 2010;81:1253–5.
13. Ubhi K, Low P, Masliah E. Multiple system atrophy: a clinical and neuropathological perspective. Trends Neurosci. 2011;34(11):581–90. https://doi.org/10.1016/j.tins.2011.08.003.
14. Ahmed Z, Asi YT, Sailer A, Lees AJ, Houlden H, Revesz T, Holton JL. The neuropathology, pathophysiology and genetics of multiple system atrophy. Neuropathol Appl Neurobiol. 2012;38:4–24.
15. Jellinger KA. Neuropathology and pathophysiology of multiple system atrophy. Neuropathol Appl Neurobiol. 2012;38:379–80. author reply 381

16. Jellinger KA, Lantos PL. Papp-Lantos inclusions and the pathogenesis of multiple system atrophy: an update. Acta Neuropathol. 2010;119:657–67.

17. Halliday GM, Holton JL, Revesz T, Dickson DW. Neuropathology underlying clinical variability in patients with synucleinopathies. Acta Neuropathol. 2011;122:187–204.

18. Jellinger KA. p25alpha immunoreactivity in multiple system atrophy and Parkinson disease. Acta Neuropathol. 2006;112:112.

19. Fellner L, Jellinger KA, Wenning GK, Stefanova N. Glial dysfunction in the pathogenesis of α-synucleinopathies: emerging concepts. Acta Neuropathol. 2011 Jun;121(6):675–93.

20. Song YJ, Lundvig DM, Huang Y, Gai WP, Blumbergs PC, Hojrup P, Otzen D, Halliday GM, Jensen PH. p25alpha relocalizes in oligodendroglia from myelin to cytoplasmic inclusions in multiple system atrophy. Am J Pathol. 2007;171:1291–303.

21. The Multiple-System Atrophy Research Collaboration. Mutations in COQ2 in familial and sporadic multiple-system atrophy. N Engl J Med. 2013;369(3):233–44.

22. Kollensperger M, Geser F, Ndayisaba JP, Boesch S, Seppi K, Ostergaard K, Dupont E, Cardozo A, Tolosa E, Abele M, Klockgether T, Yekhlef F, Tison F, Daniels C, Deuschl G, Coelho M, Sampaio C, Bozi M, Quinn N, Schrag A, Mathias CJ, Fowler C, Nilsson CF, Widner H, Schimke N, Oertel W, del Sorbo F, Albanese A, Pellecchia MT, Barone P, Djaldetti R, Colosimo C, Meco G, Gonzalez-Mandly A, Berciano J, Gurevich T, Giladi N, Galitzky M, Rascol O, Kamm C, Gasser T, Siebert U, Poewe W, Wenning GK. Presentation, diagnosis, and management of multiple system atrophy in Europe: final analysis of the European multiple system atrophy registry. Mov Disord. 2010;25:2604–12.

23. Sakakibara R, Hattori T, Uchiyama T, Kita K, Asahina M, Suzuki A, Yamanishi T. Urinary dysfunction and orthostatic hypotension in multiple system atrophy: which is the more common and earlier manifestation? J Neurol Neurosurg. Psychiatry. 2000;68: 65–9.

24. Gilman S, Wenning GK, Low PA, Brooks DJ, Mathias CJ, Trojanowski JQ, et al. Second consensus statement on the diagnosis of multiple system atrophy. Neurology. 2008;71(9):670–6.

25. Schmidt C, Berg D, Prieur S, Junghanns S, Schweitzer K, Globas C, Schols L, Reichmann H, Ziemssen T. Loss of nocturnal blood pressure fall in various extrapyramidal syndromes. Mov Disord. 2009;24:2136–42.

26. Yamaguchi M, Arai K, Asahina M, Hattori T. Laryngeal stridor in multiple system atrophy. Eur Neurol. 2003;49:154–9.

27. Sakakibara R, Odaka T, Uchiyama T, Liu R, Asahina M, Yamaguchi K, Yamaguchi T, Yamanishi T, Hattori T. Colonic transit time, sphincter EMG, and rectoanal videomanometry in multiple system atrophy. Mov Disord. 2004;19:924–9.

28. O'Sullivan SS, Massey LA, Williams DR, Silveira-Moriyama L, Kempster PA, Holton JL, Revesz T, Lees AJ. Clinical outcomes of progressive supranuclear palsy and multiple system atrophy. Brain. 2008;131:1362–72.

29. Iodice V, Lipp A, Ahlskog JE, Sandroni P, Fealey RD, Parisi JE, Matsumoto JY, Benarroch EE, Kimpinski K, Singer W, Gehrking TL, Gehrking JA, Sletten DM, Schmeichel AM, Bower JH, Gilman S, Figueroa J, Low PA. Autopsy confirmed multiple system atrophy cases: Mayo experience and role of autonomic function tests. J Neurol Neurosurg Psychiatry. 2012;83:453–9.

30. Yamashita F, Hirayama M, Nakamura T, Takamori M, Hori N, Uchida K, Hama T, Sobue G. Pupillary autonomic dysfunction in multiple system atrophy and Parkinson's disease: an assessment by eye-drop tests. Clin Auton Res. 2010;20:191–7.

31. Wenning GK, Tison F, Ben Shlomo Y, Daniel SE, Quinn NP. Multiple system atrophy: a review of 203 pathologically proven cases. Mov Disord. 1997;12:133–47.

32. Brown RG, Lacomblez L, Landwehrmeyer BG, Bak T, Uttner I, Dubois B, Agid Y, Ludolph A, Bensimon G, Payan C, Leigh NP. Cognitive impairment in patients with multiple system atrophy and progressive supranuclear palsy. Brain. 2010;133:2382–93.

33. Marconi R, Antonini A, Barone P, Colosimo C, Avarello TP, Bottacchi E, Cannas A, Ceravolo MG, Ceravolo R, Cicarelli G, Gaglio RM, Giglia L, Iemolo F, Manfredi M, Meco G, Nicoletti A, Pederzoli M, Petrone A, Pisani A, Pontieri FE, Quatrale R, Ramat S, Scala R, Volpe G, Zappulla S, Bentivoglio AR, Stocchi F, Trianni G, del Dotto P, de Gaspari D, Grasso L, Morgante F, Santangelo G, Fabbrini G, Morgante L. Frontal assessment battery scores and non-motor symptoms in parkinsonian disorders. Neurol Sci. 2012;33:585–93.

34. Colosimo C, Morgante L, Antonini A, Barone P, Avarello TP, Bottacchi E, Cannas A, Ceravolo MG, Ceravolo R, Cicarelli G, Gaglio RM, Giglia L, Iemolo F, Manfredi M, Meco G, Nicoletti A, Pederzoli M, Petrone A, Pisani A, Pontieri FE, Quatrale R, Ramat S, Scala R, Volpe G, Zappulla S, Bentivoglio AR, Stocchi F, Trianni G, del Dotto P, Simoni L, Marconi R. Non-motor symptoms in atypical and secondary parkinsonism: the PRIAMO study. J Neurol. 2010;257:5–14.

35. Boeve BF, Silber MH, Parisi JE, Dickson DW, Ferman TJ, Benarroch EE, Schmeichel AM, Smith GE, Petersen RC, Ahlskog JE, Matsumoto JY, Knopman DS, Schenck CH, Mahowald MW. Synucleinopathy pathology and REM sleep behavior disorder plus dementia or parkinsonism. Neurology. 2003;61:40–5.

36. Iranzo A, Santamaria J, Tolosa E. The clinical and pathophysiological relevance of REM sleep behavior disorder in neurodegenerative diseases. Sleep Med Rev. 2009;13:385–401.

37. Vetrugno R, Provini F, Cortelli P, Plazzi G, Lotti EM, Pierangeli G, Canali C, Montagna P. Sleep disor-

ders in multiple system atrophy: a correlative video-polysomnographic study. Sleep Med. 2004;5:21–30.

38. Gama RL, Tavora DG, Bomfi m RC, Silva CE, de Bruin VM, de Bruin PF. Sleep disturbances and brain MRI morphometry in Parkinson's disease, multiple system atrophy and progressive supranuclear palsy – a comparative study. Parkinsonism Relat Disord. 2010;16:275–9.

39. Palma J-A, Norcliffe-Kaufmann L, Kaufmann H. Diagnosis of multiple system atrophy. Auton Neurosci. 2018 May;211:15–25.

40. Burk K, Globas C, Wahl T, Buhring U, Dietz K, Zuhlke C, Luft A, Schulz JB, Voigt K, Dichgans J. MRI-based volumetric differentiation of sporadic cerebellar ataxia. Brain. 2004;127:175–81.

41. Quattrone A, Nicoletti G, Messina D, Fera F, Condino F, Pugliese P, Lanza P, Barone P, Morgante L, Zappia M, Aguglia U, Gallo O. MR imaging index for differentiation of progressive supranuclear palsy from Parkinson disease and the Parkinson variant of multiple system atrophy. Radiology. 2008;246:214–21.

42. Gilman S, Koeppe RA, Junck L, Kluin KJ, Lohman M, St Laurent RT. Patterns of cerebral glucose metabolism detected with positron emission tomography differ in multiple system atrophy and olivopontocerebellar atrophy. Ann Neurol. 1994;36:166–75.

43. Eidelberg D, Takikawa S, Moeller JR, Dhawan V, Redington K, Chaly T, Robeson W, Dahl JR, Margouleff D, Fazzini E. Striatal hypometabolism distinguishes striatonigral degeneration from Parkinson's disease. Ann Neurol. 1993;33:518–52.

44. Otsuka M, Kuwabara Y, Ichiya Y, Hosokawa S, Sasaki M, Yoshida T, Fukumura T, Kato M, Masuda K. Differentiating between multiple system atrophy and Parkinson's disease by positron emission tomography with 18F-dopa and 18F-FDG. Ann Nucl Med. 1997;11:251–7.

45. Tang CC, Poston KL, Eckert T, Feigin A, Frucht S, Gudesblatt M, Dhawan V, Lesser M, Vonsattel JP, Fahn S, Eidelberg D. Differential diagnosis of parkinsonism: a metabolic imaging study using pattern analysis. Lancet Neurol. 2010;9:149–58.

46. Bosman T, van Laere K, Santens P. Anatomically standardised 99mTc-ECD brain perfusion SPET allows accurate differentiation between healthy volunteers, multiple system atrophy and idiopathic Parkinson's disease. Eur J Nucl Med Mol Imaging. 2003;30:16–24.

47. Brooks DJ, Seppi K. Proposed neuroimaging criteria for the diagnosis of multiple system atrophy. Mov Disord. 2009;24:949–64.

48. Fanciulli A, Gobel G, Ndayisaba JP, Granata R, Duerr S, Strano S, Colosimo C, Poewe W, Pontieri FE, Wenning GK. Supine hypertension in Parkinson's disease and multiple system atrophy. Clin Auton Res. 2016;26:97–105.

49. Coon EA, Fealey RD, Sletten DM, Mandrekar JN, Benarroch EE, Sandroni P, Low PA, Singer W. Anhidrosis in multiple system atrophy involves pre- and postganglionic sudomotor dysfunction. Mov Disord. 2017;32:397–404.

50. Doppler K, Weis J, Karl K, Ebert S, Ebentheuer J, Trenkwalder C, Klebe S, Volkmann J, Sommer C. Distinctive distribution of phospho-alpha-synuclein in dermal nerves in multiple system atrophy. Mov Disord. 2015;30:1688–92.

51. Lipp A, Sandroni P, Ahlskog JE, Fealey RD, Kimpinski K, Iodice V, Gehrking TL, Weigand SD, Sletten DM, Gehrking JA, Nickander KK, Singer W, Maraganore DM, Gilman S, Wenning GK, Shults CW, Low PA. Prospective differentiation of multiple system atrophy from Parkinson disease, with and without autonomic failure. Arch Neurol. 2009;66:742–50.

52. Ogawa T, Sakakibara R, Kuno S, Ishizuka O, Kitta T, Yoshimura N. Prevalence and treatment of LUTS in patients with Parkinson disease or multiple system atrophy. Nat Rev Urol. 2017;14:79.

53. Giladi N, Simon ES, Korczyn AD, Groozman GB, Orlov Y, Shabtai H, Drory VE. Anal sphincter EMG does not distinguish between multiple system atrophy and Parkinson's disease. Muscle Nerve. 2000;23:731–4.

54. Garland EM, Raj SR, Peltier AC, Robertson D, Biaggioni I. A cross-sectional study contrasting olfactory function in autonomic disorders. Neurology. 2011;76:456–60.

55. Wenning GK, Tison F, Seppi K, Sampaio C, Diem A, Yekhlef F, et al. Multiple system atrophy study group. Development and validation of the unified multiple system atrophy rating scale (UMSARS). Mov Disord. 2004;19(12):1391–402.

56. Kim H-J, Stamelou M, Jeon B. Multiple system atrophy-mimicking conditions: diagnostic challenges. Parkinsonism Relat Disord. 2016;22:S12eS15.

57. Rohrer G, Hoglinger GU, Levin J. Symptomatic therapy of multiple system atrophy. Auton Neurosci. 2018;211:26–30.

58. Young TM, Mathias CJ. The effects of water ingestion on orthostatic hypotension in two groups of chronic autonomic failure: multiple system atrophy and pure autonomic failure. J Neurol Neurosurg Psychiatry. 2004;75:1737–41.

59. Tada M, Onodera O, Ozawa T, Piao YS, Kakita A, Takahashi H, Nishizawa M. Early development of autonomic dysfunction may predict poor prognosis in patients with multiple system atrophy. Arch Neurol. 2007;64:256–60.

60. Ben-Shlomo Y, Wenning GK, Tison F, Quinn NP. Survival of patients with pathologically proven multiple system atrophy: a meta-analysis. Neurology. 1997;48:384–93.

61. Schulz JB, Klockgether T, Petersen D, Jauch M, Muller-Schauenburg W, Spieker S, Voigt K, Dichgans J. Multiple system atrophy: natural history, MRI morphology, and dopamine receptor imaging with 123IBZM-SPECT. J Neurol Neurosurg Psychiatry. 1994;57:1047–56.

62. Petrovic IN, Ling H, Asi Y, Ahmed Z, Kukkle PL, Hazrati LN, Lang AE, Revesz T, Holton JL, Lees AJ. Multiple system atrophy-parkinsonism with slow progression and prolonged survival: a diagnostic catch. Mov Disord. 2012;27:1186–90.

Lower-Body Parkinsonism

26

Nitish Kamble and Pramod Kumar Pal

Case Scenario A 71-year-old gentleman presented with progressive difficulty walking of 2 years duration. The gait abnormality was insidious in onset and gradually progressive in nature. Initially, his walking became slow and developed short steps. Subsequently, he noticed an imbalance while walking, with a tendency to fall and difficulty turning. For 6 months he developed freezing of gait and feels as if his feet are glued to the ground and has difficulty initiating gait. For the past 1 month, he requires support to walk with frequent falls if unassisted. He also complains of urinary urgency and frequency with urge incontinence for the past 1 month. There is no cognitive impairment. There is no history of tremors, weakness of limbs, speech disturbance, orthostatic giddiness, or stiffness of limbs. He is hypertensive and diabetic for more than 10 years and is on medications. He has a past history of stroke 2.5 years back with right hemiparesis that recovered nearly completely over a period of 6 months. He is a smoker and smokes about 2–3 cigarettes per day. No history of alcohol consumption or other substance abuse. No history of coronary artery disease or any other cardiac illness. There is a family history of diabetes mellitus and hypertension in his father. On examination, the patient was conscious and oriented. Pulse rate was 78/min, regular, and BP was 164/98 mm of Hg. His cardiovascular and respiratory system examination was normal. His speech was normal. MMSE was 28/30. He had reduced facial expression with normal blink rate. His eye movement examination revealed impaired up-gaze with preserved oculocephalic movements. There was no neck or upper limb rigidity and no upper limb bradykinesia. There were mild postural tremors of both hands but no rest tremors. There was mild-to-moderate rigidity of both lower limbs and moderate bradykinesia. The deep tendon reflexes were exaggerated in both upper and lower limbs (right > left). The right plantar was extensor and the left was flexor. There was mild knee-heel in-coordination. He had difficulty in initiating gait, which improved with the sensory cue, required the support of one person to walk with short steps, reduced arm swing and en-bloc turning. His routine hemogram and biochemical investigations were normal. HbA1c was 9.9%, and his LDL cholesterol was 224 mg%. His MRI brain showed diffuse cerebral atrophy, and mild dilatation of the lateral ventricles with periventricular and subcortical white matter hyperintensities on T2W and FLAIR images. There were multiple infarcts in the basal ganglia and thalamus. MR angiography was normal. Cardiac evaluation using 2D echocardiography showed concentric left ventricular hypertrophy. Based on the history, examination and neuroimaging, the patient was diagnosed as a

N. Kamble · P. K. Pal (✉)
Department of Neurology, National Institute of Mental Health and Neuro Sciences (NIMHANS), Bengaluru, India

case of vascular parkinsonism (lower-body parkinsonism). The patient was started on antiplatelet agents (aspirin and clopidogrel), atorvastatin along with antihypertensives and oral hypoglycaemic agents. He was initiated on levodopa + carbidopa (100 + 25 mg) with a gradual increase in the drug dosage finally reaching one tablet four times a day. After about a month of treatment, the patient noticed an improvement in his symptoms and was able to walk independently with a mild increase in the walking speed. In addition to levodopa, he was advised physiotherapy and balance and gait training.

26.1 Introduction

Lower-body Parkinsonism (LBP) is a clinical condition characterized by parkinsonism features with predominant involvement of the lower limbs and sparing or minimal involvement of the upper limbs. Patients demonstrate great difficulty walking, postural instability and falls. These patients have a poor response to levodopa therapy, and resting tremor is an uncommon finding [1]. The gait is significantly affected and typically described as gait apraxia. The disturbances may include difficulty in initiating gait, freezing, unsteady gate, shuffling or festination gait. The common causes of lower-body parkinsonism include normal pressure hydrocephalus (NPH), vascular (atherosclerotic) parkinsonism (VP), Parkinson's disease—postural instability and gait difficulty (PD-PIGD), progressive supranuclear palsy—pure akinesia and gait freezing (PSP-PAGF) and frontal lobe lesions (tumours, infections and demyelination). Currently only clinical and radiological tests are available as an aid for the diagnosis of these groups of patients.

26.1.1 Vascular (Arteriosclerotic) Parkinsonism (VP)

Vascular parkinsonism (VP) is a type of atypical parkinsonism, in which the aetiology is vascular in nature and accounts for about 4.4%–12% of all cases of parkinsonism [2]. It is also called atherosclerotic parkinsonism. It was first described by Critchley in 1929 and suggested that parkinsonism can result from vascular insults to the brain and named as arteriosclerotic parkinsonism. Subsequently, it was named as vascular parkinsonism and is distinct from idiopathic (sporadic) Parkinson disease (PD) [3]. Binswanger in 1987 suggested that thickening and narrowing of cerebral arteries can lead to white matter lesions (WMLs) and cognitive impairment. There is also gait impairment in such patients and is referred to as "lower-body parkinsonism" [4]. VP is a clinical phenotype that is primarily characterized by gait impairment and is caused by pathology of the cerebral arteries and predominantly affects subcortical white matter [1]. In addition, vascular lesions other than WMLs can also lead to lower-body parkinsonism. This was initially shown in pathological observations of stroke-induced parkinsonism. In this case, unilateral parkinsonism was reported after brainstem ischaemia [5].

26.1.1.1 Epidemiology

In patients with idiopathic PD, vascular lesions are seen infrequently. These vascular lesions, when present in idiopathic PD, are most often due to age rather than a disease [6, 7]. In autopsy-confirmed idiopathic PD, vascular lesions are observed in about 1.4–3.0% [8]. VP accounts for about 3–5% of all patients with parkinsonism [9]. In some patients with VP, gait impairment is associated with cognitive impairment that makes the assessment of gait difficult. In the UK Brain Bank clinicopathological study of patients with clinically confirmed PD, 24 of 100 had additional vascular changes contributing to the clinical manifestations [10]. In another autopsy study of 400 parkinsonism cases, 6% could be classified as having vascular parkinsonism that was showing multi-infarct atrophy, Binswanger or hypertensive encephalopathy and/or multiple vascular infarcts in the brainstem and basal ganglia [8]. VP affects predominantly men with similar or later age of onset than that of idiopathic PD [11, 12]. This observation may be due to the associated vascular risk factors which are more common in men when compared to women.

26.1.1.2 Clinical Features

VP is classically characterized by lower-body parkinsonism with postural instability, shuffling or freezing of gait. Usually, there is an absence of rest tremors, poor or absent levodopa responsiveness and the presence of pyramidal and/or cerebellar signs [13]. The patient usually complains of gait abnormalities that are usually wide-based, tendency to fall and difficulty maintaining balance [14, 15]. The gait is slow and insecure and has postural instability [16]. The gait is similar to that of patients with PD, although the base (the distance between the feet) is not always as narrow in lower-body parkinsonism as it is in idiopathic PD. Posture is unstable, and postural responses to maintain balance are poor. Patients also frequently demonstrate freezing of gait, wherein they have difficulty initiating gait (gait ignition failure), as if the feet are glued to the ground and temporarily unable to move [17]. The exact pathophysiology behind the freezing of gait is not known. Bradykinesia is more in the lower limbs than the upper limbs. Spasticity with brisk deep tendon reflexes and extensor plantar have been observed [12, 15]. These patients also develop dementia, pseudobulbar palsy and urinary incontinence. Sometimes clinical features may be similar to idiopathic PD and can be attributable to lacunar infarcts in the basal ganglia. Depending on the side of WMLs, parkinsonism is seen on the contralateral side. However, ipsilateral parkinsonism has also been reported [18]. In addition, patients can have abnormal glabellar tap responses in the form of repeated and persistent eyelid blinking on repetitive tapping on the forehead. Snout and palmomental reflexes are other frontal release signs that are seen in VP [16]. There is also abnormal response in the Bender's face–hand test. In this test, the patient should be able to appreciate simultaneous touches on the face and hand with their eyes closed. Rarely, in advanced disease, these patients may also develop anosmia [19]. In some patients, the upper limbs may also be involved with bradykinesia and no or minimal tremor [12, 15].

Severe executive dysfunction in patients with vascular parkinsonism has been shown by Santangelo et al. [20]. This is in comparison to patients with PD who do not have such severe executive dysfunction. Sonia Benítez-Rivero et al. found deficits in delayed verbal recall and categorical fluency as well apart from executive dysfunction using more specific and detailed assessment [21]. The reason for such severe and more frequent occurrence of executive dysfunction is due to disruptions in frontal lobe-basal ganglia circuitry due to the location of strategic infarcts. Out of all screening questionnaires, MoCA captures executive deficits better than MMSE, while language and categorical fluency can be extensively assessed by ACE-III. A combination screen may thus be ideal and less time consuming.

26.1.1.3 Aetiology

Hypertension, hyperlipidaemia, diabetes mellitus, obstructive sleep apnoea and smoking are the risk factors associated with VP. CT and MRI brain demonstrate white matter lesions in these patients [22]. Lacunar infarcts in the basal ganglia and thalamus affect the striato-thalamocortical loops, leading to gait abnormalities and other manifestations of lower-body parkinsonism supporting vascular pathogenesis [15, 22, 23]. Unilateral parkinsonism has been reported in patients with small infarcts in the lenticulostriate arteries. Diffuse widespread periventricular white matter and subcortical white matter infarcts are associated with bilateral gait disturbances and parkinsonism.

26.1.1.4 Pathology

The hallmark features include vascular changes in the brain which are ischaemic in nature and are predominantly seen in basal ganglia, thalamus, cerebral subcortical white matter and upper brainstem [24]. These regions are relevant to the development of parkinsonism. The exact pathological changes in the blood vessels have not been described in detail. However, lipohyalinosis changes have been demonstrated in the arterioles. In one of the detailed studies comparing the brains of patients with idiopathic PD and Binswanger disease without parkinsonism, basal ganglia lacunar infarcts and extensive frontal white matter lesions were reported [25]. Similar pathologies have been observed in the brain of patients with idiopathic PD but are less severe when compared to VP and Binswanger disease. There is a severe loss of oligodendrocytes in the white matter. Multiple basal ganglia or WMLs are involved in the pathogenesis of LBP. Numerous canals and small round holes referred to as "etat crible" meaning "sieve-like" has been described in the cerebral tissue [26]. These cribriform states correspond to the dilatations of the perivascular spaces, leading to a particular type of lacunes.

26.1.1.5 Mechanism

The white matter lesions usually disrupt the interconnecting fibre between basal ganglia and the motor cortex. Also, there is a disruption of the fibre connections between the thalamus, brainstem and the cerebral cortex. Several reports have shown that lacunar infarcts in the caudate, putamen and globus pallidus externum (GPe) can result in parkinsonism [27]. In some forms, the LBP progresses more relentlessly than in a stepwise fashion [28]. Acute midbrain infarction can result in the development of hemiparkinsonism, affecting both upper and lower limbs, with good response to levodopa [29]. In patients with chronic ischaemia, the changes in the subcortical white matter are slowly progressive, leading to the development of LBP and a reduced response to levodopa [30]. The ischaemia seen in patients with VP can be both presynaptic or postsynaptic. As a result, some of the patients demonstrate levodopa responsiveness predominantly in those with presynaptic vascular insults. It has been proposed that repeated ischaemic episodes lead to the inflammatory response in the brain, which then leads to WMLs. This inflammation leads to the generation of free radicals, breakdown of the blood-brain barrier, extravasation of noxious elements and myelin breakdown [31–33].

26.1.1.6 Diagnostic Criteria

Zijlmans et al. [34] have given the diagnostic criteria for the clinical diagnosis of VP.

Following are the diagnostic criteria:

(a) Parkinsonism, defined as bradykinesia, and at least one of the three features: rest tremor, rigidity or postural instability.

(b) Cerebrovascular disease, defined as evidence of relevant cerebrovascular event by neuroimaging (CT or MRI brain) or the presence of focal signs or symptoms suggestive of stroke.

(c) A relationship between (a) and (b): acute or delayed progressive onset of parkinsonism ≤1 year after stroke with evidence of infarcts on imaging in or near areas that increase the basal ganglion motor output (GPe or SNPc) or decrease the thalamocortical drive directly (VL of thalamus or large frontal infarct), or an insidious onset of parkinsonism with extensive subcortical white matter lesions, bilateral symptoms at the onset, and the presence of early shuffling gait or early cognitive dysfunction [35].

In addition, there are some exclusion criteria: a history of repeated head injury, definite encephalitis, neuroleptic treatment at the onset of symptoms, abnormal imaging on CT/MRI (cerebral tumours, communicating hydrocephalus) and other alternative explanation for parkinsonism.

Two forms of VP have been proposed based on the above criteria: [1] acute onset related to basal ganglia infarcts and [2] insidious progression which is associated with diffuse subcortical white matter lesions [36, 37].

26.1.1.7 Imaging in VP

There is limited literature on neuroimaging in patients with VP. Computed tomography (CT), magnetic resonance imaging (MRI) and cerebral angiography (CA) can be used to ascertain lesion load and to delineate the lesions in the brain. Ischaemic lesions in VP patients are commonly seen in various vascular territories, periventricular and subcortical white matter, basal ganglia and the brainstem with significant cerebral atrophy [12]. MRI brain usually shows extensive T2 hyperintense periventricular white matter signal changes, lacunar infarcts in basal ganglia and dilatation of the lateral and third ventricles [22]. The lesions accumulate over many months and years. Normal MRI is very unlikely of VP and is against the diagnosis. These lesions are also seen in elderly patients and patients with idiopathic PD, but the lesions are very mild in comparison

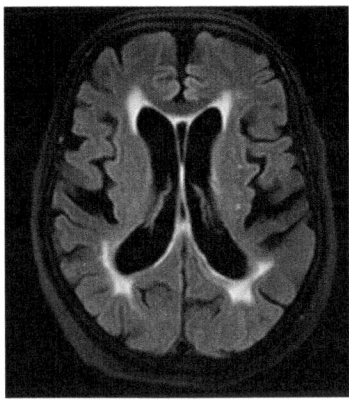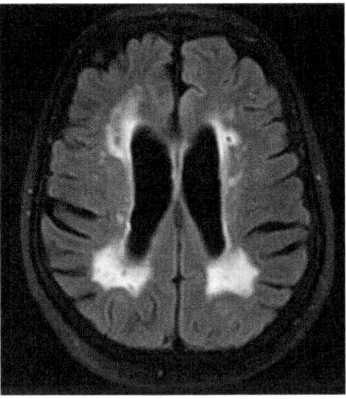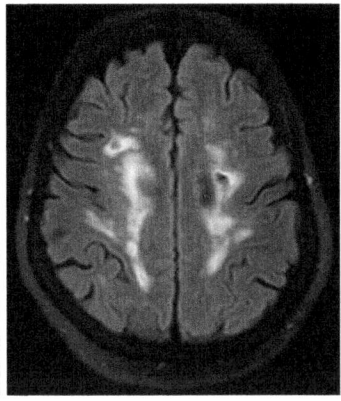

Fig. 26.1 MRI brain (FLAIR) shows diffuse cerebral atrophy with periventricular and subcortical white matter hyperintensities. Multiple small infarcts are also seen

to VP. These lesions in idiopathic PD does not well correlate with gait abnormalities [38]. Figure 26.1 shows the MRI image of a patient with vascular parkinsonism.

Single-photon emission CT (SPECT) has been used to visualize presynaptic striatal dopamine transporters in patients with PD. Patients with PD typically show asymmetric reduced uptake of dopamine markers compared to healthy controls. Patients with VP do not show similar reduction in dopamine uptake due to the preserved nigrostriatal dopaminergic pathway [19].

A vascular rating scale for VP has been developed by Winikates and Jankovic [12] (Table 26.1).

26.1.1.8 Treatment of VP

Since VP is assumed to be caused by cerebrovascular diseases, the principles of primary and secondary prevention of stroke apply to VP also. Hence good control of diabetes mellitus, hypertension and dyslipidaemia; cessation of smoking; use of antiplatelet agents; lifestyle changes and regular exercise are advocated. Plasma homocysteine levels should be reduced if the levels are increased by using folate and other medication [39]. L-Dopa therapy may be beneficial in some situations. If the vascular lesions involve the nigrostriatal pathways, L-dopa therapy is found to be effective. In patients where the other pathways involving WMLs are affected, L-dopa is ineffective. So, Levodopa, dopamine agonists and other traditional antiparkinsonian drugs are

Table 26.1 Vascular rating scale for vascular parkinsonism

Feature	Points
Pathological or angiographic evidence of vascular disease	2
Onset of parkinsonism within 1 month after stroke	1
History of two or more strokes	1
History of two or more vascular risk factors for stroke[a]	1
Neuroimaging evidence of vascular disease in two or more vascular territories	1

Vascular parkinsonism: parkinsonism with a vascular score of 2 or more.
[a]*Vascular risk factors for stroke: hypertension, smoking, diabetes mellitus, hyperlipidaemia, presence of heart disease associated with stroke (coronary artery disease, atrial fibrillation, congestive heart failure, valvular heart disease, mitral valve prolapse or other arrhythmias) and other risk factors for stroke (family history of stroke, history of gout or peripheral vascular disease)*

usually not beneficial for VP [34]. Subthalamic nucleus deep brain stimulation is also not effective [40]. Therapy to minimize the vascular risk factors is expected to slow down the rate of decline, but no studies have yet tested this hypothesis.

CSF drainage has also been suggested as a therapeutic option similar to NPH [41]. It has been noted that patients with VP also have dilated cerebral ventricles. Studies of CSF drainage in VP patients have shown positive results [41]. In most of the studies, the follow-up period was very short. Hence, large randomized studies are required with a large cohort and long follow-up periods to evaluate repeated lumbar puncture (LP) or placement of shunt tube [42].

26.1.2 Normal Pressure Hydrocephalus (NPH)

In 1965, Hakim and Adams first described normal pressure hydrocephalus (NPH). The condition is characterized by the clinical triad of gait impairment, urinary incontinence and memory loss with normal CSF pressure on LP. Neuroimaging shows enlarged cerebral ventricles and improvement of the symptoms of NPH on CSF drainage [43]. The condition is considered to be one of the reversible causes of dementia and impaired gait. NPH is now classified into idiopathic NPH (iNPH) and secondary NPH. The latter is due to subarachnoid haemorrhage, trauma or infectious meningitis [43, 44]. Idiopathic NPH is the most common form of hydrocephalus seen in adults. Ventricular shunting is now the standard of care for patients with secondary NPH [45]. Improvement following shunt surgery in idiopathic NPH is unpredictable, short-lived and associated with significant risks [45, 46].

26.1.2.1 Epidemiology
In one of the epidemiological studies, the incidence was found to be 5.5/100,000 in a Norwegian population [47]. The mean age of onset is about 70 years, and both genders are equally affected. The prevalence of iNPH was estimated at 0.2% (200 out of 100,000 individuals) in a population-based Swedish study in the age group of 70–79 years, and the prevalence increases to 5.9% (5900 out of 100,000 individuals) for the age group above 80 years [48]. In the same geographic area, the incidence of CSF shunting in patients with iNPH was only 2–3 operations per 100,000, which suggests that iNPH might have been underdiagnosed [49].

26.1.2.2 Clinical Presentation
iNPH should be suspected in any elderly patient who presents with gait impairment, cognitive dysfunction and bladder incontinence. The complete triad is not required for the diagnosis as the illness starts with gait impairment and subsequently involves urinary disturbance and cognitive impairment. In most of the patients, the symptoms start insidiously and progress over 3–6 months. iNPH is usually symmetric, and the presence of lateralizing signs should suggest other diagnoses. The presence of limb weakness and upper motor features such as spasticity and hyperreflexia are not typical for iNPH.

Gait abnormality: The gait abnormality is a higher-order gait disturbance. There is difficulty in integrating sensory signal about the position of the body in its environment, including the effect of gravity and proper selection and execution of motor plans for gait or postural reflexes [50, 51]. The gait abnormality is usually symmetric unless coexisting musculoskeletal disorders cause asymmetry. The gait abnormalities include gait initiation failure, shuffling with poor foot clearance, freezing, unstable multistep turns, tripping, falling and postural instability.

Cognitive impairment: Patients have difficulty in managing finances, driving and memory impairment. In the early stages, these patients have mild cognitive impairment, and later these patients may develop dementia. Mini-Mental State Examination (MMSE) and Montreal Cognitive Assessment (MoCA) are useful screening tools [52]. These patients on neuropsychological testing show feature suggestive of subcortical dementia with involvement of executive function causing slow processing and difficulty with problem-solving, and memory loss with poor retrieval with relatively preserved recognition memory [53, 54]. The presence of impaired naming, agnosia, memory disturbances that do not improve with cueing, delusions, hallucinations and prosopagnosia should point towards other neurodegenerative dementias. Depression is also very common, and screening test should be used in these patients [55]. Delirium is usually not a feature of iNPH and may suggest associated neurological disorder or medication side effect. Attention, executive functions, memory, visuo-spatial, visuo-constructional skills and psychomotor retardation are involved in patients with NPH [56–58]. The presence of apathy, along with a decline in executive dysfunction and psychomotor speed, characterizes frontal-subcortical dementia. In long-standing disease, both verbal and visual memory are affected and is due to loss of neurons in the hippocampus [59]. Studies have shown that following shunt surgery, the psychomotor speed improves; however, executive dysfunction rarely improves [60, 61].

Urinary incontinence: Urinary urgency and frequency with or without incontinence are the most common bladder symptoms in patients with iNPH [62]. Patients or caregivers should be asked about the bladder symptoms. Also, the enquiry should be made to the use of any diapers that may not reveal incontinence. Bladder symptoms are also very common in the elderly due to various other causes which need to be considered.

26.1.2.3 Imaging

The diagnosis of iNPH is based on the CT and/or MRI brain. MRI brain is preferable to CT brain. Neuroimaging shows an enlargement of lateral and third ventricles without obstruction to CSF flow. CSF flow studies should be done to look for any obstructive causes. Evan's ratio or index is used to assess ventricular enlargement. It is the ratio of the maximal width of frontal horn span to the maximal diameter of the brain on the same axial image [63]. Evan's ratio of more than 0.3 indicates enlarged ventricles, but not specific for the diagnosis of iNPH. Focal cerebral atrophy often denotes degenerative dementia, is asymmetric in frontotemporal dementia or is stereotypical, such as hippocampal atrophy in Alzheimer's disease. In iNPH, the Sylvian fissures are usually enlarged with ventriculomegaly, out of proportion to the cortical sulci, which are flattened termed as "high tight" convexity [64]. This is likely to impair the CSF flow over the cerebral convexity to the arachnoid granulations. This disproportionately enlarged subarachnoid space hydrocephalus (DESH) has also been reported in Japanese studies. Periventricular WMLs are seen in almost all patients with iNPH. These lesions are seen best in the fluid-attenuated inversion recovery (FLAIR) or T2 MRI sequences. In iNPH, the lesions are found predominantly in periventricular area due to the movement of fluid from the ventricles to the brain parenchyma. WMLs that are more profound in the periphery (corona radiata) or are diffuse and confluent suggest ischaemic changes. Figure 26.2 shows the MRI image of a patient with iNPH.

26.1.2.4 Comorbidities

Idiopathic NPH is a disease of elderly who may have other coexisting medical condition (i.e., comorbidities that contribute to their symptoms) [65]. NPH should be suspected in all the elderly individuals if the comorbidities doesn't clearly explain a patient's symptomatology. Hence the presence of comorbidities does not exclude the diagnosis of NPH. It is important to investigate the associated comorbid conditions as it is likely to influence the surgical outcome. Comorbid conditions such as previous stroke and the presence of neurodegenerative disease can influence the surgical outcome.

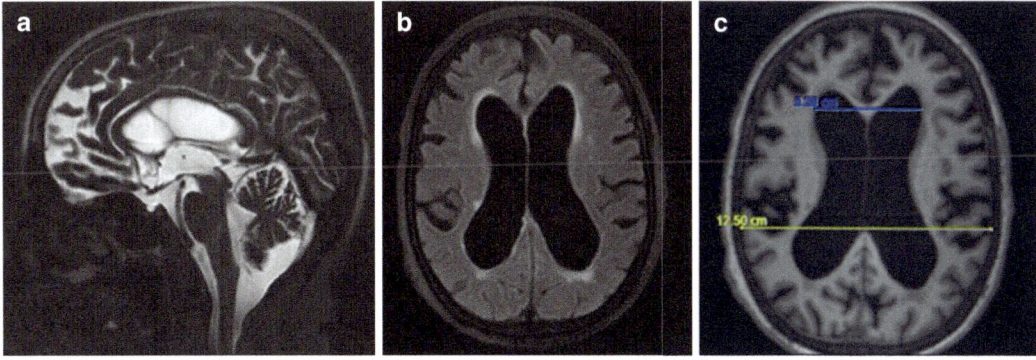

Fig. 26.2 MRI brain mild diffuse cerebral atrophy with dilated cerebral ventricles. Evan's index is 5.28/12.5, i.e., 0.42

26.1.2.5 CSF Tap Test/Lumbar Drainage

This test is performed to look for any improvement in the symptoms following CSF drainage.

It was described by Adams and Fisher. It is believed that if the patient's symptoms improve following CSF drainage, then the shunt surgery may benefit the patient [66]. The patient must be examined before and after the lumbar puncture (LP) to observe for any response and can be documented videographically. Gait impairment is most likely to respond to CSF tap. Preferably the assessments should be performed by the same person. LP should be done with an 18- or 20-gauge spinal needle, and about 30–50 mL of CSF removal is recommended. Follow-up assessment is usually done between 2 and 4 h after the LP. It has been observed that patients of iNPH do not complain of post-LP headache, and these patients need not lie down most of the time following LP. They should be encouraged to be active and can take a walk. If there is significant response following drainage, then shunt surgery can be recommended [67]. However, the lack of response to LP drainage does not exclude shunt responsiveness because the specificity of tap test ranges from 60% to 100%, with sensitivity ranging from 50% to 80%. External lumbar drainage can be another option if iNPH is still suspected even after failed response to tap test.

26.1.2.6 CSF Infusion Test

This test is rarely done to diagnose NPH. It is commonly done in Europe. In this test, Ringer's lactate solution is infused into the spinal fluid via one spinal needle, and simultaneous CSF pressure recording is done via another spinal needle [65, 68]. Various parameters such as intracranial pressure, outflow resistance, pulse pressure curve, CSF formation rate and dural venous pressure can be measured either directly or indirectly. It has been found that patients with iNPH have consistently elevated resistance to CSF outflow [69]. Studies have shown that the resistance to CSF flow of 18 mm Hg/mL per minute or higher is a good predictor of shunt surgery in these patients [70].

26.1.2.7 Treatment of NPH

Till date, the only effective treatment for iNPH is CSF diversion procedure. Symptomatic but transient relief is obtained by the use of acetazolamide and repeated lumbar punctures and can be recommended for patients with high surgical risks [71]. A ventriculoperitoneal shunt is the preferred surgical procedure in these patients, with the proximal catheter placed through the right hemisphere in the posterior parietal region and the distal catheter in the peritoneal cavity. Ventriculo-atrial shunt is placed in patients who had previous peritonitis or abdominal surgeries. The complications associated with shunt surgeries include catheter infection, peritonitis, shunt blockage, over-drainage or under-drainage. Endoscopic third ventriculostomy, another surgical procedure, is indicated in patients of NPH associated with aqueductal stenosis.

References

1. FitzGerald PM, Jankovic J. Lower body parkinsonism: evidence for vascular etiology. Mov Disord. 1989;4(3):249–60.
2. Mehanna R, Jankovic J. Movement disorders in cerebrovascular disease. Lancet Neurol. 2013;12(6):597–608.
3. Critchley M. Arteriosclerotic parkinsonism. Brain. 1929;52(1):23–83.
4. Thompson PD, Marsden CD. Gait disorder of subcortical arteriosclerotic encephalopathy: Binswanger's disease. Mov Disord. 1987;2(1):1–8.
5. Hunter R, Smith J, Thomson T, Dayan AD. Hemiparkinsonism with infarction of the ipsilateral substantia Nigra. Neuropathol Appl Neurobiol. 1978;4(4):297–301.
6. Leys D, Pruvo JP, Parent M, Vermersch P, Soetaert G, Steinling M, et al. Could Wallerian degeneration contribute to "leuko-araiosis" in subjects free of any vascular disorder? J Neurol Neurosurg Psychiatry. 1991;54(1):46–50.
7. Kyriakides TR, Leach KJ, Hoffman AS, Ratner BD, Bornstein P. Mice that lack the angiogenesis inhibitor, thrombospondin 2, mount an altered foreign body reaction characterized by increased vascularity. Proc Natl Acad Sci. 1999;96(8):4449–54.
8. Jellinger KA, Attems J. Prevalence and impact of vascular and Alzheimer pathologies in Lewy body disease. Acta Neuropathol (Berl). 2008;115(4):427–36.
9. Jellinger KA. Prevalence of cerebrovascular lesions in Parkinson's disease. A postmortem study. Acta Neuropathol (Berl). 2003;105(5):415–9.

10. Hughes AJ, Daniel SE, Blankson S, Lees AJ. A clinicopathologic study of 100 cases of Parkinson's disease. Arch Neurol. 1993;50(2):140–8.

11. Glass PG, Lees AJ, Bacellar A, Zijlmans J, Katzenschlager R, Silveira-Moriyama L. The clinical features of pathologically confirmed vascular parkinsonism. J Neurol Neurosurg Psychiatry. 2012;83(10):1027–9.

12. Winikates J, Jankovic J. Clinical correlates of vascular parkinsonism. Arch Neurol. 1999;56(1):98–102.

13. Benamer HTS, Grosset DG. Vascular parkinsonism: a clinical review. Eur Neurol. 2009;61(1):11–5.

14. Gupta D, Kuruvilla A. Vascular parkinsonism: what makes it different? Postgrad Med J. 2011;87(1034):829–36.

15. Sibon I, Fenelon G, Quinn NP, Tison F. Vascular parkinsonism. J Neurol. 2004;251(5):513–24.

16. Okuda B, Kawabata K, Tachibana H, Kamogawa K, Okamoto K. Primitive reflexes distinguish vascular parkinsonism from Parkinson's disease. Clin Neurol Neurosurg. 2008;110(6):562–5.

17. Atchison PR, Thompson PD, Frackowiak RS, Marsden CD. The syndrome of gait ignition failure: a report of six cases. Mov Disord. 1993;8(3):285–92.

18. Udagedara TB, Alahakoon AMBD, Goonaratna IK. Vascular parkinsonism: a review on management updates. Ann Indian Acad Neurol. 2019;22(1):17.

19. Navarro-Otano J, Gaig C, Muxi A, Lomeña F, Compta Y, Buongiorno MT, et al. 123I-MIBG cardiac uptake, smell identification and 123I-FP-CIT SPECT in the differential diagnosis between vascular parkinsonism and Parkinson's disease. Parkinsonism Relat Disord. 2014;20(2):192–7.

20. Santangelo G, Vitale C, Trojano L, Gaspari DD, Bilo L, Antonini A, et al. Differential neuropsychological profiles in parkinsonian patients with or without vascular lesions. Mov Disord. 2010;25(1):50–6.

21. Benítez-Rivero S, Lama MJ, Huertas-Fernández I, Álvarez de Toledo P, Cáceres-Redondo MT, Martín-Rodríguez JF, et al. Clinical features and neuropsychological profile in vascular parkinsonism. J Neurol Sci. 2014;345(1):193–7.

22. Rektor I, Goldemund D, Sheardová K, Rektorová I, Michálková Z, Dufek M. Vascular pathology in patients with idiopathic Parkinson's disease. Parkinsonism Relat Disord. 2009;15(1):24–9.

23. Balash Y, Korczyn AD. Vascular parkinsonism. Handb Clin Neurol. 2007;84:417–25.

24. Foltynie T, Barker R, Brayne C. Vascular parkinsonism: a review of the precision and frequency of the diagnosis. Neuroepidemiology. 2002;21(1):1–7.

25. Yamanouchi H, Nagura H. Neurological signs and frontal white matter lesions in vascular parkinsonism. A clinicopathologic study. Stroke. 1997;28(5):965–9.

26. Durand-Fardel M. Traite du ramollissement du cerveau (etc.). J. B. Bailliere; 1843. p. 552.

27. Park J. Movement disorders following cerebrovascular lesion in the basal ganglia circuit. J Mov Disord. 2016;9(2):71–9.

28. Vizcarra JA, Lang AE, Sethi KD, Espay AJ. Vascular parkinsonism: deconstructing a syndrome. Mov Disord. 2015;30(7):886–94.

29. Harik SI, Al-Hinti JT, Archer RL, Angtuaco EJC. Hemiparkinsonism after unilateral traumatic midbrain hemorrhage in a young woman. Neurol Clin Pract. 2013;3(1):4–7.

30. Benítez-Rivero S, Marín-Oyaga VA, García-Solís D, Huertas-Fernández I, García-Gómez FJ, Jesús S, et al. Clinical features and 123I-FP-CIT SPECT imaging in vascular parkinsonism and Parkinson's disease. J Neurol Neurosurg Psychiatry. 2013;84(2):122–9.

31. Jellinger KA. Vascular parkinsonism--neuropathological findings. Acta Neurol Scand. 2002;105(5):414–5.

32. Auriel E, Bornstein NM, Berenyi E, Varkonyi I, Gabor M, Majtenyi K, et al. Clinical, radiological and pathological correlates of leukoaraiosis. Acta Neurol Scand. 2011;123(1):41–7.

33. Rosenberg GA, Bjerke M, Wallin A. Multimodal markers of inflammation in the subcortical ischemic vascular disease type of vascular cognitive impairment. Stroke J Cereb Circ. 2014;45(5):1531–8.

34. Zijlmans JCM, Daniel SE, Hughes AJ, Révész T, Lees AJ. Clinicopathological investigation of vascular parkinsonism, including clinical criteria for diagnosis. Mov Disord. 2004;19(6):630–40.

35. Peters S, Eising EG, Przuntek H, Müller T. Vascular parkinsonism: a case report and review of the literature. J Clin Neurosci. 2001;8(3):268–71.

36. Alarcón F, Zijlmans JCM, Dueñas G, Cevallos N. Post-stroke movement disorders: report of 56 patients. J Neurol Neurosurg Psychiatry. 2004;75(11):1568–74.

37. Siniscalchi A, Gallelli L, Labate A, Malferrari G, Palleria C, Sarro GD. Post-stroke movement disorders: clinical manifestations and pharmacological management. Curr Neuropharmacol. 2012;10(3):254–62.

38. Antonini A, Vitale C, Barone P, Cilia R, Righini A, Bonuccelli U, et al. The relationship between cerebral vascular disease and parkinsonism: the VADO study. Parkinsonism Relat Disord. 2012;18(6):775–80.

39. de Vecchi AF, Novembrino C, Patrosso MC, Cresseri D, Ippolito S, Rosina M, et al. Effect of incremental doses of folate on homocysteine and metabolically related vitamin concentrations in nondiabetic patients on peritoneal dialysis. ASAIO J. 2003;49(6):655.

40. Krack P, Dowsey PL, Benabid AL, Acarin N, Benazzouz A, Künig G, et al. Ineffective subthalamic nucleus stimulation in levodopa-resistant postischemic parkinsonism. Neurology. 2000;54(11):2182–4.

41. Espay AJ, Narayan RK, Duker AP, Barrett ET, de Courten-Myers G. Lower-body parkinsonism: reconsidering the threshold for external lumbar drainage. Nat Clin Pract Neurol. 2008;4(1):50–5.

42. Korczyn AD. Vascular parkinsonism--characteristics, pathogenesis and treatment. Nat Rev Neurol. 2015;11(6):319–26.

43. Hakim S, Adams RD. The special clinical problem of symptomatic hydrocephalus with normal cerebrospinal fluid pressure. Observations on cerebrospinal fluid hydrodynamics. J Neurol Sci. 1965;2(4):307–27.

44. Ishikawa M. Guideline Committee for Idiopathic Normal Pressure Hydrocephalus, Japanese Society of Normal Pressure Hydrocephalus. Clinical guidelines for idiopathic normal pressure hydrocephalus. Neurol Med Chir (Tokyo). 2004;44(4):222–3.

45. Hebb AO, Cusimano MD. Idiopathic normal pressure hydrocephalus: a systematic review of diagnosis and outcome. Neurosurgery. 2001;49(5):1166–84; discussion 1184-1186.

46. Kahlon B, Sjunnesson J, Rehncrona S. Long-term outcome in patients with suspected normal pressure hydrocephalus. Neurosurgery. 2007;60(2):327–32; discussion 332.

47. Brean A, Eide PK. Prevalence of probable idiopathic normal pressure hydrocephalus in a Norwegian population. Acta Neurol Scand. 2008;118(1):48–53.

48. Jaraj D, Rabiei K, Marlow T, Jensen C, Skoog I, Wikkelsø C. Prevalence of idiopathic normal-pressure hydrocephalus. Neurology. 2014;82(16):1449–54.

49. Tisell M, Höglund M, Wikkelsø C. National and regional incidence of surgery for adult hydrocephalus in Sweden. Acta Neurol Scand. 2005;112(2):72–5.

50. Nutt JG, Bloem BR, Giladi N, Hallett M, Horak FB, Nieuwboer A. Freezing of gait: moving forward on a mysterious clinical phenomenon. Lancet Neurol. 2011;10(8):734–44.

51. Stolze H, Kuhtz-Buschbeck JP, Drücke H, Jöhnk K, Diercks C, Palmié S, et al. Gait analysis in idiopathic normal pressure hydrocephalus--which parameters respond to the CSF tap test? Clin Neurophysiol. 2000;111(9):1678–86.

52. Behrens A, Eklund A, Elgh E, Smith C, Williams MA, Malm J. A computerized neuropsychological test battery designed for idiopathic normal pressure hydrocephalus. Fluids Barriers CNS. 2014;11(1):22.

53. Thomas G, McGirt MJ, Woodworth G, Heidler J, Rigamonti D, Hillis AE, et al. Baseline neuropsychological profile and cognitive response to cerebrospinal fluid shunting for idiopathic Normal pressure hydrocephalus. Dement Geriatr Cogn Disord. 2005;20(2–3):163–8.

54. Hellström P, Klinge P, Tans J, Wikkelsø C. The neuropsychology of iNPH: findings and evaluation of tests in the European multicentre study. Clin Neurol Neurosurg. 2012;114(2):130–4.

55. Israelsson H, Allard P, Eklund A, Malm J. Symptoms of depression are common in patients with idiopathic Normal pressure hydrocephalus: the INPH-CRasH study. Neurosurgery. 2016;78(2):161–8.

56. Mataró M, Poca MA, Matarín MDM, Catalan R, Sahuquillo J, Galard R. CSF galanin and cognition after shunt surgery in normal pressure hydrocephalus. J Neurol Neurosurg Psychiatry. 2003;74(9):1272–7.

57. Iddon JL, Pickard JD, Cross JJ, Griffiths PD, Czosnyka M, Sahakian BJ. Specific patterns of cognitive impairment in patients with idiopathic normal pressure hydrocephalus and Alzheimer's disease: a pilot study. J Neurol Neurosurg Psychiatry. 1999;67(6):723–32.

58. Iddon J, Morgan D, Loveday C, Sahakian B, Pickard J. Neuropsychological profile of young adults with spina bifida with or without hydrocephalus. J Neurol Neurosurg Psychiatry. 2004;75(8):1112–8.

59. Golomb J, de Leon MJ, George AE, Kluger A, Convit A, Rusinek H, et al. Hippocampal atrophy correlates with severe cognitive impairment in elderly patients with suspected normal pressure hydrocephalus. J Neurol Neurosurg Psychiatry. 1994;57(5): 590–3.

60. Gustafson L, Hagberg B. Recovery in hydrocephalic dementia after shunt operation. J Neurol Neurosurg Psychiatry. 1978;41(10):940–7.

61. Goodman M, Meyer WJ. Dementia reversal in post-shunt normal pressure hydrocephalus predicted by neuropsychological assessment. J Am Geriatr Soc. 2001;49(5):685–6.

62. Sakakibara R, Kanda T, Sekido T, Uchiyama T, Awa Y, Ito T, et al. Mechanism of bladder dysfunction in idiopathic normal pressure hydrocephalus. Neurourol Urodyn. 2008;27(6):507–10.

63. Williams MA, Malm J. Diagnosis and treatment of idiopathic Normal pressure hydrocephalus. Contin Minneap Minn. 2016;22(2 Dementia):579–99.

64. Osborn AG, Salzman KL, Jhaveri MD, Barkovich AJ. Diagnostic imaging: brain E-book. Elsevier Health Sciences; 2015. p. 1237.

65. Malm J, Graff-Radford NR, Ishikawa M, Kristensen B, Leinonen V, Mori E, et al. Influence of comorbidities in idiopathic normal pressure hydrocephalus - research and clinical care. A report of the ISHCSF task force on comorbidities in INPH. Fluids Barriers CNS. 2013;10(1):22.

66. Williams MA, Relkin NR. Diagnosis and management of idiopathic normal-pressure hydrocephalus. Neurol Clin Pract. 2013;3(5):375–85.

67. Wikkelsø C, Hellström P, Klinge PM, Tans JTJ, European iNPH Multicentre Study Group. The European iNPH multicentre study on the predictive values of resistance to CSF outflow and the CSF tap test in patients with idiopathic normal pressure hydrocephalus. J Neurol Neurosurg Psychiatry. 2013;84(5):562–8.

68. Eklund A, Smielewski P, Chambers I, Alperin N, Malm J, Czosnyka M, et al. Assessment of cerebrospinal fluid outflow resistance. Med Biol Eng Comput. 2007;45(8):719–35.

69. Kim D-J, Kim H, Kim Y-T, Yoon BC, Czosnyka Z, Park K-W, et al. Thresholds of resistance to CSF outflow in predicting shunt responsiveness. Neurol Res. 2015 Apr;37(4):332–40.

70. Marmarou A, Bergsneider M, Klinge P, Relkin N, Black PM. The value of supplemental prognostic tests for the preoperative assessment of idiopathic normal-pressure hydrocephalus. Neurosurgery. 2005;57(3 Suppl):S17–28. discussion ii-v

71. Bret P, Guyotat J, Chazal J. Is normal pressure hydrocephalus a valid concept in 2002? A reappraisal in five questions and proposal for a new designation of the syndrome as "chronic hydrocephalus". J Neurol Neurosurg Psychiatry. 2002;73(1): 9–12.

Childhood Dystonia

Anjali Chouksey and Sanjay Pandey

Case Scenario An 8-year-old male child was referred to our movement disorder clinic with a history of abnormal involuntary posturing of both lower limb and neck first noticed by his parents when he started walking with support at 1 year of age. It gradually progressed to involve both of his upper limbs over the next 1 year. He was a full-term normal vaginal delivery with prolonged labour leading to birth asphyxia and delayed crying with 2 episodes of seizures on day 1 of life. There was no history of diurnal variation of symptoms or any trigger factors or worsening of symptoms with stress fatigue or action. Cognitive development was normal, but he left school because of restriction of physical ability. Parents denied any history of other abnormal movement disorder in the form of myoclonic jerks or tremors. There was no history suggestive of acute febrile encephalopathy in early childhood or any evidence of drug or toxin exposure. There was no associated history of hearing loss or vision problems, painful muscle spasm, alopecia, diarrhoea, or endocrinal and skeletal abnormalities, or history suggestive of gastroesophageal reflux. There was no similar family history or parental consanguinity. On general physical examination, there was no pallor, icterus, Kayser-Fleischer ring or organomegaly. Central nervous system examination revealed normal mentation. Tone, power and deep tendon reflex were also normal. The planters were bilateral extensor. On extrapyramidal examination, upper limb and lower limb dystonia and left torticollis were present. Sensory examination was normal. Investigations showed normal hemogram, liver and renal function tests. Serum ceruloplasmin level was normal. Urine for organic acids was also negative. Magnetic resonance imaging (MRI) of the brain revealed no significant intracranial abnormality.

27.1 Introduction

In 1911, Oppenheim provided the initial account of dystonia by introducing the term "dystonia musculorum deformans". He documented the experiences of four young individuals, describing their condition as a fluctuation between reduced muscle tone and prolonged muscle spasms, often occurring when they moved voluntarily, but not exclusively limited to those instances [1]. Subsequently, Oppenheim coined the term "dystonia", which continues to be used today.

In 2013, an international Consensus Committee was formed with the support of the Dystonia Medical Research Foundation, the Dystonia Coalition, and the 'European Dystonia

A. Chouksey
Department of Neurology, Govind Ballabh Pant Postgraduate Institute of Medical Education and Research, New Delhi, India

S. Pandey (✉)
Department of Neurology, Amrita Hospital, Faridabad, Delhi National Capital Region, India

© Springer Nature Singapore Pte Ltd. 2024
K. K. Oli et al. (eds.), *Case-based Approach to Common Neurological Disorders*,
https://doi.org/10.1007/978-981-99-8676-7_27

Cooperation in Science and Technology (COST) Action.' This committee put forth a revised definition of dystonia, stating that it is a movement disorder characterized by sustained or intermittent muscle contractions causing abnormal, often repetitive, movements, postures, or both. Dystonic movements are typically characterized by twisting patterns and may exhibit tremors. Dystonia is often triggered or aggravated by voluntary actions and is associated with overflow muscle activation [2].

The categorization of dystonia based on the age of onset is significant for both diagnostic assessments and prognostic implications. In previous classification systems, three age groups were taken into account: childhood (0–12 years), adolescence (12–20 years), and adult onset (above 20 years) [3]. In the 2013 Consensus Committee's proposal, various categories of dystonia were suggested, each corresponding to a specific range of age at onset. These categories include:

- Infancy: from birth to 2 years of age
- Childhood: from 3 to 12 years of age
- Adolescence: from 13 to 20 years of age
- Early adulthood: from 21 to 40 years of age
- Late adulthood: above 40 years of age

Dystonia that appears during the initial 1–2 years of life is associated with underlying causes such as inherited metabolic disorder with specific diagnostic approach and carries poor prognostic implications [4]. Therefore, it is proposed to divide dystonia in the paediatric age group into two further classes, namely infancy and childhood.

Correct identification of dystonia in paediatric patients requires good knowledge about the phenomenology of dystonia, as the characteristic features of dystonia seen in the adult population may not be present. Features such as sensory tricks and overflowing should be interpreted in the context of the age of the patient with dystonia. For example, sensory tricks are often not seen in paediatric dystonia patients, because they are more commonly observed in cranial or cervical dystonia, while in children, dystonia is more often generalized with limb and trunk predomi-

nance. Similarly, overflowing can be a normal physiological process seen in young children which disappears with normal motor development [5].

In some cases, children may exhibit transient dystonic movements and postures, such as benign paroxysmal torticollis and benign idiopathic dystonia of infancy, which are often attributed to temporary neuronal dysfunction. However, it is important to note that these conditions usually resolve on their own without any long-lasting dystonic effects [6].

The Consensus Committee also put forth a suggestion to replace the terms "primary" and "secondary" dystonia with "inherited", "acquired", or "idiopathic" dystonia. Under this proposed framework, the classifications are defined as follows:

- Inherited dystonia: Dystonia with a confirmed genetic origin
- Acquired dystonia: Dystonia linked to a specific non-genetic cause that has been identified
- Idiopathic dystonia: Dystonia with an unknown or yet-to-be-identified cause

27.2 Common Causes of Acquired Dystonia

1. *Cerebral palsy*: Dyskinetic cerebral palsy (CP) is the predominant form of acquired dystonia observed in children, and it is characterized by the coexistence of choreoathetosis and dystonia. It is more prevalent in children born at full term who have a history of birth asphyxia or perinatal trauma. In dyskinetic CP, the hyperkinetic movements typically manifest bilaterally and typically commence after the first year of life. These movements tend to progress gradually over the course of several years [7].

2. *Infection:* Occasional isolated cases have been reported where childhood dystonia has been associated with infections, including viral infections, tuberculosis, mycoplasma, or toxoplasmosis. Among these, dystonia caused by flaviviruses, particularly Japanese enceph-

alitis, is a significant factor in the development of childhood dystonia [8]. The primary bacterial infections linked to dystonia include tuberculosis and mycoplasma pneumoniae [9]. In children presenting with dystonia accompanied by symptoms of meningoencephalitis or encephalitis, it is crucial to investigate the possibility of an underlying infection.

3. *Acquired structural lesions:* Structural lesions, such as stroke, trauma, or neoplasms involving caudate, lenticular nucleus, or thalamus may result in unilateral childhood dystonia (focal or hemi-dystonia). In such cases, the dystonia develops months or even years after the incident [10].

4. *Autoimmune encephalitis*: Several autoantibody-associated disorders can lead to childhood dystonia but are usually combined with other signs of encephalopathy like behavioural changes or epilepsy. Antibodies against N-methyl-D-aspartate, glutamic acid decarboxylase, collapsin response mediator protein, Ma2, and Yo are identified to be associated with autoimmune encephalitis in children [11]. Rubio-Agusti et al. and Mohammad et al. reported cases of children and young adults with NMDAR antibodies having hemi-dystonia and craniocervical dystonia as the most prominent feature respectively [12, 13].

5. *Drug and toxin*: Dystonia can be attributed to a diverse range of drug groups, such as neuroleptics, antiemetics (dopamine receptor blocking drugs), dopamine receptor stimulants, anticonvulsants (specifically phenytoin and carbamazepine), antimalarials, antihistamines, stimulants, or calcium channel blockers, as well as exposure to substances like carbon monoxide and cyanide.

6. *Metabolic causes*: Metabolic causes of dystonia can be categorized into the following groups:
   (a) *Metal and Mineral Metabolism:* This includes conditions such as Wilson's disease, neurodegeneration with brain iron accumulation type I, neuroferritinopathy, and idiopathic basal ganglia calcification (Fahr disease).
   (b) *In-born Errors of Metabolism:* Disorders such as Lesch-Nyhan syndrome, triosephosphate isomerase deficiency, and glucose transport defects are part of this group.
   (c) *Lysosomal Storage Disorders:* Conditions like Niemann-Pick disease type C, GM1 and 2 gangliosidosis, metachromatic leukodystrophy, Krabbe disease, Pelizaeus-Merzbacher disease, and Fucosidosis fall under this category.
   (d) *Amino and Organic Acidurias:* Conditions like glutaric aciduria type 1, homocystinuria, propionic acidemia, methylmalonic aciduria, 4-hydroxybutyric aciduria, 3-methylglutaconic aciduria, 2-oxoglutaric aciduria, and Hartnup's disease are included in this category.

27.3 Dystonia Mimics

- Tics, stereotypies
- Functional
- Myotonia, neuromyotonia
- Cramp, rigidity, spasticity, spasms (hypocalcaemia, hypomagnesaemia, alkalosis)
- Focal tonic seizures
- Syndromes like spasmus nutans, Sandifer syndrome, Satoyoshi syndrome, etc.

27.3.1 Spasmus Nutans

Spasmus nutans is a syndrome that typically manifests during early childhood. It is characterized by a triad of symptoms, including rhythmic head nodding, oscillations of the eyes, and an abnormal head position. Other ophthalmological and neurological examinations yield normal results. This syndrome is considered benign and tends to resolve spontaneously over time [14].

27.3.2 Sandifer Syndrome

Sandifer syndrome refers to a condition where gastro-oesophageal reflux disease is accompanied by spastic torticollis and dystonic body movements, sometimes occurring with or without hiatal hernia. One hypothesis suggests that the unusual positioning of the head provides relief from abdominal discomfort caused by acid reflux [15].

27.3.3 Satoyoshi Syndrome

Satoyoshi syndrome is an uncommon condition that affects multiple systems and is believed to have an autoimmune cause. It is characterized by gradually worsening muscle spasms accompanied by pain, hair loss (alopecia), persistent diarrhea, and skeletal and endocrine irregularities. These symptoms often lead to early disability and, in severe cases, even death. Treatment options for patients have included immunoglobulins and glucocorticoids, although the outcomes have varied [16].

27.4 Genetic Dystonia

Genetic dystonias consist of three main categories [17] (Tables 27.1 and 27.2):
1. Isolated or pure dystonia
2. Combined (formerly "dystonia-plus"), in which dystonia is accompanied by myoclonus or parkinsonism
3. Complex, in which dystonia is one feature of a complex neurological syndrome

Table 27.1 New phenotypic group of genetic dystonias

New phenotypic group	Subgroups	Loci	Gene involved	Clinical features	Hereditary pattern
Isolated	Generalized	DYT 1	TOR1A	• Onset as a focal *lower limb dystonia in childhood* • Average age of onset is 13 years • More than 60% of patients will progress to generalized or multifocal dystonia • *Robust response to pallidal deep brain stimulation (GPi DBS)* • Sparing of larynx and neck; can be jerky	AD
		DYT 2	HPCA	• *Mainly upper limb* and cervical dystonia that presented within the first decade of life and gradually progressed	AR
		DYT 4	TUBB4A	• *Prominent laryngeal dysphonia*, with craniocervical, segmental, or generalized dystonia • A characteristic *"hobby horse" gait* • Onset is mostly in the second to third decade • TUBB 4 A gene mutations also associated with disorder of hypomyelination with atrophy of the basal ganglia and cerebellum (H-ABC syndrome), characterized by infantile to childhood onset, developmental delay with cerebellar ataxia, dystonia, progressive spastic tetraplegia, and epilepsy	AD
		DYT 6	THAP1	• Average age of onset is in *late adolescence (16.1 years)* but can range from 2 to 54 years • 50% of patients initially present with cranial or cervical dystonia and have *prominent laryngeal involvement* • DBS therapy less effective in this type	AD
	Focal or segmental	DYT 23	CIZ1	• Age of onset ranging from the second to the seventh decade • Cervical dystonia sometimes with tremor • Awaiting confirmation	AD
		DYT 24	ANO3	• *Tremor* is a key feature, mostly as head and arm tremor, and sometimes manifesting before clinically overt dystonia • Cranial and laryngeal dystonia as well as mild dystonia of the arms noted in some cases • Generalized dystonia is almost never seen • 2 reported cases of ANO3-related *childhood onset generalized dystonia with myoclonus* • Age at onset ranges from 3 to 40 years	AD
		DYT 25		• Cervical dystonia which progresses to segmental dystonia • Average age of onset is 31 years • *Hyposmia* may be a clue to diagnosis in the respective clinical setting, present in 0–36% cases	AD
Combined	Myoclonus	DYT11	Epsilon sarcoglycan (SGCE)	• Onset usually in the first or second decade, although can be as late as the fifth decade • *Myoclonic jerks, sometimes alcohol responsive*, affecting principally the proximal limb musculature • Dystonia, typically cervical dystonia and writer's cramp • Psychiatric morbidity • Inter- and intra-familial clinical heterogeneity due to a maternal imprinting mechanism	
		DYT 5a	GTP cyclohydrolase 1	• Typical age of presentation 5–9 years • *Focal limb-onset (leg > arm) dystonia* • Diurnal fluctuation • Brisk deep tendon reflexes and ankle clonus may be present on examination • Higher penetrance in females with ratio of *1:2.5–4 boys to girls* • Improvement with levodopa treatment	AD
		DYT5b	Tyrosine hydroxylase deficiency	• Type A—Progressive hypokinetic–rigid syndrome with dystonia • Type B—complex encephalopathy, tremor, ptosis, autonomic disturbance, spasticity, hypotonia, delayed motor developmental milestones, intellectual disability	AR
			Sepiapterin reductase deficiency	• Axial hypotonia, delays in the development of motor function and language, *oculogyric crises*, muscle weakness, and action dystonia • Onset of symptoms is usually before the age of 12 months	AR
		BHC	NKX2.1 gene	• Onset of chorea is usually in early childhood (median age 2.5–3 years) • Generalized chorea, affecting all body parts (face, limbs, trunk) and tends to worsen with stress or excitement • In the majority of cases, the chorea remain static, or improve in later life with other movement disorders like ataxia, upper limb intention tremor, limb dystonia, and motor and vocal tics becoming more prevalent and disabling	AD

(continued)

Table 27.1 (continued)

New phenotypic group	Subgroups	Loci	Gene involved	Clinical features	Hereditary pattern
	Parkinsonism	DYT 3 OR XDP OR LUBAG	TAF 1	• XDP or Lubag affects primarily adult *Filipino men* and, rarely, women • Male-to-female ratio 99:1 • Mean age of onset in men is 39 years • *Initial presenting sign is almost universally parkinsonism* • The dystonia develops focally, mostly in the jaw, neck, trunk, and eyes, and less commonly in the limbs, tongue, pharynx, and larynx • Most characteristic dystonia *is jaw dystonia*, more commonly presenting as jaw opening difficulty as compared to jaw closing • Jaw dystonia often progresses to neck dystonia, with *retrocollis > torticollis*	X-linked
		DYT 16	PRKRA	• Early-onset generalized dystonia • Age of onset-2-18 years, and • The condition manifests as a focal, predominantly limb dystonia that causes gait and writing problems and then becomes generalized • Prominent oro– mandibular involvement, dystonic sardonic smile, dysarthria, dysphagia, retrocollis and dystonic opisthotonus, and psychiatric changes • Pyramidal signs (hyperreflexia and ankle clonus) are present in most of the patients • In all the cases the dystonia spreads to involve facial, cervical, or laryngeal regions, differentiating from another early-onset dystonia, DYT1, starting in the limbs • Parkinsonism, if present, is usually mild, and mostly unresponsive to levodopa	AR
		DYT 5a and 5b		As explained	
		YOPD	PARKIN; PINK1; DJ-1	• Focal dystonia involving mainly lower limb can be presenting feature	AR

		ROPD/ DYT 12	ATP1A3	• Mutations in ATP1A3 cause a spectrum of neurological disorders, which includes
				  1. *ROPD* (rapid onset dystonia parkinsonism)
				  2. *AHC* (alternating hemiplegia of childhood), and
				  3. *CAPOS* syndrome (cerebellar ataxia, areflexia, pes cavus, optic atrophy, and sensorineural hearing loss)
				• Onset of RDP typically occurs in adolescence or early adulthood, rare after the age of 40
				• *Asymmetric dystonia and parkinsonism with prominent bulbar symptoms of abrupt onset, often associated with triggering factors* (stress, alcohol, exercise, hyperthermia and hypothermia, childbirth)
				• *Rostrocaudal gradient of severity of bulbar symptoms* >upper limbs, >lower limbs
				• RDP stops progressing within weeks, after which there is little or no improvement
				• Patients with RODP do not respond to levodopa
				• Imaging studies do not show any decrease of dopamine reuptake sites or striatal dopamine transporters
					AD

		DTDS	SLC63	• Usually infantile-onset parkinsonism-dystonia with a rapidly progressive disease course, but may have a later onset (childhood–adulthood) and a slower disease course • Oculogyric crisis may be seen similar to other dopa-responsive dystonia due to defects of the dopamine synthesis pathway • DTDS responds poorly to dopaminergic medication • The DAT SPECT scan in DTDS is grossly abnormal • Characteristic cerebrospinal fluid abnormality with a ratio of homovanillic acid to 5-hydroxyindoleacetic acid (HVA:5-HIAA) > 4	AR
Paroxysmal	Paroxysmal kinesigenic dyskinesia	PKD; DYT10	PRRT2	• Childhood onset • Episodic dystonia induced by rapid movement to an unexpected stimulus; spells decrease in adulthood • Last for seconds in duration, around 100 times a day • Responds well to anticonvulsants	AD
	Paroxysmal non-kinesigenic dyskinesia	PNKD1; DYT8	MR-1	• Infancy onset • Episodic, last longer (10mins), and less frequent • Episodes precipitated by stress, caffeine, and ethanol • Does not respond to anticonvulsants	AD
	Paroxysmal exercise-induced dyskinesia	PED; DYT18	SLC2A1, encoding the Glut1 glucose transporter	• Episodes of involuntary movements that are triggered by exercise, such as sustained period of walking • Spasticity, ataxia, dystonia, seizures, and intellectual disability • Symptom onset is usually in infancy or early childhood • Hallmark of the disease is a *low CSF glucose concentration in the setting of normoglycemia* • Ketogenic diet leads to significant improvement in symptoms and may improve long-term outcome	AD

Table 27.2 Complex Dystonias

S No	Disorder	Pathogenesis	Gene involved
1	Biotin-responsive basal ganglia disease	Thiamine transporter-2 (hTHTR2) deficiency	SLC19A3 gene
2	Lesch-Nyhan syndrome	Disorder of purine metabolism resulting from deficiency of enzyme hypoxanthine–guanine phosphoribosyl transferase	X-linked (HGPRT)
3	Niemann-Pick disease type C	Lipid storage disorder- impaired intracellular cholesterol homeostasis and defective cholesterol trafficking through the late endosomal / lysosomal system	(NPC1)
4	Glutaric aciduria and other organic acidemias with dystonia		
5	Dystonia with brain manganese accumulation (DBMA)		SLC30A10 mutation
6	Mitochondrial encephalopathies		various mitochondrial DNA and nuclear DNA genes
7	Homocystinuria	Different enzymatic defects. The most common is cystathionine— synthase deficiency	
8	Hartnup disease	Defect in amino acid transport	SLC6A19
9	NBIA		PLA2G6, PANK2, WDR45, ATP13A2 and others
10	Wilson's disease	Defect of copper metabolism leading to deposition of copper in the liver, brain, and other tissues	ATP7B

27.5 Approach to Childhood Dystonia

Considering the patient's history and examination, it appears that dyskinetic cerebral palsy (DCP) is the most likely diagnosis in this case. DCP is the leading cause of acquired dystonia in childhood. It tends to be more prevalent in full-term infants who have experienced perinatal insults, as is the case here, since the basal ganglia are susceptible to pathogenic events during the later stages of pregnancy [13]. In DCP, the hyperkinetic movements are usually bilateral and mostly begin after the first year of life, and are slowly progressive over years as was the case in our patient. Other common secondary causes are less likely as there is no history of preceding febrile illness, drug or toxin exposure, or trauma during infancy. Insidious onset and slowly progressive nature of the disease in this case also negates the likelihood of infectious, demyelinating, or traumatic cause of dystonia. Most of the cases of DCP are characterized by the presence of both dystonia and choreoathetosis, although both movement disorders occur independently and dystonia predominates in most patients with DCP [18] (Fig. 27.1).

Each child with suspected dyskinetic cerebral palsy should undergo appropriate evaluation and investigation to establish a specific cause and to rule out any underlying treatable cause. Various neurological or metabolic disorder increases the risk of perinatal stress; therefore investigation should be done to rule out such etiology even when a history of perinatal trauma is present.

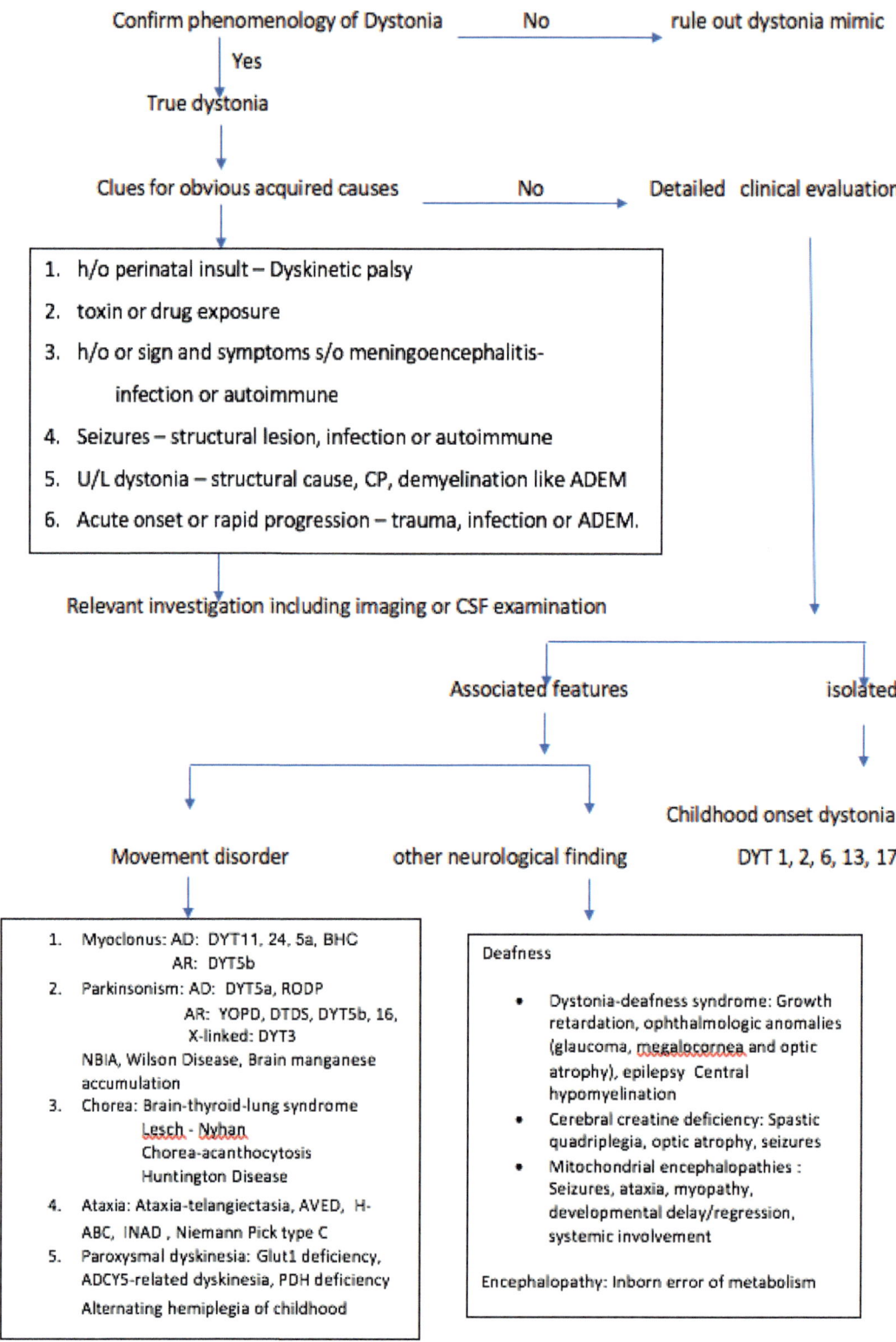

Fig. 27.1 Flow chart: Approach to childhood dystonia

Apart from considering the history of birth asphyxia, other possible differential diagnoses in this patient include glutaric aciduria and other organic acidemias associated with dystonia. Typically, clinical symptoms in such cases manifest between 5 and 14 months of age, although mild signs such as slight motor delay and hypotonia may be observed earlier. Around 70% of cases exhibit macrocephaly at birth or develop it during infancy [19]. In most cases, symptoms present abruptly with focal seizures or generalized convulsions, vomiting, altered sensorium, or lethargy, often following an acute infectious illness. Following the acute episode, there is a subsequent onset of psychomotor regression and dystonic or choreo-athetoid movements. Generalized dystonia is a distinctive neurological manifestation, while cognitive function tends to remain relatively preserved. [20] Roughly 50% of patients with these conditions do not survive beyond the age of four due to complications during intercurrent illnesses. However, in the case of our patient, no significant head enlargement was observed by the parents. Additionally, the gradual onset of the disease without a preceding history of triggers such as acute febrile illness also makes the possibility of glutaric aciduria or other acidurias less likely. The potential clinical complications associated with glutaric aciduria can be prevented through the oral administration of L-carnitine and proactive treatment during episodes of intercurrent illness. With this in mind, we conducted tests to detect the presence of organic acids in the patient's urine, but the results were negative.

Infantile-onset dystonia can also be attributed to Lesch-Nyhan syndrome, which typically emerges at between 6 and 18 months of age. Patients with this condition often exhibit delayed psychomotor development, as well as hypotonia or spasticity. Initially, abnormal movements manifest as fine athetoid movements in the hands and feet, but later become predominantly dystonic, occasionally accompanied by chorea and tremor. An identifying characteristic is the presence of aggressive behaviour and self-mutilation, particularly affecting the lips and fingers, which commonly starts with the eruption of teeth.

Furthermore, patients may experience extra-neurological symptoms such as hematuria, crystalluria, and signs of hyperuricemia, including renal stones, gouty arthritis, and tophi [21]. Since there was no such history of behavioural abnormality and absence of features suggestive of hyperuricemia, the probability of Lesch-Nyhan syndrome is low in our case. However, Lesch-Nyhan variants can also manifest in the form of a dystonic gait, speech difficulties, spasticity, less severe dystonia with normal cognitive function, and behavioural abnormality without self-mutilation. To exclude this condition, plasma uric acid was tested in our patient, which was in normal range.

Considering the genetically isolated dystonias, it is worth considering the possibility of DYT1 dystonia in this case. DYT1 dystonia is the most prevalent form of genetic dystonia, inherited in an autosomal-dominant pattern. Typically, DYT1-TOR1A manifests as focal limb dystonia during childhood. The average age of onset is around 13 years, although it can vary widely from 1 to 28 years. Over 60% of patients with DYT1 dystonia will eventually progress to generalized or multifocal dystonia. Importantly, DYT1 dystonia has shown highly positive responses to pallidal deep brain stimulation (GPi DBS). Therefore, it should be considered as a potential diagnosis in patients presenting with isolated dystonia characterized by focal limb onset without any associated neurological deficits [22, 23].

Since our patient had gradually progressive persistent dystonias without any fluctuation or paroxysmal episodes triggered by exercise, stress, caffeine, or any particular task, primary paroxysmal syndromes like DYT 8, 10, and 18 were not considered.

Dopa-responsive dystonia (DRD) may have a presentation similar to DCP. There is higher penetrance in females, with a ratio of 1:2.5–4 (boys to girls). Dystonia in DRD usually starts as focal limb onset (leg > arm), which usually worsens as the day progresses, with sleep benefit. The typical age of presentation is 5–9 years. DRD usually shows a dramatic response to small doses of levodopa [24, 25].

27.6 Treatment

Limited clinical trials are available for the treatment of childhood dystonia, resulting in a scarcity of established therapeutic protocols. Consequently, treatment guidelines primarily rely on consensus or expert opinions in this field [26].

Currently, treatment options for childhood dystonia encompass physical and supportive therapies, oral medications, botulinum toxin injections, and surgery. In cases of dopa-responsive dystonia, levodopa serves as the first-line treatment. Levodopa administration yields significant improvements, including reduced abnormal movements, postures, and gait in affected patients. Due to the notably positive response to levodopa therapy, it is recommended as the initial treatment approach for any child suspected of having dopa-responsive dystonia or presenting with unexplained dystonia. Levodopa can also provide symptom relief in non-dopa-responsive dystonia cases. The recommended starting dosage of levodopa is 1 mg/kg/day, which can be gradually increased until maximum benefit is achieved or until dose-limiting side effects manifest. Most individuals typically respond to doses of 4–5 mg/kg/day, divided into multiple doses. It is advised to administer levodopa for a minimum of 3 months before deeming the trial unsuccessful [24, 27].

Botulinum toxin is the primary treatment option for focal and segmental dystonias. Its effects are typically temporary, necessitating repeated injections at intervals, typically every 12–16 weeks. The most frequent side effects are dose-dependent weakness and localized spread of the toxin. In cases of cervical dystonia, patients may experience temporary difficulty swallowing (dysphagia), particularly when the botulinum toxin is injected into the sternomastoid muscles. Ptosis, drooping of the eyelid, is a common complication of injections for blepharospasm [28, 29].

Functional neurosurgical stereotactic procedures encompass deep brain stimulation (DBS) targeting the globus pallidus internus (GPi) and thalamus. DBS is recommended for primary generalized and segmental dystonia that has not responded to drug treatment and botulinum toxin therapy. This option is applicable for patients who are at least 7 years of age [30]. Overall, individuals with primary dystonia, particularly those with DYT1 dystonia, tend to exhibit better responses to deep brain stimulation (DBS) therapy compared to secondary cases. However, it is important to note that not all primary dystonias consistently respond to DBS treatment. The most promising outcomes with DBS are typically observed in children diagnosed with primary DYT1 dystonia [23].

References

1. Oppenheim H. About a rare spasm disease of childhood and young age (Dysbasia lordotica progressiva, dystonia musculorum deformans). Neurologische Centralblatt. 1911;30:1090–107.
2. Albanese A, Bhatia K, Bressman SB, et al. Phenomenology and classification of dystonia: a consensus update. Mov Disord. 2013;28:863–73.
3. Fahn S. Concept and classification of dystonia. Adv Neurol. 1988;50:1–8.
4. Sanger TD. Pathophysiology of pediatric movement disorders. J Child Neurol. 2003;18(Suppl 1):S9–S24.
5. Mink JW. Special concerns in defining, studying, and treating dystonia in children. Mov Disord. 2013;28:921–5.
6. Calado R, Monteiro JP, Fonseca MJ. Transient idiopathic dystonia in infancy. Acta Paediatr. 2011;100:624–7.
7. Himmelmann K, McManus V, Hagberg G, et al. SCPE collaboration. Dyskinetic cerebral palsy in Europe: trends in prevalence and severity. Arch Dis Child. 2009;94:921–6.
8. Misra UK, Kalita J. Spectrum of movement disorders in encephalitis. J Neurol. 2010;257:2052–8.
9. Donaldson IM, Marsden CD, Schneider SA, et al. Marsden's book of movement disorders. Oxford: Oxford University Press; 2012.
10. Singer HS, Jankovic J, Mink JW, et al. Movement disorders in childhood. Philadelphia: Saunders Elsevier; 2010.
11. Gulati S, Sondhi V, Chakrabarty B, Prashant Jauhari RD. Autoimmune encephalitis in children: clinical profile and outcome from a single tertiary care Centre in India. Neurology. 2018;90(15):P2.313.
12. Rubio-Agusti I, Dalmau J, Sevilla T, Burgal M, Beltran E, Bataller L. Isolated hemidystonia associated with NMDA receptor antibodies. Mov Disord. 2011;26:351–2.
13. Mohammad SS, Fung VS, Grattan-Smith P, Gill D, Pillai S, Ramanathan S, et al. Movement disorders in children with anti- NMDAR encephalitis and

other autoimmune encephalopathies. Mov Disord. 2014a;29:1539–42.

14. Doummar D, Roussat B, Beauvais P, Billette de Villemeur T, Richardet JM. Spasmus nutans: apropos of 16 cases. Arch Pediatr. 1998;5:264–8.

15. Olguner M, Akgur FM, Hakguder G, et al. Gastroesophageal reflux associated with dystonic movements: Sandifer's syndrome. Pediatr Int. 1999;41(3):321–2.

16. Ashalatha R, Kishore A, Sarada C, Nair MD. Satoyoshi syndrome. Neurol India. 2004;52:94–5.

17. Klein C. Genetics in dystonia. Parkinsonism Relat Disord. 2014;20(Suppl 1):S137–42.

18. Monbaliu E, De Cock P, Ortibus E, Heyrman L, Klingels K, Feys H. Clinical patterns of dystonia and choreoathetosis in participants with dyskinetic cerebral palsy. Dev Med Child Neurol. 2016;58:138–44.

19. Iafolla AK, Kahler SG. Megaloencephaly in the neonatal period as the initial manifestation of glutaric aciduria type I. J Pediatr. 1989;114:1004–6.

20. Hoffmann GF, Athanassopoulos S, Burlina AB, et al. Clinical course, early diagnosis, treatment, and prevention of disease in glutaryl-CoA dehydrogenase deficiency. Neuropediatrics. 1996;27:115–23.

21. Jinnah HA, De Gregorio L, Harris JC, et al. The spectrum of inherited mutations causing HPRT deficiency: 75 new cases and a review of 196 previously reported cases. Mutat Res. 2000;463:309–26.

22. Ozelius L, Lubarr N. DYT1 early-onset isolated dystonia. In: Adam MP, Ardinger HH, Pagon RA, et al., editors. . Seattle (WA): GeneReviews((R)); 1993.

23. Bruggemann N, Kuhn A, Schneider SA, et al. Short- and long-term outcome of chronic pallidal neurostimulation in monogenic isolated dystonia. Neurology. 2015;84:895–903.

24. Tadic V, Kasten M, Bruggemann N, et al. Dopa-responsive dystonia revisited: diagnostic delay, residual signs, and nonmotor signs. Arch Neurol. 2012;69:1558–62.

25. Roubertie A, Mariani LL, Fernandez-Alvarez E, et al. Treatment for dystonia in childhood. Eur J Neurol. 2012;19:1292–9.

26. Thenganatt MA, Jankovic J. Treatment of dystonia. Neurotherapeutics. 2014;11:139–52.

27. Albanese A, Asmus F, Bhatia KP, et al. EFNS guidelines on diagnosis and treatment of primary dystonias. Eur J Neurol. 2011;18(1):5–18.

28. Borggraefe I, Mehrkens JH, Telegravciska M, et al. Bi- lateral pallidal stimulation in children and adolescents with primary generalized dystonia–report of six patients and literature-based analysis of predictive outcomes variables. Brain and Development. 2010;32(3):223–8.

29. Comella CL, Pullman SL. Botulinum Toxin in neurological disease. Muscle Nerve. 2004;29:628–44.

30. Tintner R, Jankovic J. Botulinum toxin. In: Warner TT, Bressman SB, editors. Clinical diagnosis and management of dystonia. Informa Press; 2007. p. 188–207.

Neurodegeneration with Brain Iron Accumulation

Roopa Rajan

Case Scenario A 12-year-old girl presented with abnormal posturing of limbs and trunk, recurrent falls, and abnormal facial movements for the past 3 years. Over the past 2 years, she had progressive difficulties at school due to lack of attention and impaired ability to retain new information. These worsened over the past 6 months, and she stopped attending school. She developed speech disturbances, spells of inappropriate laughter, and swallowing difficulty for the past 1 year. There were no history of seizures, myoclonic jerks, visual or hearing disturbances. She was the first-born child of non-consanguineous parents, and there was no history of similar illness in any family member. Examination revealed generalized dystonia involving all four limbs, neck, and trunk (opisthotonus). Blepharospasm and jaw-opening dystonia were also prominent.

There was spasticity in all four limbs with ankle clonus bilaterally. All deep tendon jerks were brisk, and plantars were extensor bilaterally. Extraocular movements were normal. Fundus examination revealed pigmentary retinopathy.

Routine hematological and biochemical investigations were normal. The workup for Wilson's disease was negative. Peripheral blood smear revealed acanthocytosis. Cranial MRI revealed hypointensities in the globus pallidus bilaterally on T2-weighted sequences with central T2-hyperintensities (Fig. 28.1). The possibility of neurodegeneration with brain iron accumulation (NBIA) and probable pantothenate kinase-associated neurodegeneration (PKAN) was considered. Genetic testing revealed a pathogenic variant in the *PANK2* gene consistent with the diagnosis of PKAN.

R. Rajan (✉)
Department of Neurology, All India Institute of
Medical Sciences, New Delhi, India
e-mail: rooparajan@aiims.edu

© Springer Nature Singapore Pte Ltd. 2024
K. K. Oli et al. (eds.), *Case-based Approach to Common Neurological Disorders*,
https://doi.org/10.1007/978-981-99-8676-7_28

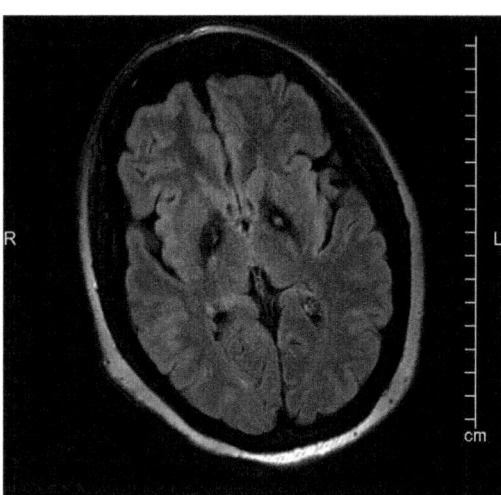

Fig. 28.1 Cranial MRI T2-FLAIR sequence showing hypointensities in the bilateral globus pallidus with anteromedial T2-hyperintensities consistent with "eye of the tiger" sign

28.1 Introduction

Neurodegeneration with brain iron accumulation (NBIA) is an umbrella term for a group of clinically and etiologically heterogeneous disorders, all of which involve pathological iron deposition in the brain [1]. The mineral deposition is usually most prominent in the deep gray matter nuclei of basal ganglia, but may additionally involve the midbrain structures like substantia nigra and the red nucleus. NBIAs are relentlessly progressive degenerative disorders that present with a spectrum of neurological involvement ranging from movement disorders to cognitive impairment, spasticity, ataxia, and others. Typically, neurological deficits exist across multiple domains in most patients and can range from progressive neurodevelopmental regression in infancy to milder forms of parkinsonism or dystonia in adulthood. Genetic defects have been linked to specific clinical manifestations, which aids in the diagnosis; however, significant variability exists among carriers of similar genetic defects.

28.2 Epidemiology

Data regarding community prevalence of NBIA is unavailable; however, NBIAs are thought to be very rare disorders. Within the group of NBIA, certain types are more common—specifically, pantothenate kinase-associated neurodegeneration (PKAN), phospholipase A2-associated neurodegeneration (PLAN), mitochondrial membrane protein-associated neurodegeneration (MPAN), and beta-propeller protein-associated neurodegeneration (BPAN). The commonest NBIA, PKAN, is estimated to affect approximately 1 in 500,000–1,000,000 persons worldwide [2]. There may be region-specific differences in the distribution, for instance, up to 25% of a Japanese cohort with intellectual disability and young-onset parkinsonism had BPAN. Unusual phenotypes, including Parkinson's disease-like presentations and late-onset tremors, have been reported from the Indian subcontinent.

28.3 Etiology

In addition to the four common NBIAs (PKAN, PLAN, MPAN, and BPAN) discussed above, the other disorders considered under this term include fatty acid hydroxylase-associated neurodegeneration (FAHN), coenzyme A synthase protein-associated neurodegeneration (CoPAN), Kufor-Rakeb syndrome, Woodhouse-Sakati syndrome, neuroferritinopathy, and aceruloplasminemia. The genes and proteins associated with these disorders and their mode of inheritance are given in Table 28.1. As a group, these are genetic disorders with varying modes of inheritance.

Table 28.1 The ten diseases considered NBIA and the genes, proteins, and modes of inheritance associated with them

Disease	Gene	Protein	Mode of inheritance
Pantothenate kinase-associated neurodegeneration (PKAN)	*PANK2*	Pantothenate kinase 2	Autosomal recessive
Phospholipase A2-associated neurodegeneration (PLAN)	*PLA2G6*	Calcium-independent phospholipase A2	Autosomal recessive
Mitochondrial membrane protein-associated neurodegeneration (MPAN)	*C19orf12*	C19orf12	Autosomal recessive
Beta-propeller protein-associated neurodegeneration (BPAN)	*WDR45*	WD40-repeat protein 45	X-linked dominant
Fatty acid hydroxylase-associated neurodegeneration (FAHN)	*FA2H*	Fatty acid 2 hydroxylase	Autosomal recessive
Coenzyme A synthase protein-associated neurodegeneration (CoPAN)	*COASY*	Coenzyme A synthase	Autosomal recessive
Kufor-Rakeb syndrome	*ATP13A2*	Cation-transporting ATPase 13A2	Autosomal recessive
Neuroferritinopathy	*FTL*	Ferritin light chain	Autosomal dominant
Aceruloplasminemia	*CPL*	Ceruloplasmin	Autosomal recessive
Woodhouse-Sakati syndrome	*DCAF17*	DDB1 and CUL4 associated factor 17	Autosomal recessive

28.4 Pathogenesis

The unifying pathogenic feature in all NBIA disorders is degeneration of the globus pallidus and substantia nigra with abnormal iron accumulation in these regions. Additional brain regions are affected variably in different subtypes. It is not clearly known whether the iron deposition is a primary feature resulting in degeneration or it is an epi-phenomenon of neurodegeneration in these naturally iron-rich regions of the brain [3]. The proteins encoded by the majority of the NBIA-associated genes are involved in mitochondrial function. Only a few (ferritin light chain, ceruloplasmin) are directly related to iron metabolism. These proteins are widely expressed in other brain as well as body regions, but the defects in NBIA are limited to specific brain regions. Current understanding is limited; however, it points toward mitochondrial membrane functional disruptions, lipid metabolism defects, and associated defects in energy and autophagy pathways as contributory pathogenic mechanisms.

28.5 Clinical Features

NBIA disorders are suspected by the presence of typical clinical features and characteristic brain magnetic resonance imaging (MRI) findings. The specific phenotypic features of each subtype are briefly discussed below.

28.6 Pantothenate Kinase-Associated Neurodegeneration (PKAN)

Typical PKAN is a childhood-onset, rapidly progressive disease with onset in the early first decade in most patients. Early symptoms include abnormal gait, falls, and cognitive decline. Neurological examination reveals dystonia and pyramidal signs (spasticity, brisk reflexes, and up-going plantars). Opisthotonus and pseudobulbar effects are often seen. Ophthalmological evaluation may reveal pigmentary retinopathy and, occasionally, abnormal pursuits and saccades. Acanthocytosis may be seen on peripheral smear examination. The MRI brain is pathognomonic, with the "eye of the tiger" sign seen in the majority of early-onset, "typical" PKAN patients. This classic sign consists of a T2-weighted hypointensity in the globus pallidus with an anteromedial hyperintensity. PKAN may progress in a stepwise manner with periods of rapid deterioration interspersed with clinical stability. Majority of patients with typical PKAN develop speech and swallowing disturbances and are wheelchair dependent by the second decade of life. Some succumb to aspiration pneumonia or other complications of immobility in the first/second decade; those who survive to adulthood are left with significant disability.

PKAN presenting after the first decade is known as "atypical" PKAN. Patients present in the second or third decade with speech disturbances and craniobulbar dystonia. Tics, parkinsonism, dystonia, and spasticity are often encountered. Younger patients tend to present with dystonia as the prominent feature, whereas adults present with akinetic-rigid parkinsonism and significant gait disturbance. Cranial dystonia may be action induced, occurring only while eating or speaking. Behavioral symptoms may be prominent including mood changes and obsessive-compulsive behaviors. Pigmentary retinopathy is less common in atypical PKAN. Atypical form progresses much slower compared to typical PKAN, and individuals may remain into adulthood without worsening disability. MRI findings are similar to typical PKAN. Although the "eye of the tiger" sign is highly suggestive of *PANK2* mutations, it is not absolutely sensitive or specific. Some patients who harbor pathogenic *PANK2* mutations do not reveal the classic sign, and conversely it has been reported in other conditions like MPAN, neuroferritinopathy, multiple system atrophy, organic acidurias, Leigh disease, and carbon monoxide poisoning.

28.7 Phospholipase A2-Associated Neurodegeneration (PLAN)

Among the NBIA, PLAN is associated with the widest range of clinical presentations [4]. Infantile neuroaxonal dystrophy is the variant of PLAN that presents between the age of 6 months and 3 years. It is characterized by relentless neurodevelopmental regression and loss of previously attained milestones. Children present with axial hypotonia in the initial stages, which progresses to spastic tetraplegia over a period of few years. Visual disturbances are marked consisting of optic atrophy, strabismus, and nystagmus. Seizures may be present in a minority. Nerve biopsy reveals dystrophic neurons with "axonal spheroids." Children with classic INAD usually succumb to the disease in the first decade. PLAN with onset in later childhood is termed atypical infantile neuroaxonal dystrophy (aNAD). This variant has a slower progression, and the clinical picture is dominated by cerebellar involvement (gait ataxia, dysarthria). Hypotonia and areflexia remain for longer durations. Dystonia may be present, and the cognition is progressively impaired. Adult-onset forms of PLAN are characterized by dystonia, parkinsonism, and spasticity, often with cognitive impairment. Cerebellar signs are less prominent in adult-onset PLAN. The parkinsonism in PLAN may be levodopa responsive initially, although motor fluctuations appear quickly.

Cerebellar atrophy is a prominent feature on MRI in all forms of PLAN, particularly the childhood-onset variants. Additionally, diffuse T2 hyperintensities in the white matter, thin corpus callosum, and cerebral atrophy may be seen. T2 hypointensities, the imaging hallmark of any NBIA, are notably absent or subtle early on in the disease course of PLAN. Specifically, the infantile and childhood variants often do not demonstrate iron deposition in the pallidum. The adult-onset PLAN usually reveals iron deposition in the globus pallidus along with variable cerebellar atrophy [5].

28.8 Mitochondrial Membrane Protein-Associated Neurodegeneration (MPAN)

MPAN presents in the first to third decades. Spasticity is a prominent feature in MPAN, and children often present with a spastic gait along with speech disturbances, optic atrophy, and neuropsychiatric problems. Dystonia is usually subtle in childhood MPAN. Adults present with parkinsonism, gait disturbances, spasticity, and cognitive impairment. Both variants may develop lower motor neuron signs, including atrophy and areflexia, as the disease progresses. MPAN is slow to progress in majority of patients, especially with the childhood-onset variant. Dysphagia and severe cognitive impairment complicate the later stages of this disease. MRI brain reveals T2 hypointensities in the globus pallidus and substantia nigra. T2 hyperintense streaking of the medial medullary lamina within the pallidum is often seen and can be mistaken for "eye of the tiger" sign.

28.9 Beta-Propeller Protein-Associated Neurodegeneration (BPAN)

BPAN, earlier known as static encephalopathy with neurodegeneration in adulthood (SENDA), is characterized by a cerebral palsy-like illness in childhood followed by progressive decline in adulthood. In the initial phase, children suffer from global developmental delay without obvious regression, autistic features, spasticity, and seizures, leading to a diagnosis of static encephalopathy. Sleep disorders like hypersomnolence, hyposomnolence, and abnormal REM sleep are seen in some children. Hand stereotypies akin to Rett syndrome may be prominent in others. This state of static deficits is followed by the development of dystonic posturing, parkinsonism, and

cognitive impairment in adolescence or early adulthood. Parkinsonism may be levodopa responsive in the initial stages; however, effects are short lasting, and motor and behavioral complications may emerge. Due to its unusual inheritance pattern (X-linked dominant) majority of the patients are female. During the static phase in childhood, MRI brain is usually normal. During the later deterioration phase, typical features are seen consisting of T2 hypointensities in the globus pallidus, substantia nigra, and cerebral peduncles. The substantia nigra is markedly involved, and on T1, a hyperintense "halo" is seen around the substantia nigra, extending to the cerebral peduncles.

28.10 Fatty Acid Hydroxylase-Associated Neurodegeneration (FAHN)

FAHN presents in the first decade of life with spastic gait, dystonia, and cerebellar signs. It progresses rapidly to loss of ambulation, speech, and swallowing disturbances. Optic atrophy, seizures, and cognitive decline are frequent accompaniments. *FA2H* gene mutations were initially described as being associated with leukodystrophy and complicated hereditary spastic paraplegia (HSP35). MRI brain reveals T2 hyperintense lesions in the white matter, thin corpus callosum, and widespread atrophy of the cerebellum, brainstem, and spinal cord. T2 hypointensities may be seen in the globus pallidus but are not universally present.

28.11 Coenzyme A Synthase Protein-Associated Neurodegeneration (CoPAN)

CoPAN is a rare NBIA that presents in the first few years of life with gait problems and cognitive decline. As the disease progresses craniobulbar dystonia, parkinsonism, speech disturbances, spasticity, and peripheral neuropathy predominate. MRI brain reveals non-homogeneous T2 hypointensities in the globus pallidus with medial T2 hyperintensity.

28.12 Kufor-Rakeb Syndrome

Kufor-Rakeb syndrome is a classic example of a pallidopyramidal syndrome with prominent akinetic-rigid parkinsonism and spasticity (PARK9) [6]. Prominent supranuclear gaze involvement is seen, and juvenile progressive supranuclear palsy is another descriptive term used for this disorder. Distal myoclonic jerks over the face, fingers, and tremors are also seen in some patients. Generalized cortical atrophy is a prominent finding on the MRI brain, and T2 hypointensities in the basal ganglia may not be prominent, especially in the early stages of the disease.

28.13 Neuroferritinopathy

Neuroferritinopathy is classically a late-onset NBIA which presents beyond the third decade of life. In addition to orofacial dystonia, parkinsonism, and cognitive decline common to most NBIA, chorea is often a prominent feature. Investigations reveal a low serum ferritin. MRI brain reveals T2 hypointensities in the caudate, putamen, globus pallidus, thalamus, substantia nigra, and red nucleus.

28.14 Aceruloplasminemia

Aceruloplasminemia presents in late adulthood with the classic triad, including extrapyramidal movement disorder, diabetes, and retinitis pigmentosa [7]. Most patients also have microcytic anemia and cognitive decline. The movement disorder phenotype is heterogeneous, with cranial dystonia, parkinsonism, ataxia, tremor, and chorea present often. Investigations reveal low or absent serum ceruloplasmin, elevated ferritin, low serum copper, low serum iron, and normal urinary copper. MRI reveals extensive iron accumulation and T2 hypointensities in the globus pallidus, substantia nigra, putamen, red nucleus, thalamus, and dentate nucleus of the cerebellum. Iron accumulation can also be seen in the liver on MRI.

28.15 Woodhouse-Sakati Syndrome

Woodhouse-Sakati syndrome is a multisystem disorder with endocrine, dermatological, and neurological manifestations. Patients present with hypogonadism, diabetes mellitus, alopecia, intellectual disability, and sensorineural hearing loss. Neurological manifestations include dystonia, speech, and swallowing problems. MRI brain reveals T2 hypointensities in the basal ganglia and T2 hyperintensities in the white matter.

28.16 Idiopathic NBIA

In 5–15% of patients in research cohorts, underlying etiology cannot be identified with existing genetic study techniques. These patients with progressive neurological impairment and evidence of iron deposition in the basal ganglia are currently grouped as idiopathic NBIA.

28.17 Diagnosis

In patients with the typical clinical features, NBIA is often suspected when an MRI of the brain reveals the characteristic pattern of iron accumulation. The addition of MRI sequences specifically sensitive to iron-such as gradient echo sequences (GRE) or susceptibility-weighted imaging (SWI) in addition to the routine T2-weighted and T1 sequences will increase the yield of MRI in a patient with suspected NBIA. Sometimes, repeat MR imaging as the disease progresses may demonstrate iron deposition that was absent in the initial scans. In addition to a detailed neurological examination all patients should undergo an ophthalmologic evaluation to detect optic atrophy, pigmentary retinopathy, or saccadic and gaze abnormalities. Serum levels of ceruloplasmin, ferritin, iron, and copper as well as urinary copper need to be estimated. Peripheral smear may reveal acanthocytes in PKAN. Electrophysiological testing may include nerve conduction studies for coexisting peripheral neuropathy (FAHN, CoPAN, and neuroferritinopathy) and electroencephalography for high-frequency anteriorly dominant discharges in INAD. Final diagnosis is usually achieved by genetic testing. A step-wise approach using targeted sequencing of suspected genes individually or a broader approach using whole exome or genome sequencing may be adopted. Genetic testing for the major NBIA is now available commercially in the Indian subcontinent.

28.18 Differential Diagnosis

Differential diagnoses are among the NBIA once MRI reveals definite mineral deposition [8]. In subjects without definite iron deposition or prior to availability of imaging differential diagnoses include Wilson's disease, leukodystrophies, complicated hereditary spastic paraplegia, mitochondrial disorders, and lysosomal storage disorders. In adult patients, other degenerative movement disorders like progressive supranuclear palsy, multiple system atrophy, and corticobasal degeneration may be suspected. Neuroferritinopathy may raise suspicion of Huntington's disease or neuroacanthocytosis syndromes.

28.19 Treatment

Treatment remains symptomatic management of the movement disorders and other problems. Parkinsonism may respond to levodopa transiently, soon followed by the emergence of motor fluctuations and dyskinesias. There are reports of longer duration responses in a few patients. Dystonia and spasticity are treated with anticholinergics, baclofen, benzodiazepines, and tetrabenazine. Botulinum toxin may be offered for focal dystonia. Seizures can be managed by standard antiseizure medications. Patients at all stages of disease may benefit from physiotherapy and speech therapy. At advanced stages, percutaneous gastrostomy tube insertion may be considered for nutrition. Deep brain stimulation of the globus pallidus interna has been used in patients with NBIA, particularly PKAN, with modest improvements (26%) in dystonia at 1-year follow-up [9]. Patients with atypical PKAN and severe dystonia responded better than patients with typical PKAN. There is no curative or disease-modifying treatment available currently for any of the NBIA. Iron-chelating agents like deferiprone have been shown to reduce T2 hypointensities in the globus pallidus in a few patients; however, evidence of clinical improvement is not documented [10].

References

1. Hayflick SJ, Kurian MA, Hogarth P. Neurodegeneration with brain iron accumulation. Handb Clin Neurol. 2018;23(3):293–305. https://doi.org/10.1016/b978-0-444-63233-3.00019-1.
2. Hogarth P. Neurodegeneration with brain iron accumulation: diagnosis and management. J Mov Disord. 2015;8(1):1–13.
3. Ndayisaba A, Kaindlstorfer C, Wenning GK. Iron in neurodegeneration - cause or consequence? Front Neurosci. 2019;13:180.
4. Aggarwal A, Schneider SA, Houlden H, Silverdale M, Paudel R, Paisan-Ruiz C, Desai S, Munshi M, Sanghvi D, Hardy J, Bhatia KP, Bhatt M. Indian-subcontinent NBIA: unusual phenotypes, novel PANK2 mutations, and undetermined genetic forms. Mov Disord. 2010;25(10):1424–31.
5. Darling A, Aguilera-Albesa S, Tello CA, Serrano M, Tomás M, Camino-León R, et al. PLA2G6-associated neurodegeneration: new insights into brain abnormalities and disease progression. Parkinsonism Relat Disord. 2019;61:179–86.
6. Kruer MC, Paudel R, Wagoner W, Sanford L, Kara E, Gregory A, et al. Analysis of ATP13A2 in large neurodegeneration with brain iron accumulation (NBIA) and dystonia-parkinsonism cohorts. Neurosci Lett. 2012;523(1):35–8.
7. Marchi G, Busti F, Lira Zidanes A, Castagna A, Girelli D. Aceruloplasminemia: a severe neurodegenerative disorder deserving an early diagnosis. Front Neurosci. 2019;13:325.
8. Lee JH, Lee MS. Brain iron accumulation in atypical parkinsonian syndromes: in vivo MRI evidences for distinctive patterns. Front Neurol. 2019;10:74. https://doi.org/10.3389/fneur.2019.00074.
9. De Vloo P, Lee DJ, Dallapiazza RF, Rohani M, Fasano A, Munhoz RP, et al. Deep brain stimulation for pantothenate kinase-associated neurodegeneration: a meta-analysis. Mov Disord. 2019;34(2):264–73.
10. Cossu G, Abbruzzesse G, Matta G, Murgia D, Melis M, Ricchi V, et al. Efficacy and safety of deferiprone for the treatment of pantothenate kinase-associated neurodegeneration (PKAN) and neurodegeneration with brain iron accumulation (NBIA): results from a four years follow-up. Parkinsonism Relat Disord. 2014;20(6):651–4.

29

R. Subasree and Suvarna Alladi

Case Vignette

A 60-year-old woman, homemaker, right-handed, educated till primary school, who speaks Kannada and Telugu, was brought by her husband with complaints of change in behaviour for the past 3 years. A premorbidly well-adjusted, empathetic extrovert personality was noticed to gradually behave abnormally. The first time, the husband noticed that the wife was careless about her valuables and jewellery which she wore at a family gathering. Subsequently, she was found to forget to switch off the gas stove, adding too much salt in food, not able to plan for a meal or cook, and having difficulty in mingling with relatives. She was also found to have irritability, anger outbursts, hoarding of plastics, pins, and garments underneath her bed, and developed increased craving for sweets. She was often seen to perform pooja and repeatedly lighting the lamp and was not interested in talking or playing with grandchildren. She was not able to plan her packing when they went on a pilgrim trip. She was not bothered when her son got ill and sick. She was not interested in social gatherings, stopped seeing and following her TV serials, and had sleep disturbances. She began to occasionally forget names of son and daughter as well. She also was found to have difficulty in identifying the rupee notes and in transacting the money bills in groceries. Gradually, she also had difficulty in remembering recent conversations and would forget if she had breakfast and would quarrel with her daughter for not feeding her. She missed all her medications and misplaced them, and kept on searching her dentures.

Over the next 1 year, as per the caretakers, she was found to be unkempt and was not interested in keeping herself clean; she had to be coaxed to brush and bathe. She was not able to bathe herself, was wearing one blouse over the other, and forgot to flush her washroom. She had a newfound interest in painting her sarees and pillow covers. She was eating very hurriedly, and her eating pattern had changed. She was, however, able to identify the places and never got lost. There was no family history of dementia, psychiatric illness, or motor weakness. Gradually over the next 6 months, when the couple came for follow-up, she was found to be slow in all activities, spoke very less, was not interested, amotivated to do all her daily activities. She occasionally uttered few words and was mute most of the times. She also had developed occasional unconcerned urinary incontinence. There was no family history of psychoses, dementia, motor weakness or movement disorders.

A detailed neurological examination revealed an elderly woman with poor personal hygiene. She lacked insight about her illness and was quiet most of the times, trying to touch and handle

R. Subasree · S. Alladi (✉)
Department of Neurology, National Institute of
Mental Health and Neurosciences, Bangalore, India

most objects in the room. On repeated coaxing, she could only understand simple commands and she could only utter few words; she had difficulty in reading, naming, and was often referring things as "it" and "that". She was not able to perform Luria tests; she had verbal and motor perseveration. She had early parkinsonian features and was slow with reduced blink rate, expressionless face, and had slow gait with reduced arm swing. There were no tremors, and she had primitive reflexes like grasp reflex, palmomental reflex, and snout reflex present.

With this history and examination, in view of the late onset of behavioural symptoms, personality changes, loss of insight, apathy, amotivation, loss of empathy, difficulty in decision making, dysexecution, loss of personal hygiene, incontinence and parkinsonian features with release reflexes, the possibility of frontotemporal dementia-behavioural variant evolving to primary progressive aphasia was considered. Neuropsychological assessment showed dysfunction of dorsolateral prefrontal cortex and medial temporal lobe. MRI of her brain revealed significant frontotemporal atrophy, especially of the orbitofrontal region and also cerebellum. Her CSF analysis and other workup for dementia, including vitamin B_{12} and thyroid function, were all normal. Whole exome sequencing did not reveal any abnormal genetic mutations. Repeat primer PCR (RP-PCR) analysis revealed heterozygous mutation in expanded GGGGCC hexanucleotide repeat in *C9ORF72*.

Caregivers were explained about the nature and prognosis of the disease, and she was started on tablet fluoxetine along with appropriate behavioural therapy and was advised regular follow-up. Speech therapy, physical therapy, and cognitively stimulating activities were started. Caregiver burden was assessed and addressed.

29.1 Introduction

Frontotemporal dementia (FTD) is a heterogeneous neurological disorder that involves a range of behavioural, cognitive, and motor weakness. It is associated with selective degeneration of the prefrontal and anterior temporal cortex. FTD commonly affects individuals at a younger age than Alzheimer's dementia and frequently has a familial history, presenting with intricate and overlapping clinical symptoms, psychiatric manifestations, and varying patterns of genetic expression and imaging biomarkers. Consequently, the diagnosis and treatment of FTD pose significant challenges [1].

29.2 Epidemiology of Frontotemporal Dementia

Frontotemporal dementia is one of the leading causes of early-onset dementia, typically occurring before the age of 65. Its prevalence is estimated to be 15 cases per 100,000 individuals between 45 and 64 years. The average age of onset is around 56 years, and survival rates range from 3 to 14 years following diagnosis. Approximately 40% of FTD cases have a familial component, and about 10–15% of cases exhibit an autosomal dominant inheritance pattern. In a study conducted in India, out of 347 dementia patients assessed at a memory clinic, 65 individuals (18.7%) were diagnosed with frontotemporal dementia. Among these patients, 24 had behavioural-variant FTD (bvFTD), 14 had progressive nonfluent aphasia (PNFA), 14 had semantic dementia (SD), 5 had corticobasal degeneration (CBD), and 8 had FTD-motor neuron disease [2–4].

29.3 Clinical Features of FTD

FTD is characterized by a wide range of clinical variations, often accompanied by early-onset behavioural disturbances that can be mistakenly attributed to psychiatric disorders. Furthermore, there is increasing evidence of connections between FTD and other neurodegenerative conditions such as motor neuron disease (MND), corticobasal degeneration (CBD), and progressive supranuclear palsy (PSP). This overlap expands the clinical spectrum of FTD syndromes, further complicating the diagnosis and understanding of the disorder [5].

29.4 Behavioural-Variant Frontotemporal Dementia (bvFTD)

The most common form of FTD is behavioural-variant FTD (bvFTD), characterized by noticeable and early alterations in personality and behaviour, even in the absence of significant cognitive decline. Dysfunction in the reciprocal neural connections between the orbitofrontal, dorsolateral prefrontal, and medial prefrontal cortices, as well as subcortical brain nuclei are implicated in same. Positive symptoms of bvFTD encompass perseverative or compulsive behaviours, disinhibition, impulsivity, stereotypic and ritualistic behaviour, food fixation, and hyperorality. On the other hand, negative symptoms include diminished empathy and motivation, as well as impaired planning and decision-making abilities [5, 6].

Patients with bvFTD commonly experience profound deficits in understanding and processing the emotional states of others, leading to a lack of empathy and sympathy towards both strangers and close relationships. This impairment in social cognition is associated with the involvement of the right anterior temporal lobe, right medial orbitofrontal cortex (OFC), and anterior insula. Another striking feature is disinhibition, due to the involvement of the orbitofrontal cortex, which can manifest as engaging in socially inappropriate behaviours such as cursing, spitting, hugging strangers, public urination, engaging in inappropriate sexual acts, or sharing offensive jokes. Furthermore, behavioural disinhibition may extend to criminal behaviours, impulsivity, reckless driving, the onset of gambling or substance abuse, or unnecessary excessive purchasing. In addition to emotional and behavioural changes, patients with bvFTD may exhibit repetitive motor actions or verbalizations, including clapping, tapping, rubbing, humming, throat clearing, and other similar behaviours. They often engage in more complex repetitive movements and utterances, such as repetitive counting, elaborate cleaning routines, frequent trips to the bathroom, or repeatedly vocalizing specific phrases. Importantly, individuals with bvFTD are typically unaware of how their behaviours affect others, a phenomenon known as a loss of "theory of mind". Another consequence of bvFTD is dysexecutive functioning, resulting from the involvement of the dorsolateral prefrontal cortex. This can manifest as difficulties in multitasking, poor working memory, inflexibility in thinking, and imitation and utilization behaviours. It is essential to recognize that these various features can occur within the same individual at different stages of the disease progression [7, 8].

Neurological examination may reveal poor personal hygiene, loss of insight, lack of proper manners, dull affect, restlessness, environmental dependency and frontal release signs. Extrapyramidal or motor neuron signs can also manifest [9]. Indian patients are reported to present with advanced and florid disease. Utilization, imitation, and environmental dependency behaviours were observed in a significant proportion [10, 11]. Social cognition deficits characterized by loss of empathy, poor emotion recognition, and impaired theory of mind have also been reported in FTD patients in the Indian context using culturally adapted tests. Caregiver-based questionnaires and the application of behavioural scales that include Neuropsychiatric Inventory and Cambridge Behavioural Inventory assist in diagnosing bvFTD. Addenbrooke's Cognitive Examination detects majority of cases at presentation and discriminates FTD from Alzheimer dementia more than MMSE [12, 13]. The Frontotemporal Dementia Rating Scale aids in staging the severity of FTD and in determining disease progression. The cross cultural adapted Indian semantic battery is sensitive to detect semantic memory impairment in subjects with FTD.

29.5 Diagnostic Criteria

Multiple diagnostic criteria have been established, including the Lund Manchester criteria (1994), Neary criteria (1998), and the criteria proposed by McKhann et al. (2001). Although the Neary criteria were initially widely adopted, the International Behavioural Variant FTD Criteria Consortium (FTDC) has since revised the diagnostic guidelines for bvFTD, as outlined by Rascovsky et al. (2011) (Table 29.1) [14]. The criteria for diagnos-

Table 29.1 Rascovsky criteria for BvFTD 2011

I. Neurodegenerative disease
The following symptom must be present to meet criteria for bvFTD
A. Shows progressive deterioration of behaviour and/or cognition by observation or history (as provided by a knowledgeable informant)
II. Possible bvFTD
Three of the following behavioural/cognitive symptoms (A–F) must be present to meet criteria. Ascertainment requires that symptoms be persistent or recurrent, rather than single or rare events
A. Early* behavioural disinhibition [one of the following symptoms (A.1–A.3) must be present]:
1. Socially inappropriate behaviour
2. Loss of manners or decorum
3. Impulsive, rash, or careless actions
B. Early apathy or inertia [one of the following symptoms (B.1–B.2) must be present]:
1. Apathy
2. Inertia
C. Early loss of sympathy or empathy [one of the following symptoms (C.1–C.2) must be present]:
1. Diminished response to other people's needs and feelings
2. Diminished social interest, interrelatedness, or personal warmth
D. Early perseverative, stereotyped, or compulsive/ritualistic behaviour [one of the following symptoms (D.1–D.3) must be present]:
1. Simple repetitive movements
2. Complex, compulsive, or ritualistic behaviours
3. Stereotypy of speech
E. Hyperorality and dietary changes [one of the following symptoms (E.1–E.3) must be present]:
1. Altered food preferences
2. Binge eating, increased consumption of alcohol or cigarettes
3. Oral exploration or consumption of inedible objects
F. Neuropsychological profile: Executive/generation deficits with relative sparing of memory and visuospatial functions [all of the following symptoms (F.1–F.3) must be present]:
1. Deficits in executive tasks
2. Relative sparing of episodic memory
3. Relative sparing of visuospatial skills
II. Probable bvFTD
All of the following symptoms (A–C) must be present to meet criteria:
A. Meets criteria for possible bvFTD
B. Exhibits significant functional decline (by caregiver report or as evidenced by Clinical Dementia Rating Scale or Functional Activities Questionnaire scores)
C. Imaging results consistent with bvFTD [one of the following (C.1–C.2) must be present]:
1. Frontal and/or anterior temporal atrophy on MRI or CT
2. Frontal and/or anterior temporal hypoperfusion or hypometabolism on PET or SPECT
III. Behavioural-variant FTD with definite FTLD pathology
Criterion A and either criterion B or C must be present to meet criteria:
A. Meets criteria for possible or probable bvFTD
B. Histopathological evidence of FTLD on biopsy or at post-mortem
C. Presence of a known pathogenic mutation
IV. Exclusionary criteria for bvFTD
Criteria A and B must be answered negatively for any bvFTD diagnosis. Criterion C can be positive for possible bvFTD but must be negative for probable bvFTD.
A. Pattern of deficits is better accounted for by other non-degenerative nervous system or medical disorders
B. Behavioural disturbance is better accounted for by a psychiatric diagnosis
C. Biomarkers strongly indicative of Alzheimer's disease or other neurodegenerative process

ing bvFTD establish a hierarchical classification into three categories: possible, probable, and definite. This classification is determined by considering a range of factors, including clinical presentation, neuroimaging findings, molecular analyses, and histopathological data.

29.6 Molecular Pathology

The description of frontotemporal dementia dates back to 1892 when it was first documented by neuropsychiatrist Arnold Pick. In 1911, Alois Alzheimer confirmed the presence of distinct neuronal inclusions called Pick bodies, which exhibited intense argyrophilic staining. Macroscopically, frontotemporal lobar degeneration (FTLD) results in focal atrophy of limbic, paralimbic, and associated cortices of frontal and temporal lobes, insular cortex, and subcortical nuclei. It is associated with the accumulation of abnormal protein inclusions in the neurons and/or glial cells of the brain. These abnormal protein inclusions include tau protein (FTLD-tau), transactive response DNA-binding protein 43 (FTLD-TDP), fused-in sarcoma (FTLD-FUS) protein, and dipeptide proteins derived from mutated forms of the C9ORF72 gene. The majority of pathologically confirmed cases of FTLD are characterized by the presence of tau protein (FTLD-tau) or TDP-43-positive (FTLD-TDP) inclusions that can be visualized using ubiquitin staining [15]. Several biofluid biomarkers like assays for $A\beta_{42}$, p-tau$_{181}$, t-tau, TDP-43, Progranulin levels, Neurofilament estimation helps in discriminating FTD from other neurodegenerative dementias.

29.7 Genetics in FTD

Currently, the majority of familial cases of FTLD have been associated with mutations in three genes that exhibit nearly 100% penetrance: microtubule-associated protein tau (MAPT), granulin (GRN), and C9 open reading frame 72 (C9ORF72). Additionally, five other genes have been identified to be linked with a small number of families affected by FTLD: valosin-containing protein, charged multivesicular body protein 2b, fused-in sarcoma (FUS), TAR DNA-binding protein, and the UBQLN2 gene [16]. In the Indian context, around 9.5–20% of patients have a family history of dementia which is much lesser than reported in Caucasian population (30-50%). MAPT and C9orf72 have not so far been detected in the dementia groups, and only one novel PGRN mutation was detected, contributing to the heterogeneity of FTD in India [17]. More studies focusing on newer FTD genes/mutations are required in the Asian population.

29.8 Clinical, Pathological, and Genetic Correlations in FTD

The identification of genes associated with FTLD has brought together various aspects of knowledge, including neuropathology, neuroimaging, and clinical syndromes. This convergence of information has broadened our understanding of the different phenotypes associated with both hereditary and sporadic forms of FTLD (Table 29.2).

Table 29.2 Genetics of FTD

Gene	Chromosome	Protein	Inheritance	
Microtubule-associated protein tau (MAPT)	17q21.32	Microtubule-associated tau protein	AD	bvFTD, PSP, CBSbvFTD with parkinsonism, semantic PPA
C9ORF72	9p21.2	Unknown	Uncertain	bvFTD, ALS, FTLD-ALS, PPA
GRN	17q21.31	Progranulin	AD	bvFTD, PPA, semantic-variant PPA, CBS
TAR DNA-binding protein (TARDBP)	1q36	TDP-43	AD/AR	ALS, FTLD-ALS, FTD, semantic PPA
VCP	9p13.3	Valosin-containing protein	AD	Multisystem proteinopathy IBM-FTD, bvFTD, semantic PPA, FTD-ALS
CHMP2B	3p11.2	Charged multivesicular body protein 2B	AD	bvFTD, bvFTD with parkinsonism, FTD-ALS
DCTN1	2p13	Dynactin	AD	Perry syndrome, bvFTD, PSPs, FTD-ALS
FUS	16p11.2	Fused-in sarcoma	AD/AR	FTD-ALS (more rarely bvFTD)
SIGMAR1	9p13.3	Sigma non-opioid intracellular receptor 1	AD/AR	FTD-ALS
TBK1	12q14	TANK-binding kinase 1	AD	FTD-ALS
UBQLN2	Xp11.21	Ubiquilin-2	Dominant (X-linked)	FTD-ALS
CHCHD10	22q11.23	Coiled-coil-helix-coiled-coil-helix domain containing 10	AD with incomplete penetrance	FTD-ALS

AD, autosomal dominant; *AR*, autosomal recessive (Adapted from Finger 2016 and Fillipi 2016)

29.9 Imaging in bvFTD

Coronal imaging of patients with behavioural-variant FTD reveals noticeable atrophy in the mesial frontal, orbitofrontal, and anterior insula cortices. Frontal or anterior temporal lobe hypoperfusion on SPECT and right temporal/right or bilateral frontal lobe hypometabolism on FDG-PET imaging help in discriminating FTD from AD. The role of tau tracer imaging is under investigation currently. Second generation Tau tracers like 18F-MK-6240 has shown to be potential biomarker for tau in FTD especially in those with genetic tau mutations. Voxel-based morphometry, cortical thickness mapping, arterial spin labelling, diffusion tensor imaging, and functional MRI also show specific changes in early bvFTD [16, 18]. MRI studies have demonstrated specific neuroanatomical patterns associated with the different FTD pathologies, which could potentially be useful biomarkers in FTD. There are

specific imaging atrophy patterns described in relation to specific mutations by visual rating scales. MAPT mutations typically result in symmetrical involvement of the anterior and medial temporal lobes, while GRN mutations are associated with asymmetric loss in the frontal and parietal regions. In contrast, C9ORF72 mutations tend to exhibit a more widespread pattern of brain involvement and also atrophy of thalamus and cerebellum [19]. Multimodal MRI features and atrophy patterns are also described for presymptomatic genetic carriers in FTD [19].

29.10 Patient Management and Future Challenges

Currently, there are no approved treatments specifically designed to cure frontotemporal dementia (FTD). The primary management strategy for FTD focuses on increasing awareness, providing education, and addressing behavioural issues in patients. This includes implementing physical therapy, gait and balance training, as well as occupational therapy to support the individual's functional abilities. The management of FTD involves establishing a social support network that includes psychiatric and voluntary services. It is important to provide a range of care options, such as day care, respite care, and residential care, to meet the specific needs of patients. Additionally, caregiver stress management is an essential component of FTD management, as caregivers play a crucial role in the overall well-being of the affected individuals.

Trials of modulation of serotonin in FTD using selective serotonin reuptake inhibitors (SSRI) such as citalopram, paroxetine, sertraline, or trazodone have shown benefits. They are used to treat disinhibition, irritability, or compulsive behaviours. Randomized controlled trials have shown that SSRIs, trazodone, and amphetamines are useful in behavioural symptoms in FTD and are well tolerated. Use of antipsychotics like risperidone and quetiapine for behavioural issues is reserved for severe cases, along with behavioural management, and for a short duration.

In the last decade, there has been an enormous understanding of genetics, molecular pathology, and radiology, increasing the scope for developing disease-modifying drugs for FTD. The contribution of Next generation sequencing, whole exome sequencing and genome wide association studies along with pathological studies has helped us understand the entanglements of the overlap syndromes of FTD and has opened up new pathways for clinical trials and management options. There are ongoing clinical trials using anti-tau antibodies and vaccines with tau peptides. FOXY study is exploring the role of intranasal oxytocin for improving social cognition in FTD. Several antisense oligonucleotides (ASO) which reduce RNA accumulation have been identified in C9orf72-induced pluripotent stem cells. Drugs like nimodipine and FRM-0334, a histone deacetylase inhibitor, have been tried to enhance PGRN expression in those with GRN mutations [20]. Dozens of disease-causing progranulin mutations have been identified, and most result in lowered levels of progranulin. Understanding how exactly low progranulin levels cause neurodegeneration is the central focus of the Bluefield Research Consortium. Intrathecal ASO targeting expanded c9orf RNA are in trials for those with FTD and ALS spectrum due to C9orf mutations.

References

1. Neary D, Snowden J, Mann D. Frontotemporal dementia. Lancet Neurol. 2005;4:771–80.
2. Ratnavalli E, Brayne C, Dawson K, Hodges JR. The prevalence of frontotemporal dementia. Neurology. 2002;58:1615–21.
3. Rohrer JD, Guerreiro R, Vandrovcova J, Uphill J, Reiman D, Beck J, et al. The heritability and genetics of frontotemporal lobar degeneration. Neurology. 2009;73:1451–6.
4. Alladi S, Mekala S, Chadalawada SK, Jala S, Mridula R, Kaul S. Subtypes of dementia: a study from a memory clinic in India. Dement Geriatr Cogn Disord. 2011;32(1):32–8.
5. Onyike CU, Diehl-Schmid J. The epidemiology of frontotemporal dementia. Int Rev Psychiatry. 2013;25(2):130–7.
6. Lanata SC, Miller BL. The behavioural variant frontotemporal dementia (bvFTD) syndrome in psychiatry. J Neurol Neurosurg Psychiatry. 2016;87(5):501–11.
7. Piguet O, Hornberger M, Mioshi E, et al. Behavioural-variant frontotemporal dementia: diagnosis, clinical staging, and management. Lancet Neurol. 2011;10:162–72.
8. Kirshner HS. Frontotemporal dementia and primary progressive aphasia, a review. Neuropsychiatr Dis Treat. 2014;10:1045–55.
9. Warren JD, Rohrer JD, Rossor MN. Clinical review. Frontotemporal dementia. BMJ. 2013;347:f4827.
10. Ghosh A, et al. Genetic study on frontotemporal lobar degeneration in India. Parkinsonism Relat Disord. 2013;19:487–9.
11. Ghosh A, Dutt A. Utilisation behaviour in frontotemporal dementia. J Neurol Neurosurg Psychiatry. 2010;81:154–6.
12. Mathuranath PS, Nestor PJ, Berrios GE, et al. A brief cognitive test battery to differentiate Alzheimer's disease and frontotemporal dementia. Neurology. 2000;55:1613–20.
13. Yew B, Alladi S, Shailaja M, et al. Lost and forgotten? Orientation versus memory in Alzheimer's disease and frontotemporal dementia. J Alzheimers Dis. 2013;33:473–81.
14. Rascovsky K, Hodges JR, Knopman D, et al. Sensitivity of revised diagnostic criteria for the behavioural variant of frontotemporal dementia. Brain. 2011;134(Pt 9):2456–77.

15. Mackenzie IRA, Neurmann M. Molecular neuropathology of frontotemporal dementia: insights into disease mechanisms from postmortem studies. J Neurochem. 2016;138(Suppl. 1):54–70.
16. Filippi M, Agosta F, Ferraro PM. Charting frontotemporal dementia: from genes to networks. J Neuroimaging. 2016;26:16–27.
17. Aswathy PM, Jairani PS, Raghavan SK, et al. Progranulin mutation analysis: identification of one novel mutation in exon 12 associated with frontotemporal dementia. Neurobiol Aging. 2016;39:218.
18. Rohrer JD, Rosen HJ. Neuroimaging in frontotemporal dementia. Int Rev Psychiatry. 2013;25:221–9.
19. Fumagalli GG, Basilico P, Arighi A, et al. Distinct patterns of brain atrophy in genetic frontotemporal dementia initiative (GENFI) cohort revealed by visual rating scales. Alzheimers Res Ther. 2018;10:46.
20. Tsai RM, Boxer AL. Therapy and clinical trials in frontotemporal dementia: past, present, and future. J Neurochem. 2016;138(Suppl 1):211–21.

Parkinson's Disease

30

Ragesh Karn

Case Scenario

A 70-year-old ex-army officer, presented with progressive slowness of movement and resting tremor of hands (right > left) for 12 years. He was being treated with medicines along with physiotherapy and had been doing well until 3 years earlier. Then, he developed additional progressive difficulty in walking characterized by sudden stopping while walking and tendency to fall while turning around. There were abnormal movements in the form of slow jerky and tonic posturing of upper limbs, neck and trunk which were prominent during the period of off-medicines. These symptoms had significantly increased in last 2–3 months. He gave history of erectile dysfunction. There was no abnormal movement of jaw or tongue, fall, imbalance, dizziness, diplopia on upgaze, or impaired smell and taste sensations. He had no recent stress, fever, cough, burning micturition, or other systemic diseases like hypertension, diabetes mellitus, or pulmonary tuberculosis. He was non-vegetarian, an ex-smoker, and had given up alcohol consumption 3 years before.

On examination, his vitals and other general physical condition were normal without postural drop in blood pressure. On neurological examination, there was no nystagmus or restriction of eye movements. He had generalized increased tone with lead pipe rigidity in bilateral elbow movement and cogwheel rigidity in bilateral wrist movement with normal power of limbs. There were normal bilateral deep tendon reflexes and bilateral planter was down-going. He had abnormal gait with difficulty in initiation of walking, turning around, freezing, and positive pull test. He had positive glabellar tap and palmomental reflexes, with normal cerebellar, sensory, superficial reflexes, and absent meningeal signs. On investigation, his laboratory investigations and neuroimaging of the brain were normal. He was diagnosed with Parkinson's disease and was treated with increased frequency of levodopa along with addition of dopamine agonist. At 1-month follow-up, he was doing well and was able to walk independently without periodic fluctuation in symptoms.

30.1 Introduction

Parkinson's disease (PD) is a chronic neurodegenerative disorder that has slow progressive motor and non-motor symptoms. Tremor, rigidity, bradykinesia, and postural instability are the common clinical manifestations of PD. Depression and anxiety are frequent non-motor symptoms seen in PD. Dementia usually develops in the advanced stage of PD [1]. Other symptoms are hyposmia or anosmia, pain and

R. Karn (✉)
Department of Neurology, Tribhuvan University Institute of Medicine, Kathmandu, Nepal

K. K. Oli et al. (eds.), *Case-based Approach to Common Neurological Disorders*,
https://doi.org/10.1007/978-981-99-8676-7_30

abnormal sensory symptoms, sleep-related disorders, and dysautonomia [1].

Although the causes of PD are usually unknown, both genetic and environmental factors contribute to its pathogenesis [2]. Certain pesticides and prior head injuries increase the risk, while reduced risk has been found to be associated with tobacco and tea or coffee consumption [2]. The motor dysfunctions are due to decreased dopamine-containing cells in the substantia nigra secondary to intracellular accumulation of Lewy bodies [2]. Diagnosis is usually done by clinical features and neuroimaging is used to rule out other diseases.

30.2 Classification

Parkinson's disease, also known as "idiopathic parkinsonism," is the most common form of parkinsonism [3]. Some identifiable causes of parkinsonism are toxins, infections, drug effects, metabolic abnormality, and stroke. Many degenerative disorders of the brain are also associated with parkinsonism and are termed "Parkinson's plus" syndromes or "atypical parkinsonism," for example multiple system atrophy (MSA), progressive supranuclear palsy (PSP), corticobasal degeneration (CBD), and Lewy body dementia (DLB) [3].

30.3 Clinical Features

30.3.1 Motor

The commonest motor sign is low frequency, resting, and pill-rolling hand tremor, where the index finger and thumb have a tendency to repeatedly touch each other in a circular fashion, which disappears with voluntary movement and in deeper sleep [4]. Bradykinesia is the most common feature of PD, and is due to disturbances in initiation and execution of motor planning. Rigidity is caused by increased muscle tone leading to resistance to limb movement, which can be uniform (lead-pipe) or ratchety (cogwheel) [3, 4]. The combination of tremor and increased tone

leads to cogwheel rigidity. There is also associated reduced arm swing and sometimes rigid and painful shoulder joints and spine. Postural impairment is frequently observed during presentation due to abnormal postural reflexes, which is further worsened by rigidity and bradykinesia. Later, it can lead to imbalance and repeated falls, decreased mobility, and even fractures [5].

Other recognized motor clinical features include abnormal gait and postural instability such as festination (fast shuffling steps and a forward-bending posture with decreased arm swing). Freezing of gait is characterized by transient arrests while walking, and feet appear to get stuck to the floor, especially while turning. A monotonous hypophonic voice, masked facies, and micrographic handwriting that gets progressively smaller are some other common features [6].

30.3.2 Non-Motor

Neuropsychiatric disturbances in PD range from mild to severe cognitive, mood and behavioral disorders [4]. Executive dysfunction is frequently observed in PD patients, involving planning difficulty, impairment of abstract thinking, poor working memory, and reduced attention [7]. In comparison to the general population, they have a 2- to 6-fold higher risk of dementia [4, 7]. Increase in age and duration of illness are associated with the prevalence of dementia in PD. Dementia in PD causes reduction in quality of life in both patients and their caregivers, raises complications and mortality, and increases the need for in-hospital care [7]. Behavior and mood disorders are usually present in PD patients with dementia. Depression, apathy, and anxiety are other neuropsychiatric features seen in PD patients [4]. Hallucinations or delusions occur in about half of PD patients, which are usually seen in the later stage. Punding, which is a repetitive aimless stereotyped behavior seen in PD, is caused by anti-Parkinson's drugs.

Sleep disorders are frequently present in PD and are often associated with active motor movements in sleep and sleep apnea [4]. Common symptoms can be fatigue, daytime somnolence, REM sleep disorders, and insomnia [4]. REM behavior disorder (RBD) is dream-enacting behavior, occasionally injurious to a patient or their spouse, usually reported a few years before the onset of motor symptoms [8]. Autonomic dysfunction is also commonly reported, and can lead to orthostatic hypotension, oily skin, increased sweating, urinary symptoms, and sexual dysfunction [4]. Constipation is usually seen from a few years before the onset of motor symptoms and can have severe complications leading to frequent hospital admission. Hyposmia or anosmia, blurred vision, pain, and paresthesia can occur years before PD diagnosis [4].

30.4 Causes

30.4.1 Environmental Factors and Genetics

PD is caused by a complex interaction of genetic and environmental factors [2]. Pesticides exposure and history of head injury have been found to be associated with Parkinson's disease (PD) with modest risks. Smoking cigarettes and drinking coffee are associated with a small decrement in the risk of developing PD. However, low blood urate level has been found to be associated with an increased PD risk [9]. About 15% of PD patients have a first-degree relative affected with the disease [3]. Various genes related to PD have been identified such as SNCA, LRRK2, GBA, PRKN, PINK1, PARK7, VPS35, EIF4G1, DNAJC13, and CHCHD2, and the number is increasing [10].

30.5 Epidemiology

PD ranks second among neurodegenerative brain disorders after Alzheimer's disease, [2]. Prevalence in Western countries is found to be higher, with predominance in white populations [2, 11]. It affects about 0.3% of the general population and men are predominantly affected with a male-female ratio of 3:2 [11]. PD prevalence increases with age and rates increases from 1% in those over 60 years to 4% in people over 80 years [12]. PD in patients below the age of 45 is likely to be associated with hereditary forms.

30.6 Pathophysiology

The main pathological characteristic of PD is dopamine-secreting cell death in substantia nigra due to accumulations of alpha-synuclein protein (Lewy bodies) [13]. The five major pathways connecting cortical areas with the basal ganglia are motor, oculo-motor, associative, limbic, and orbitofrontal networks. All of them are affected in PD, while the motor pathway is most severely involved. Thus, varieties of symptoms manifest and lead to impairment in movement, attention, and learning [14].

30.7 Diagnosis

A detailed clinical history and neurological examination are needed to assess for Parkinson's disease. According to the MDS-PD criteria, the core features of the disease are classical motor signs of parkinsonism, which are described as bradykinesia with rest tremor (4–6 Hz) or rigidity, or both [15]. A trial of levodopa with any significant improvement in motor dysfunction may further help in the confirmation of PD diagnosis. Autopsy showing Lewy bodies in the midbrain is usually considered diagnostic. The clinical presentation of PD should be periodically reviewed to confirm the accuracy of the diagnosis [4, 16].

Vascular and drug-induced parkinsonisms are the common secondary parkinsonisms [16]. Similarly, Parkinson's plus syndromes like progressive supranuclear palsy, corticobasal degeneration, and multiple system atrophy also need to be excluded [4]. Although some improvement may be seen in the early drug initiation phase, anti-Parkinson's drugs are not very effective in prolonged control of symptoms in Parkinson's plus syndromes [4]. Rapid progression, early cognitive disturbance or postural problem, dysautonomia, absence of resting tremor, or symmetry at onset may point to Parkinson's plus syndrome instead of PD [17]. In case of young-onset parkinsonism or multiple PDs in the family, genetic PD with autosomal-dominant or recessive pattern of inheritance should be taken into account [3].

30.8 Imaging

MRI is more specific in diagnosing PD, specifically if iron-sensitive T2 and SWI sequences have been done in at least 3T MRI. It shows absence of the "swallow tail," which is the hyperintense signal within the substantia nigra that has very high sensitivity and specificity. It also helps in distinguishing it from Parkinson's plus disease [18]. In both PD and PD plus syndrome, there is less dopamine-related activity in the basal ganglia, elicited by PET and SPECT, which can help to rule out drug-induced parkinsonism [16].

30.9 Management

Parkinson's disease is not curable but drugs, surgery, and physiotherapy can help improve the symptoms. The main drugs effective for motor symptoms are levodopa (in combination with dopamine decarboxylase inhibitor), catechol-O-methyltransferase (COMT) inhibitors, dopamine agonists, and monoamine oxidase B (MAO-B) inhibitors. Drug effectiveness depends on disease stage and patient age at disease onset [19].

PD patients usually undergo three different stages: an initial stage, where some disability has already developed and they require drug therapy; a second stage associated with various complications of levodopa usage; and the final stage, where symptoms are unrelated to levodopa therapy [20]. In the first stage, proper drug titration is needed for adequate control of symptoms and treatment-related side effects. Initial use of MAO-B inhibitors and dopamine agonists is suggested; this may be helpful to delay the likely complications of early levodopa use [21]. However, levodopa is regarded as the most effective option for the motor symptoms and there

should be no delay in starting this medicine for better quality of life in patients. Disease duration and its severity are more responsible for levodopa-related dyskinesias than time period of levodopa therapy, so delayed use of levodopa may not provide longer dyskinesia-free time [22].

In the second stage, the main aim of treatment is to reduce symptoms and control fluctuations in PD patients. Rapid withdrawals or higher drug dosages need to be controlled [21]. When oral medications are not enough to control symptoms, lesioning surgery, deep brain stimulation (DBS), subcutaneous apomorphine infusion, and enteral dopamine pumps can be suitable [23]. DBS of the internal globus pallidus (GPi) and the subthalamic nucleus (STN) were found to be effective and safe targets in PD patients. Randomized control trials on DBS have shown better functional outcomes with minimal adverse effects, and therefore DBS has recently replaced lesioning surgery in developed nations [24, 25].

The third and final stage presents many challenging problems like psychiatric symptoms, orthostatic hypotension, and bladder dysfunction requiring a variety of treatments [23]. Palliative care is usually offered to patients in the final stages of the disease to improve quality of life [26].

30.10 Gene Therapy

Enzymes produced by the used gene help to control its symptoms or protect the cerebral tissue from further damage. Four clinical trials related to gene therapy in Parkinson's disease were done in 2010 [27]. There were no severe adverse events, but also no greater effectiveness of gene therapy was reported [27].

30.11 Prognosis

PD is a neurodegenerative disease and patient symptoms progress with time. The Unified Parkinson's Disease Rating Scale (UPDRS) is commonly used for measuring the clinical severity of the disease. The Modified Hoehn and Yahr Scale is a PD staging method which is commonly used. Since current therapies are quite effective to control motor symptoms, non-motor features cannot be adequately managed with available therapy [27]. Without adequate treatment, motor symptoms progress rapidly in the early stages of the disease and more slowly later. Consequently, patients become wheelchair bound after about 8 years and become bedridden after 10 years of disease onset [28].

References

1. Sveinbjornsdottir S. The clinical symptoms of Parkinson's disease. J Neurochem. 2016;139:318–24.
2. Kalia LV, Lang AE. Parkinson's disease. Lancet. 2015;386(9996):896–912.
3. Mosley AD. The encyclopedia of Parkinson's disease. 2nd ed. New York: Facts on File; 2010. p. 89.
4. Ling H, Massey LA, Lees AJ, Brown P, Day BL. Hypokinesia without decrement distinguishes progressive supranuclear palsy from Parkinson's disease. Brain. 2012;135(Pt 4):1141–53.
5. Aarsland D, Londos E, Ballard C. Parkinson's disease dementia and dementia with Lewy bodies: different aspects of one entity. Int Psychogeriatr. 2009;21(2):216–9.
6. Charcot J-M, Sigerson G. Lectures on the diseases of the nervous system. 2nd ed. Philadelphia: Henry C. Lea; 1879. p. 113.
7. Jankovic J. Parkinson's disease: clinical features and diagnosis. J Neurol Neurosurg Psychiatry. 2008;79(4):368–76.
8. Fung VS, Thompson PD. Rigidity and spasticity. In: Tolosa E, Jankovic J, editors. Parkinson's disease and movement disorders. Hagerstown, MD: Lippincott Williams & Wilkins; 2007. p. 504–13.
9. Yao SC, Hart AD, Terzella MJ. An evidence-based osteopathic approach to Parkinson disease. Osteopath Fam Physician. 2013;5(3):96–101.
10. Hoehn MM, Yahr MD. Parkinsonism: onset, progression and mortality. Neurology. 1967;17(5):427–42.
11. de Lau LML, Giesbergen PCLM, de Rijk MC, et al. Incidence of parkinsonism and Parkinson disease in a general population. Neurology. 2004;63:1240–4.
12. de Lau LM, Breteler MM. Epidemiology of Parkinson's disease. Lancet Neurol. 2006;5(6):525–35.
13. Rajesh P, Lyons KE. Handbook of Parkinson's disease. 3rd ed. CRC Press; 2003. p. 76.
14. Shergill SS, Walker Z, Le K, C. A preliminary investigation of laterality in Parkinson's disease and susceptibility to psychosis. J Neurol Neurosurg Psychiatry. 1998;65(4):610–1.
15. Postuma RB, Berg D, Stern M, Poewe W, Olanow CW, Oertel W, et al. MDS clinical diagnostic criteria for Parkinson's disease. Mov Disord. 2015;30:1591–601.
16. Chahine LM, Stern MB, Chen-Plotkin A. Blood-based biomarkers for Parkinson's disease. Parkinsonism Relat Disord. 2014;20(Suppl 1):S99–103.
17. Lesage S, Brice A. Parkinson's disease: from monogenic forms to genetic susceptibility factors. Hum Mol Genet. 2009;18(R1):R48–59.
18. Jubault T, Brambati SM, Degroot C, Gendelman H. Regional brain stem atrophy in idiopathic Parkinson's disease detected by anatomical MRI. PLoS One. 2009;4(12):e8247.
19. Gibb WR, Lees AJ. The relevance of the Lewy body to the pathogenesis of idiopathic Parkinson's disease. J Neurol Neurosurg Psychiatry. 1988;51(6):745–52.
20. Rizzo G, Copetti M, Arcuti S, Martino D, Fontana A, Logroscino G. Accuracy of clinical diagnosis of Parkinson disease: a systematic review and meta-analysis. Neurology. 2016;86(6):566–76.
21. Postuma RB, Berg D, Stern M, Poewe W, Olanow CW, Oertel W, et al. MDS clinical diagnostic criteria for Parkinson's disease. Mov Disord. 2015;30(12):1591–601.
22. Berg D, Postuma RB, Adler CH, Bloem BR, Chan P, Dubois B, et al. MDS research criteria for prodromal Parkinson's disease. Mov Disord. 2015;30(12):1600–11.
23. Brooks DJ. Imaging approaches to Parkinson disease. J Nucl Med. 2010;51(4):596–609.
24. Esselink RAJ, de Bie RMA, de Haan RJ, Lenders MWPM, Nijssen PCG, Staal MJ, et al. Unilateral pallidotomy versus bilateral subthalamic nucleus stimulation in PD. Neurology. 2004;62:201–7.
25. Schuurmann PR, Bosch DA, Bossuyt PMM, Bonsel GJ, van Someren EJW, De Bie RMA. A comparison of continuous thalamic stimulation and thalamotomy for suppression of severe tremor. N Engl J Med. 2000;342:461–8.
26. Schwarz ST, Afzal M, Morgan PS, Bajaj N, Gowland PA, Auer DP. The 'swallow tail' appearance of the healthy nigrosome - a new accurate test of Parkinson's disease: a case-control and retrospective cross-sectional MRI study at 3T. PLoS One. 2014;9(4):e93814.
27. Friedman JH. Parkinson's disease psychosis 2010: a review article. Parkinsonism Relat Disord. 2010;16(9):553–60.
28. Poewe W. The natural history of Parkinson's disease. J Neurol. 2006;253(Suppl 7):VII2–6.

Part VII
Others

Trigeminal Neuralgia

31

Bibhukalyani Das and Supriyo Choudhury

Case Scenario

A 52-year-old hypertensive female presented with a lancinating pain in right side of face for 15 years, frequently affecting her daily life activity. Chewing food or brushing teeth would precipitate into severe facial pain, which radiated towards forehead and ears. Her sleep was also severely affected due to facial pain. She was initially treated with carbamazepine 100 mg/day that was later increased up to 400 mg/day. Her pain was controlled inadequately despite the additional administration of gabapentin at 450 mg/day. As a result of difficulty in taking food, she had lost a lot of weight in the past 1 year. The pain was distributed in all the three zones of trigeminal nerve. Routine blood tests and MRI of the trigeminal nerve were done. The trigger of pain was found to be confined to zone 2. We planned to perform transcutaneous transovale radiofrequency ablation (RFA) of the trigeminal root entry zone. Patient was counselled for possible complications, and her consent was taken. The whole procedure was done under sedation with propofol, and vitals were constantly monitored. Oxygen was given through a nasal cannula. The position of the patient was supine with head-end raised up

to 30°. The procedure was performed in a cathlab under C-Arm. C-Arm was focused on sub-mental view, and ipsilateral foramen ovale was identified. The RFA cannula was then introduced approximately 2 cm lateral to ipsilateral angle of mouth and directed towards the foramen of ovale. Upon penetration of foramen ovale, the patient experienced extreme pain. The RF lesion generator was checked, and ground electrode was attached. RFA electrode was introduced through the cannula, and correct impedance was monitored to ensure its correct placement (Fig. 31.1). Stimulation was given, and the patient experienced pain similar to her facial pain due to trigeminal neuralgia. Three consecutive lesions were made at 60, 70, and 80 centigrade for 60 s each. During lesioning, the corneal reflex was examined by the assistant. Ice pack was placed over the affected side of the face, and prophylactically, a single dose of 1 g of ceftriaxone was administered. In the first follow-up, 15 days after the intervention, the patient reported a reduction in pain and mild heaviness of the face, with no fever, an absence of Kernig's sign, and an intact corneal reflex. She did not report or notice any complications, for example, an increase in the threshold of pain, corneal anaesthesia, or anaesthesia dolorosa. The dose of the medication was tapered and gradually stabilised at carbamazepine 200 mg/day over a month. On her second follow-up (after 2 months), she was relatively free from facial pain.

B. Das (✉)
Neuroscience Critical Care Unit and Pain Clinic, Institute of Neurosciences, Kolkata, India

S. Choudhury
Department of Neurology, Institute of Neurosciences, Kolkata, India

© Springer Nature Singapore Pte Ltd. 2024
K. K. Oli et al. (eds.), *Case-based Approach to Common Neurological Disorders*,
https://doi.org/10.1007/978-981-99-8676-7_31

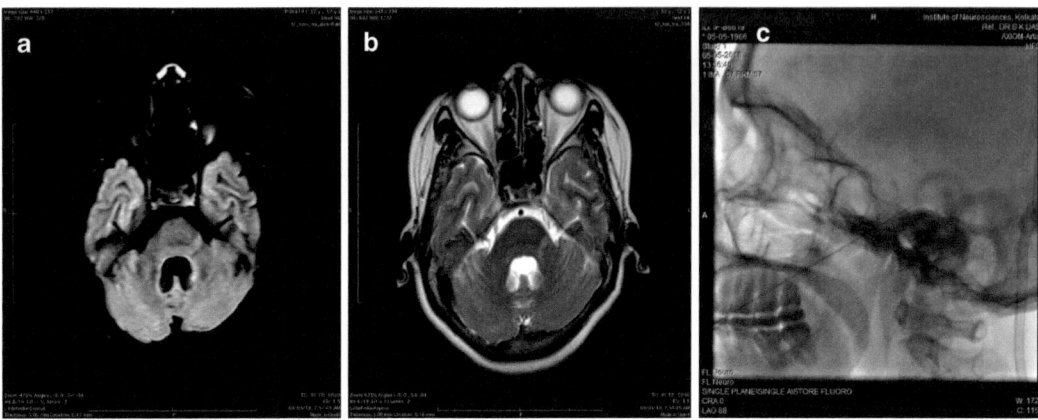

Fig. 31.1 (**a, b**) A well-defined T2 FLAIR hyperintense oval lesion noted at left side of the pons along the intraparenchymal course of the left trigeminal nerve. The TOF MRA and 3D CLGS images (not shown here) didn't reveal any neurovascular conflict. The imaging suggested of a focal demyelinating plaque. (**c**) RFA canula and electrode in the vicinity of the trigeminal nerve root

31.1 Introduction

Trigeminal neuralgia (TN), the most common of all cranial neuralgias [1], manifests with moderate-to-severe pain in the areas of the head and face. This clinical condition was first mentioned in ancient medical literature by a Greek physician, Aretaeus of Cappadocia (circa 150 AD book 1), who described it as 'hemicrania' [2]. Persian scholar and physician Ibn Sina or Avicenna (980–1037) also described a similar infirmity which appears to be a combination of facial palsy and TN. However, the first convincing and clear description of TN was found in the eulogy of Dr Johannes Bausch (1605–1665), who, unfortunately, expired due to complications of TN [3]. He was the first president of German Academy of Sciences Leopoldina (the oldest continuously existing and learned society in the world) [4]. Nicolaus Andre, a French physician, in 1756 had coined the term "tic douloureux" (facial grimace in response to pain) [2]. This term is still used in modern medical literature, although rarely. Another British physician, John Fothergill, had described the features of TN in his paper; till date TN is also known as the 'Fothergill disease' [2].

31.2 Clinical Picture

The pain of TN is classically characterised by paroxysmal pain attacks (sudden, unexpected, and short-lasting). The nature of pain is usually stabbing, electrical shock-like, or shooting. A single pain paroxysm could last for a few seconds to hours, appearing intermittently [5]. The pain-free interval is known as the refractory period, which could last for minutes to hours. The pain attack could appear several times in a day. These attacks could seem continuous when the intermittent intervals are extremely short. Half of the patients complain of continual aches or dull or burning background pain of lower intensity in the same area as the paroxysmal pain [6]. This particular type of pain is more common in women [7]. The refractory period could be due to hyperpolarisation of sensory neurons, and pain is often triggered by intraoral/extraoral sensory stimulus, such as light touching, talking, chewing, brushing teeth, or simply a cold wind blowing against the face. Even a subtle sensory stimulus can potentially trigger spontaneous pain [8]. The pain is localised more towards the right side, most frequently at the second (maxillary) and third (mandibular) divisions of trigeminal nerve [6]. Bilateral involvement is very rare and should raise suspicion of secondary TN.

Classically, TN was thought to be a progressive disease. However, recent studies have revealed that the intensity of pain and morphological changes do not increase with age or the duration of the disease. The duration of refractory period is unpredictable and could be due to partial remyelination. Certain specific autonomic symptoms could be associated with TN, such as tearing, rhinorrhoea, or sialorrhoea, and probably result from excessive pain-induced trigeminovascular reflex [5].

31.3 Epidemiology

It is difficult to estimate the incidence of TN due to misdiagnosis and underreporting. As a result, TN has been reported quite variably across studies ranging from 4.3 to 27 new cases per 100,000 people per year [9–11]. Female gender and increased age are the known risk factors for TN. The average age of onset is 53 years for classical TN and 43 years for secondary TN. It is uncommon in younger age group [11].

31.4 Pathophysiology

Trigeminal nerve is a sensory nerve which carries sensation from its three branches. These sensory fibres are myelinated, and in TN the myelin sheath could be damaged either due to multiple sclerosis or as a result of continuous pressure at the nerve root.

Damaged insulation leads to abnormal connectivity and transmission between the sensory fibres, resulting in barraging the brain with signals (perceived as TN pain). More precisely, these demyelinated sensory fibres could either generate ectopic spontaneous impulses due to hyper-excitability or initiate unnatural cross-talk with the healthy ones [12, 13]. The compression is by a blood vessel, usually an artery, in the cerebellopontine cistern and is termed neurovascular conflict with compression. Morphological changes resulting from neurovascular conflict are commonly associated with TN. Studies have also shown that a simple contact between a blood vessel and the nerve, without any significant morphological changes, could result in symptoms of TN (Fig. 31.2) [14]. As a matter of fact, decompression in such situations had demonstrated improvement in selected cases. A recent study suggests a 'gain in function' of the voltage-gated sodium channel, resulting from a missense mutation, in TN patients [15].

31.5 Diagnostic Criteria and Sub-classification as per International Association for the Study of Pain (IASP)

Following are the diagnostic criteria for TN:

- Orofacial pain distributed within the trigeminal facial or intraoral territory
- Paroxysmal character of pain
- Pain triggered by typical manoeuvres

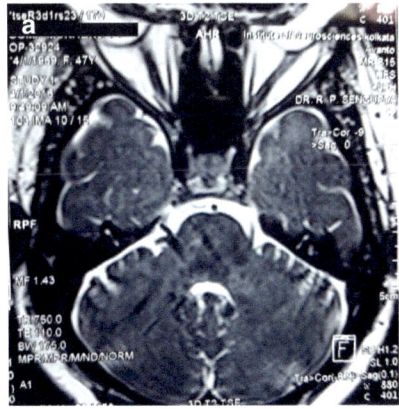 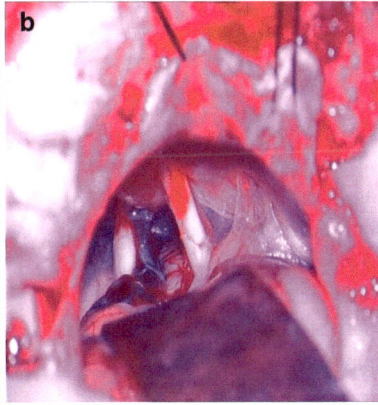

Fig. 31.2 (**a**) T2-weighted image demonstrates a vascular loop around the root of the right trigeminal nerve. (**b**) Image showing microvascular decompression surgery in the same patient

TN can be sub-classified as (a) idiopathic TN, where there is no apparent cause; (b) classical TN, which is caused by vascular compression of the trigeminal nerve root resulting in morphological changes of the nerve root; and (c) secondary TN, which is caused by major neurological disease, e.g., a tumour of the cerebellopontine angle or multiple sclerosis [16].

Alternatively, the diagnosis and classification could be made according to the beta-version of the third edition of the International Classification of Headache Disorders (ICHD3-beta) [17].

31.6 Differential Diagnosis of TN

The clinical diagnosis of TN is quite straightforward in most cases. However, at times clinicians might also consider some other clinical conditions which have similar presenting features. If the patient has a history of skin rash resembling varicella zoster, then one should consider the diagnosis of post-herpetic neuralgia. Similarly, in patients with a history of tooth extraction or trauma in the temporo-mandibular region, post-traumatic neuralgia should be excluded. In both conditions, gain and loss of function should usually coexist. Sensory abnormality in the form of tingling sensation is frequent. Dental conditions like dental caries or cracked tooth could mimic TN. Thus, selective aggravation of pain following chewing of hard, cold, or sweet food should raise the suspicion of dental problems and should be referred to a dental surgeon to exclude any such possibilities. Glossopharyngeal neuralgia can present with evoked stabbing pain located at the back of the tongue, the pharynx, or deep in the ear. Trigger factors are somewhat different from TN and might include swallowing, coughing, or sneezing. In conditions like short-lasting unilateral neuralgiform headache attacks with autonomic symptoms (SUNA) or short-lasting unilateral neuralgiform headache attacks with conjunctival injection and tearing (SUNCT), the affected side can change, unlike TN, and each pain attack is accompanied by autonomic symptoms such as conjunctival injection, miosis, or lacrimation.

31.7 Management

The diagnosis of TN should be based on a medical history and physical examination, yet for classification and assessment of the vascular loop, an MRI scan should be advised early. MRI can detect or exclude conditions like MS or cerebellopontine tumour (two common causes of secondary TN). Serum sodium, potassium, renal and liver function tests, and ECG should be assessed before initiation of pharmacotherapy because antiepileptic drugs can aggravate or precipitate dyselectrolytaemia, hepatic, or renal toxicity. Drugs like carbamazepine or oxcarbazepine are contraindicated in patients with atrioventricular block.

The first line of treatment for TN is pharmacotherapy; sodium channel blockers like carbamazepine or oxcarbazepine are the drugs of choice. Monotherapy with both the drugs is quite effective in most cases. However, sometimes due to their adverse effects it is challenging to reach the therapeutic dose of these drugs. Carbamazepine is discontinued more often compared to oxcarbazepine due to the side effects like skin rash, tremor, dizziness, drowsiness, somnolence, etc. However, the incidence of electrolyte imbalance is more frequent with the use of oxcarbazepine. Lamotrigine, baclofen, pregabalin, or gabapentin could be used in combination with carbamazepine or oxcarbazepine if the first-line agents show a lack of efficacy or reduced tolerance as adverse effects. The second-line drugs are likely to be effective as monotherapy, although the evidence remains weak.

In medically refractory cases with neurovascular conflict, microvascular decompression is the treatment of choice. This surgical procedure involves craniotomy and exploration of the posterior fossa for the identification of an abnormal blood vessel loop pressing against the nerve root [18, 19]. This gives significant pain relief in more than 70% of the patients after 5 years: higher than other surgical techniques. The complication is rare but may include new aches or burning pain, sensory loss, mild or transient cranial nerve dysfunction (2–7%), major cranial nerve dysfunction (2%), stroke (0.3%), and death [18, 19]. Therefore, it is essential to inform the patients regarding the possible complications before surgery. Other less invasive procedures include chemical lesioning of the trigeminal ganglion, glycerol blockade, mechanically by balloon compression, or thermally by radiofrequency thermo-coagulation. Stereotactically, the radiation beam (gamma knife) is focused to ablate the trigeminal ganglia. In this radio-intervention, 50% patients remain pain-free, even after 5 years. Minor complications such as sensory loss (12–50%), masticatory problems (balloon compression, up to 50%), and new burning or aching pain (12%) are reported following these less invasive procedures [20].

References

1. Zakrzewska J. Differential diagnosis of facial pain and guidelines for management. Br J Anaesth. 2013;111(1):95–104.
2. Rose FC. Trigeminal neuralgia. Arch Neurol. 1999;56(9):1163–4.
3. Johnson MC, Salmon JH. Arteriovenous malformation presenting as trigeminal neuralgia: case report. J Neurosurg. 1968;29(3):287–9.
4. Siviero M, Teixeira M, De Siqueira J, Siqueira S. Somesthetic, gustatory, olfactory function and salivary flow in patients with neuropathic trigeminal pain. Oral Dis. 2010;16(5):482–7.
5. Cheshire WP. Trigeminal neuralgia: diagnosis and treatment. Curr Neurol Neurosci Rep. 2005;5(2):79–85.
6. Maarbjerg S, Gozalov A, Olesen J, Bendtsen L. Trigeminal neuralgia—a prospective systematic study of clinical characteristics in 158 patients. Headache. 2014;54(10):1574–82.
7. Maarbjerg S, Gozalov A, Olesen J, Bendtsen L. Concomitant persistent pain in classical trigeminal neuralgia–evidence for different subtypes. Headache. 2014;54(7):1173–83.
8. Rasmussen P, Facial pain. IV. A prospective study of 1052 patients with a view of: precipitating factors, associated symptoms, objective psychiatric and neurological symptoms. Acta Neurochir. 1991;108(3–4):100–9.
9. Katusic S, Beard CM, Bergstralth E, Kurland LT. Incidence and clinical features of trigeminal neuralgia, Rochester, Minnesota, 1945–1984. Ann Neurol. 1990;27(1):89–95.
10. Mueller D, Obermann M, Yoon M-S, Poitz F, Hansen N, Slomke M-A, et al. Prevalence of trigeminal neuralgia and persistent idiopathic facial pain: a population-based study. Cephalalgia. 2011;31(15):1542–8.
11. MacDonald B, Cockerell O, Sander J, Shorvon S. The incidence and lifetime prevalence of neurological disorders in a prospective community-based study in the UK. Brain. 2000;123(4):665–76.
12. Calvin WH, Loeser JD, Howe JF. A neurophysiological theory for the pain mechanism of tic douloureux. Pain. 1977;3(2):147–54.
13. Burchiel KJ. Abnormal impulse generation in focally demyelinated trigeminal roots. J Neurosurg. 1980;53(5):674–83.
14. Maarbjerg S, Wolfram F, Gozalov A, Olesen J, Bendtsen L. Association between neurovascular contact and clinical characteristics in classical trigeminal neuralgia: a prospective clinical study using 3.0 Tesla MRI. Cephalalgia. 2015;35(12):1077–84.
15. Huang J, Han C, Estacion M, Vasylyev D, Hoeijmakers JG, Gerrits MM, et al. Gain-of-function mutations in sodium channel NaV1. 9 in painful neuropathy. Brain. 2014;137(6):1627–42.
16. Cruccu G, Finnerup NB, Jensen TS, Scholz J, Sindou M, Svensson P, et al. Trigeminal neuralgia new classification and diagnostic grading for practice and research. Neurology. 2016;87(2):220–8.
17. Arnold M. Headache Classification Committee of the International Headache Society (IHS) the international classification of headache disorders. Cephalalgia. 2018;38(1):1–211.
18. Zhang H, Lei D, You C, Mao B-Y, Wu B, Fang Y. The long-term outcome predictors of pure microvascular decompression for primary trigeminal neuralgia. World Neurosurg. 2013;79(5):756–62.
19. Sandell T, Eide PK. Effect of microvascular decompression in trigeminal neuralgia patients with or without constant pain. Neurosurgery. 2008;63(1):93–100.
20. Cruccu G, Gronseth G, Alksne J, Argoff C, Brainin M, Burchiel K, et al. AAN-EFNS guidelines on trigeminal neuralgia management. Eur J Neurol. 2008;15(10):1013–28.

Hypoxic Ischemic Encephalopathy

32

Masoom J. Desai, Roohi Katyal, Pratik Agrawal, and Gentle Sunder Shrestha

Case Scenario

A 58-year-old man with a history of hypertension was found unconscious at his home for an unknown duration of time. He was noted to have pulseless electrical activity (PEA) by the time of arrival of paramedics. Cardiopulmonary resuscitation (CPR) was initiated and return of spontaneous circulation was achieved in 12 min. Subsequently, he was transferred to our hospital for further care.

Upon arrival, the patient was afebrile, blood pressure was 149/95 mmHg, pulse rate ranged from 61 to 78 beats/min, and oxygen saturation was 100% while on mechanical ventilation (assist control/volume controlled mode, FiO2 40%, tidal volume 400 mL, and respiratory rate 16/min). Upon initial examination, performed 30 min after holding sedation, the patient was in a comatose state. There was no response to verbal and noxious stimulation. Pupillary assessment showed 5 mm pupils with minimal reactivity to light bilaterally. No spontaneous eye movements were noted. He had an absent vestibulo-ocular reflex. Corneal reflex was intact. There was no facial muscle weakness bilaterally. Cough and gag reflexes were absent on assessment and he was breathing with a ventilator. He had sudden, involuntary movements consistent with myoclonic jerks involving bilateral upper and lower extremities.

The patient was treated with lorazepam and subsequently with levetiracetam for myoclonus, which alleviated the myoclonic jerks. Initial laboratory testing revealed normal white cell count of 6.73 K/mm^3 (range 4–11 K/mm^3), acute renal failure (serum creatinine 1.35 mg/dL, range 0.7–1.1 mg/dL), and elevated creatine kinase 476 units/L (range 37–264 units/L). Urine drug screen analysis was positive for cannabinoids. CT of the head without contrast showed adequate gray–white matter differentiation. Midline structures were non-displaced. The ventricles and basilar cisterns were of normal size and configuration. Structures of the posterior fossa were unremarkable.

Targeted temperature management (TTM) was initiated with a temperature goal of 36 °C which was continued for 24 h. The patient underwent slow rewarming at 0.1 °C per hour over 24 h after completion of TTM. Repeat neurological

M. J. Desai (✉)
Department of Neurology,
University of New Mexico, Albuquerque, NM, USA
e-mail: mdesai@salud.unm.edu

R. Katyal
Department of Neurology, Ochsner-LSU Health Shreveport, Shreveport, LA, USA

P. Agrawal
Division of Cardiology, Ochsner-LSU Health Shreveport, Shreveport, LA, USA

G. S. Shrestha
Tribhuvan University Teaching Hospital,
Institute of Medicine, Kathmandu, Nepal

© Springer Nature Singapore Pte Ltd. 2024
K. K. Oli et al. (eds.), *Case-based Approach to Common Neurological Disorders*,
https://doi.org/10.1007/978-981-99-8676-7_32

examination was performed post rewarming and after holding sedation for 2 h. The patient remained unresponsive to verbal or noxious stimuli. His pupils were dilated (7 mm) and non-reactive to light reflex bilaterally. Vestibulo-ocular reflex response was absent. Corneal reflex was present. There was no facial muscle weakness bilaterally. Cough and gag reflexes were absent and he was breathing with a ventilator. There were no myoclonic jerks or any voluntary movement.

Video-electroencephalography (vEEG) showed generalized background slowing in the frequency range of 1–3 Hz alternating with periods of generalized voltage attenuation (Fig. 32.1a, b). MRI of the brain obtained on day five after presentation demonstrated extensive diffusion restriction involving the entire cerebral cortex bilaterally extending to the sub-cortical regions, including diffusion restriction in the basal ganglia and thalami bilaterally. This was associated with diffuse cerebral edema resulting in effacement of cortical sulci and basal cisterns. There was also mild bilateral uncal herniation (Fig. 32.2a–c).

vEEG did not demonstrate any change in frequency and amplitude of waves in reaction to verbal and noxious stimulation. In the absence of any confounders to explain the patient's current examination findings, he was diagnosed with hypoxic ischemic encephalopathy due to out-of-hospital cardiac arrest (OHCA). Given the findings on MRI of the brain, lack of reactivity on EEG, and repeat neurological examination without any improvement after completion of TTM protocol, a family discussion was held and the decision was made to pursue comfort care measures only.

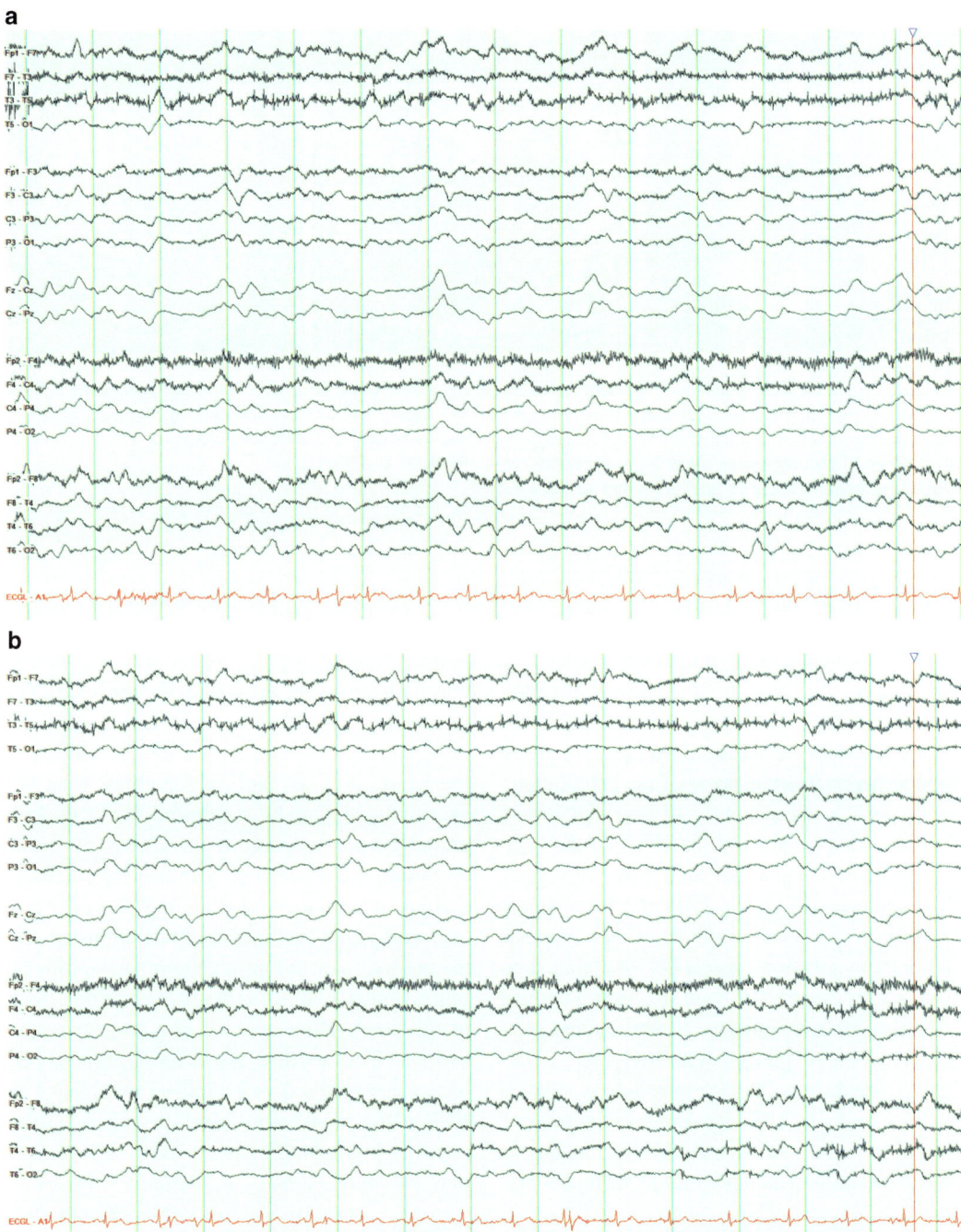

Fig. 32.1 (**a**) This abnormal EEG is consistent with severe, generalized, non-specific cerebral dysfunction. During this period, frequent right upper extremity myoclonic jerks were observed without any associated EEG change. Sensitivity 10 μV/mm, LFF 1 Hz, HFF 70 Hz, notch filter: 60 Hz. (**b**) External noxious stimulation on left lower extremity at the beginning of this page was not associated with any EEG change, thus demonstrating a lack of reactivity. There was absence of both posterior dominant rhythm (PDR) and well-formed sleep architectures throughout the study. Sensitivity 10 μV/mm, LFF 1 Hz, HFF 70 Hz, notch filter: 60 Hz

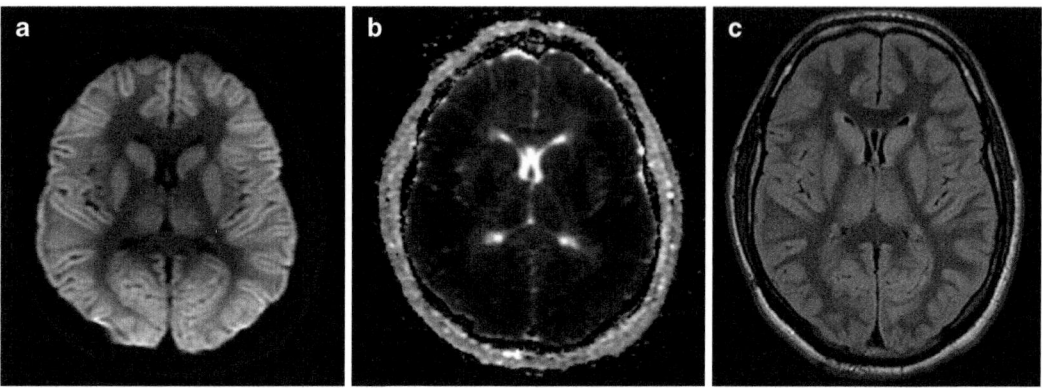

Fig. 32.2 (a) MRI DWI sequence demonstrating extensive marked restricted diffusion involving the entire cerebral cortex bilaterally extending to the subcortical regions; (b): MRI ADC sequence demonstrating hypointense cortical and subcortical regions corresponding to the DWI hyperintensities; (c): MRI T2-FLAIR sequence demonstrating diffuse cortical and subcortical hyperintensities and associated diffuse edema, resulting in effacement of the cortical sulci

32.1 Introduction

Hypoxic ischemic encephalopathy (HIE) is a major cause of neurologic disabilities in cardiac arrest patients. It is a type of brain insult that occurs secondary to reduced oxygen supply or hypoperfusion. Certain areas of the cerebral cortex (especially the parietal and occipital lobes), the hippocampi, the basal ganglia, and the cerebellum are more vulnerable to hypoxic injury [1]. The outcome of hypoxic ischemic brain injury depends on age, severity, and duration of hypoxia and/or hypoperfusion episode [2]. Moderate therapeutic hypothermia has been shown in a number of clinical trials to improve morbidity and mortality outcomes in patients with HIE [3–5]. In this chapter, we discuss the pathophysiology, clinical manifestations of HIE, its prognostication, and current evidence on management strategies to improve neurological outcomes in such patients.

32.2 Epidemiology

The commonest cause of hypoxic ischemic encephalopathy is cardiac arrest. The estimated annual incidence of sudden cardiac arrest (SCA) ranges between 180,000 and 250,000 cases per year in the United States (total population 300 million), while it is estimated to be between 4 and 5 million cases per year worldwide (total population 6.54 billion) [6]. Approximately 80% of SCAs are attributed to coronary artery disease and its sequelae. The remaining 15–20% cases are associated with either structural or electrical abnormalities of the heart, such as cardiomyopathies, long QT syndrome, Brugada syndrome, or catecholaminergic polymorphic ventricular tachycardia. Although the prevalence of pulseless electrical activity as presenting rhythm of SCA is increasing, ventricular tachycardia/fibrillation remains the predominant symptom. Owing to significant improvements in bystander resuscitation efforts in the twenty-first century, the rate of overall survival from cardiac arrest has increased and hence has resulted in increased prevalence of HIE in the population. Mortality after cardiac arrest is high. Studies have shown a mortality rate as high as 64% in patients with post-hypoxic coma. Among survivors, 9% remained comatose while 27% regained consciousness in 4 weeks [7]. Furthermore, long-term functional assessment after cardiac arrest can be carried out using the Cerebral Performance Category (CPC) scale. CPC is a five-point scale which includes functional and cognitive domain assessment and can help predict long-term survival in cardiac arrest patients when administered at hospital discharge [8].

32.3 Pathophysiology

Several mechanisms have been proposed to explain the complex pathophysiology of HIE. As the brain consumes nearly 20–25% of cardiac output, a hypoxic event can result in neuronal loss within minutes after a cardiac arrest event. This is caused by cessation in adenosine triphosphate production and subsequent cytotoxic edema and anerobic metabolism with resultant cerebral lactate accumulation. This results in cell death, which further causes influx of Ca^{2+} ions, thus activating lytic enzymes. The calcium entry likely takes place via N-methyl-D-aspartate receptors [9]. This has been described as the primary insult after cardiac arrest.

In addition, accumulation of Ca^{2+} ions results in functional changes via mitochondrial dysfunction and overproduction of free radicals. The increase in intracellular calcium activates the calpain system, which plays an integral role in altering the cytoskeletal structure as well as in apoptosis [10, 11].

Despite the return of spontaneous circulation (ROSC) after a hypoxic ischemic event, the processes of cell repair continue to remain impaired. Given the highly metabolic state of the cerebral cortex, hypothalami, striatum, and thalami, these structures are more easily susceptible to reperfusion injury with the achievement of ROSC and a resultant increase in free radicals. Further damage is caused by microvascular dysfunction, cerebral edema, anemia, impaired autoregulation, hyperoxia, and hyperthermia at this stage [9].

32.4 Clinical Manifestations

The severity of the hypoxic episode determines the clinical signs and symptoms of HIE [12]. In cases of cerebral hypoxia, the most common clinical manifestation is a comatose state [13]. It is important to consider the effect of confounding factors such as sedative and paralytic medications, hypothermia or hyperthermia, and persistent metabolic abnormalities, among others, while interpreting the presentation of a patient with suspected hypoxic ischemic brain injury.

Clinical presentation can range from complete recovery after a hypoxic event, to a persistent vegetative state, to a comatose state [12]. Impairment in memory and executive dysfunction are common with HIE [14]. Additionally, psychosocial difficulties have a significant impact on the health of patients who experience hypoxic brain injury [14].

Involvement of globus pallidus, cerebellum, and frontal lobes may result in significant loss of motor control and increase in extensor tone [13]. Such disturbances can affect posture and gait and can result in akinetic-rigid and dystonia syndromes [15]. Patients with impaired speech and language function due to HIE commonly have expressive dysphasia, dysarthria, and speech dyspraxia. Frontal lobe injury secondary to hypoxia can present with behavioral disturbances, loss of insight, apathy, and loss of executive function. Additionally, seizures, tremor, and myoclonus have been described [16].

32.5 Management and Prognostication

Supportive care remains the mainstay of management of hypoxic ischemic injury. For patients who are comatose after cardiac arrest related to initial shockable cardiac rhythm (either pulseless ventricular tachycardia or ventricular fibrillation), therapeutic hypothermia (TH) has strong evidence in improving neurological outcome according to American Academy of Neurology (AAN) guidelines [4]. Prognostic benefit of TH in cardiac arrest patients with initial non-shockable cardiac rhythm (e.g., pulseless electrical activity or asystole) remains debated due to limited evidence (Level C) [4], although a recent randomized controlled trial comparing TH (33 °C during the first 24 h) to targeted normothermia (37 °C) in comatose patients after cardiac arrest due to non-shockable cardiac rhythm has reported a favorable neurologic outcome at 90 days with TH [5]. It is worth adding that a study by TTM Trial Investigators [3] showed no significant difference in all-cause mortality or composite outcome of poor neurological function or death when targeted hypothermia at 33 °C was compared to 36 °C, both intended to prevent fever, in post-cardiac arrest patients irrespective of initial cardiac rhythm. Furthermore, targeted hypothermia did not result in decreased mortality by 6 months compared to targeted normothermia in comatose individuals following an out-of-hospital cardiac arrest [17]. Hemodynamic stability is crucial for post-resuscitation care. Studies have shown that a mean arterial pressure (MAP) of <65 mmHg is inadequate for cerebral perfusion. Another observational study, which monitored patients with near-infrared spectroscopy, reported that a MAP between 85 and 100 mm Hg is needed to achieve optimal cerebral oxygenation [18].

A systemic review of 73 studies examining prognostication is such patients reported low to very low quality of evidence along with a relatively small sample size in almost all studies [19]. Hence, when determining prognosis after cardiac arrest, a multimodal approach including neurological examination, neuroimaging, electrophysiological studies, and biomarkers is recommended. In terms of neurological examination, a Glasgow Coma Scale (GCS) motor score of ≤ 2 at 72-h post ROSC has been shown to have low specificity but relatively high sensitivity of 70–80% in predicting poor neurological outcome, while pupillary light reflex and corneal reflex testing has high specificity and low sensitivity [19]. Evidence of hypoxic injury to other organs, for example acute liver injury (transaminitis), acute kidney injury (elevated creatinine), and cardiac injury (elevated troponins), may further aid in diagnosis and outcome prediction [20].

Certain biomarkers have been studied for their outcome-predicting capabilities. These include ubiquitin carboxyl-terminal esterase L1 (UCH-L1), glial fibrillary acidic protein (GFAP) [21], and neuron-specific enolase (NSE) [22]. Biomarker testing with NSE has shown > 95% specificity and 63% sensitivity at 72 h post ROSC [19].

CT of the head findings may include hypodensities in cortical and subcortical regions as well as a reduced gray-white matter ratio (GWR). GWR is calculated as the ratio of Hounsfield units (HU) between gray and white matter. With regard to neuro-prognostication, a GWR between 1.16 and 1.22 on CT of the brain detected within 24 h from ROSC predicted poor neurological outcome with a specificity of 100% and sensitivities ranging between 28 and 76% [19]. T2-weighted MRI brain images typically depict hyperintense signal changes in the involved regions and are often associated with cytotoxic edema resulting in compression of cisterns and sulci [23, 24]. A meta-analysis study has demonstrated a specificity of 92% and sensitivity of 77% of diffusion-weighted imaging (DWI) on MRI in predicting outcomes [25]. In patients with hypoxic ischemic injury, unfavorable outcomes have been associated with significantly more signal abnormalities on MRI DWI and FLAIR imaging [24]. Additionally, signal changes found in the cortex and subcortical gray nuclei predicted poor outcome. A low gray-white matter ratio (less than 1.10 in at least 10% of the brain) predicted poor outcome within hours to up to 3 days after cardiac arrest, while ADC measurements may predict outcome after 2–5 days. Patients with poor outcome after cardiac arrest have been noted to have MRI abnormalities in the cerebral cortex (occipital and temporal lobes particularly), the putamen, and cerebellum that approached a nadir between 3 and 5 days after cardiac arrest [26]. Poor outcome was also associated with decreased network strengths in the default mode network using functional MRI (fMRI) [27]. In a prospective, observational study of 57 patients, a prognostic model based on diffusion tensor imaging (DTI) seemed to accurately predict 1-year functional outcome after cardiac arrest [28]; however, the current generalized application of DTI for prognostication is lacking.

Another modality in neuro-prognostication in comatose post-cardiac arrest patients is electroencephalography (EEG), which serves as a useful adjunct. A continuous or reactive EEG background predicts good recovery after cardiac arrest compared to patients with unreactive EEG background or a burst-suppression EEG pattern [22]. Changes in reactivity in EEG during different stages of management, from therapeutic hypothermia and rewarming to normothermia, may help predict functional outcome [29]. EEG has a specificity of 100% with sensitivity of 50% in predicting poor neurological outcomes if there is presence of at least two malignant features, described as status epilepticus, burst suppression over an unreactive background, or suppressed background with or without periodic discharges [19]. Due to limitations in interrater agreement among electroencephalographers, prognostication in cardiac arrest can further be supported by quantitative EEG reactivity methods using machine-learning methods. In a retrospective study, long-term outcome prediction after cardiac arrest was comparable between expert assessment and quantitative EEG assessment [30].

Electrophysiological study with somatosensory evoked potential (SSEP) with an amplitude ≤ 0.62 µV has shown 100% specificity and 57% sensitivity in predicting poor neurological outcomes [19]. According to American Academy of Neurology (AAN) guidelines, absent cortical SSEPs (N20 response) bilaterally is predictive of poor outcome [31].

Several important questions regarding the management of cardiac arrest remain unanswered and a number of trials are underway to address these questions. Controversy remains regarding the optimal duration of TTM and its utilization in patients with non-shockable rhythms. A favorable approach to temperature management in cardiac arrest patients who undergo extracorporeal life support is yet to be established [32].

Neuro-prognostication after cardiac arrest is complex and can be limited by several confounding factors. Several tests have high specificity for determining poor outcome after cardiac arrest. These include absent pupillary light reflex at 72 h, bilaterally absent N20 cortical responses on SSEPs, and increasing NSE levels. The sensitivity of these tests, however, is limited. As a result, physicians must rely on integrating several pieces of information when prognosticating. Furthermore, when interpreting these test results, physicians must realize that cognitive biases can result in errors in judgment [33]. Hence, it is of paramount importance to be fully aware of the prognostic accuracy and shortcomings of each tool. It is also important to take into account a qualitative component to prognostication influenced by patient age, established goals of care, premorbid conditions, and other organ failures [34].

Returning to our case, after ensuring lack of confounding factors, the determination of poor prognosis was based on the use of a combination of tools (multiple neurological examinations, video-EEG, and neuroimaging). There is uncertainty around predicting outcomes when using these tools individually. However, using a multimodal approach at an optimal time and with the help of a multidisciplinary team, it was felt that there was a low likelihood of meaningful functional recovery in our patient. Hence, taking into consideration the patient's previously established goals of care, it was decided to withdraw further life-sustaining measures using a shared decision-making process.

References

1. Nolan JP, Neumar RW, Adrie C, et al. Post-cardiac arrest syndrome: epidemiology, pathophysiology, treatment, and prognostication: a scientific statement from the International liaison Committee on Resuscitation; the American Heart Association Emergency cardiovascular Care Committee; the Council on Cardiovascular Surgery and Anesthesia; the Council on cardiopulmonary, Perioperative, and Critical Care; the Council on clinical cardiology; the Council on Stroke. Resuscitation. 2008;79:350–79.
2. Schaaf KPW, Artman LK, Peberdy MA, et al. Anxiety, depression, and PTSD following cardiac arrest: a systematic review of the literature. Resuscitation. 2013;84:873–7.
3. Nielsen N, Wetterslev J, Cronberg T, et al. Targeted temperature management at 33 C versus 36 C after cardiac arrest. N Engl J Med. 2013;369:2197–206.
4. Geocadin RG, Wijdicks E, Armstrong MJ, Damian M, Mayer SA, Ornato JP, et al. Practice guideline summary: reducing brain injury following cardiopulmonary resuscitation: report of the guideline development, dissemination, and implementation Subcommittee of the American Academy of Neurology. Neurology. 2017;88(22):2141–9.
5. Lascarrou J-B, Merdji H, Le Gouge A, Colin G, Grillet G, Girardie P, et al. Targeted temperature management for cardiac arrest with nonshockable rhythm. N Engl J Med. 2019;381:2327.
6. Chugh SS, Reinier K, Teodorescu C, et al. Epidemiology of sudden cardiac death: clinical and research implications. Prog Cardiovasc Dis. 2008;51(3):213–28.

7. Heinz UE, Rollnik JD. Outcome and prognosis of hypoxic brain damage patients undergoing neurological early rehabilitation [published correction appears in BMC Res Notes. 2016;9:396]. BMC Res Notes. 2015;8:243.

8. Phelps R, Dumas F, Maynard C, Silver J, Rea T. Cerebral performance category and long-term prognosis following out-of-hospital cardiac arrest. Crit Care Med. 2013;41(5):1252–7.

9. Sekhon MS, Ainslie PN, Griesdale DE. Clinical pathophysiology of hypoxic ischemic brain injury after cardiac arrest: a "two-hit" model. Crit Care. 2017;21:90.

10. Goll DE, Thompson VF, Li H, Wei W, Cong J. The calpain system. Physiol Rev. 2003;83(3):731–801.

11. Busl KM, Greer DM. Hypoxic-ischemic brain injury: pathophysiology, neuropathology and mechanisms. NeuroRehabilitation. 2010;26:5–13.

12. Vendrame M, Azizi SA. Pyramidal and extrapyramidal dysfunction as a sequela of hypoxic injury: case report. BMC Neurol. 2007;27(7):18.

13. Merrill MS, Wares CM, Heffner AC, Shauger KL, Norton HJ, Runyon MS, et al. Early neurologic examination is not reliable for prognostication in post-cardiac arrest patients who undergo therapeutic hypothermia. Am J Emerg Med. 2016;34(6):975–9.

14. Wilson M, Staniforth A, Till R, das Nair R, Vesey P. The psychosocial outcomes of anoxic brain injury following cardiac arrest. Resuscitation. 2014;85(6):795–800.

15. Bhatt MH, Obeso JA, Marsden CD. Time course of postanoxic akinetic-rigid and dystonic syndromes. Neurology. 1993;43:314–7.

16. Fitzgerald A, Aditya H, Prior A, McNeill E, Pentland B. Anoxic brain injury: clinical patterns and functional outcomes. A study of 93 cases. Brain Inj. 2010;24(11):1311–23.

17. Dankiewicz J, Cronberg T, Lilja G, Jakobsen JC, Levin H, Ullén S, Rylander C, et al. TTM2 trial investigators. Hypothermia versus normothermia after out-of-hospital cardiac arrest. N Engl J Med. 2021;384(24):2283–94.

18. Grand J, Lilja G, Kjaergaard J, Bro-Jeppesen J, Friberg H, Wanscher M, et al. Arterial blood pressure during targeted temperature management after out-of-hospital cardiac arrest and association with brain injury and long-term cognitive function. Eur Heart J Acute Cardiovasc Care. 2019;9:S122.

19. Sandroni C, D'Arrigo S, Nolan J. Prognostication after cardiac arrest. Crit Care. 2018;22(1):150.

20. Guneś T, OzturkMA KSM, Narin N, Koklu E. Troponin-T levels in perinatally asphyxiated infants during the first 15 days of life. Acta Paediatr. 2005;94(11):1638–43.

21. Douglas-Escobar M, Weiss MD. Hypoxic-ischemic encephalopathy: a review for the clinician. JAMA Pediatr. 2015;169:397–403.

22. Oddo M, Rossetti AO. Predicting neurological outcome after cardiac arrest. Curr Opin Crit Care. 2011;17(3):254–9.

23. Godinho MV, Pires CE, Hygino da Cruz LC Jr. Hypoxic, toxic, and acquired metabolic encephalopathies at the emergency room: the role of magnetic resonance imaging. Semin Ultrasound CT MR. 2018;39(5):481–94.

24. Keijzer HM, Hoedemaekers CWE, Meijer FJA, Tonino BAR, Klijn CJM, Hofmeijer J. Brain imaging in comatose survivors of cardiac arrest: pathophysiological correlates and prognostic properties. Resuscitation. 2018;133:124–36.

25. Lopez Soto C, Dragoi L, Heyn CC, et al. Imaging for neuroprognostication after cardiac arrest: systematic review and meta-analysis. Neurocrit Care. 2020;32:206–16.

26. Mlynash M, Campbell DM, Leproust EM, Fischbein NJ, Bammer R, Eyngorn I, et al. Temporal and spatial profile of brain diffusion-weighted MRI after cardiac arrest. Stroke. 2010;41(8):1665–72.

27. Koenig MA, Holt JL, Ernst T, Buchthal SD, Nakagawa K, Stenger VA, et al. MRI default mode network connectivity is associated with functional outcome after cardiopulmonary arrest. Neurocrit Care. 2014;20(3):348–57.

28. Luyt C, Galanaud D, Perlbarg V, Vanhaudenhuyse A, Stevens RD, Gupta R, et al. Diffusion tensor imaging to predict long-term outcome after cardiac arrest - a bicentric pilot study. Anesthesiology. 2012;117(6):1311.

29. Crepeau AZ, Rabinstein AA, Fugate JE, et al. Continuous EEG in therapeutic hypothermia after cardiac arrest: prognostic and clinical value. Neurology. 2013;80(4):339–44.

30. Amorim E, van der Stoel M, Nagaraj SB, Ghassemi MM, Jing J, O'Reilly UM, et al. Quantitative EEG reactivity and machine learning for prognostication in hypoxic-ischemic brain injury. Clin Neurophysiol. 2019;130(10):1908–16.

31. Wijdicks EF, Hijdra A, Young GB, et al. Practice parameter: prediction of outcome in comatose survivors after cardiopulmonary resuscitation (an evidence-based review): report of the Quality Standards Subcommittee of the American Academy of Neurology. Neurology. 2006;67:203–10.

32. Walker AC, Johnson NJ. Targeted temperature management and postcardiac arrest care. Emerg Med Clin North Am. 2019;37(3):381–93.

33. Steinberg A, Elmer J. Prognostication after cardiac arrest: are we thinking fast or thinking slow? Resuscitation. 2020;149:228–9.

34. Seder DB. Management of comatose survivors of cardiac arrest. Continuum (Minneap Minn). 2018;24(6):1732–52.

Coma and Vegetative State

Krishna Kumar Oli and Aashish Shrestha

Case Scenario

A 19-year-old woman with G2P0A1 38 + 6 weeks of gestation status had a history of prolonged second stage of labor, for which she presented to a local hospital, and emergency cesarean section was done 6 months back due to the presence of signs of fetal distress. Perioperatively, she went to sudden cardiac arrest without any known perioperative complications after the delivery of a healthy baby. Four cycles of cardiopulmonary resuscitation (CPR) were given following which she was revived. However, due to continuous unconscious state and uncontrolled seizure episodes, she was referred to higher.

Patient was then taken to another hospital where she was treated in intensive care unit (ICU) with the provisional diagnosis of post-CPR status with probable amniotic fluid embolism with refractory status epilepticus secondary to hypoxic ischemic encephalopathy. Tracheostomy was also done on the seventh day of admission. But patient's seizure was not controlled, and her conscious level was not improving despite 1 and ½ months of hospital stay. So, patient was further referred to our center. She was treated in the ICU, and a percutaneous endoscopic gastrostomy feeding tube was placed, and the dose of antiepileptic drugs was adjusted.

During admission at our center, examinations showed her vitals were stable without any significant abnormal findings on general and systemic examinations. Her Glasgow Coma Scale (GCS) was $E_1V_TM_3$, which later improved to spontaneous but purposeless eye opening without visual fixation and tracking. Pupils were bilaterally equal and normally reacting to light. Patient had normal awake and sleep cycle with no evidence of purposeful or voluntary behavioral responses to external stimuli. However, random movements of limbs and trunk were present. Brainstem reflexes such as corneal reflexes, gag reflex, and vestibulo-ocular reflex were preserved. There was the presence of snout, glabellar, and palmomental reflexes. The muscle bulk of all extremities was reduced, and tone was increased with brisk deep tendon reflexes and bilaterally upgoing plantar reflexes.

The patient developed a grade II bed sore during the hospital stay, which has healed now and also has a bilateral foot drop. During the hospital stay, the patient once developed urinary tract infection but well responded to tazobactam-piperacillin. Her routine investigations, such as complete blood count, renal and liver function test, viral serology, abdominal and pelvis ultrasonography, were normal. Electroencephalography findings showed persistent bilateral generalized slow waves without sharps and spikes. Computed tomography of the head, which was done after 1 week of post-CPR

K. K. Oli (✉) · A. Shrestha
Department of Neurology, Tribhuvan University Teaching Hospital, Kathmandu, Nepal

© Springer Nature Singapore Pte Ltd. 2024
K. K. Oli et al. (eds.), *Case-based Approach to Common Neurological Disorders*,
https://doi.org/10.1007/978-981-99-8676-7_33

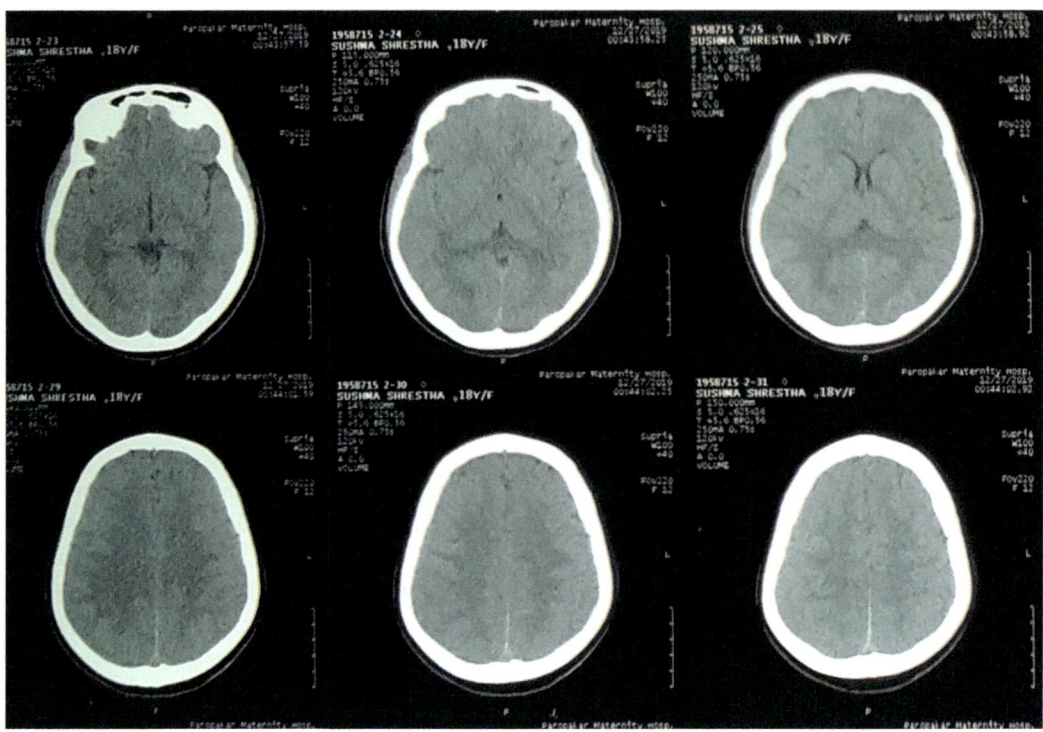

Fig. 33.1 Plain CT head showed periventricular hypodense lesion with narrow ventricles with mild impairment of gray white matter interphase

event, showed features of bilateral cerebral edema (Fig. 33.1). Magnetic resonance imaging (MRI) brain was done then, which showed FLAIR hyperintense bilateral cerebral cortex and posterior putamen (Fig. 33.2). An MRI brain that was repeated 3 months later showed significant cerebral atrophy with gliotic changes over bilateral occipital lobes and a hyperintense lesion on the bilateral frontal lobe and posterior putamen (Fig. 33.3).

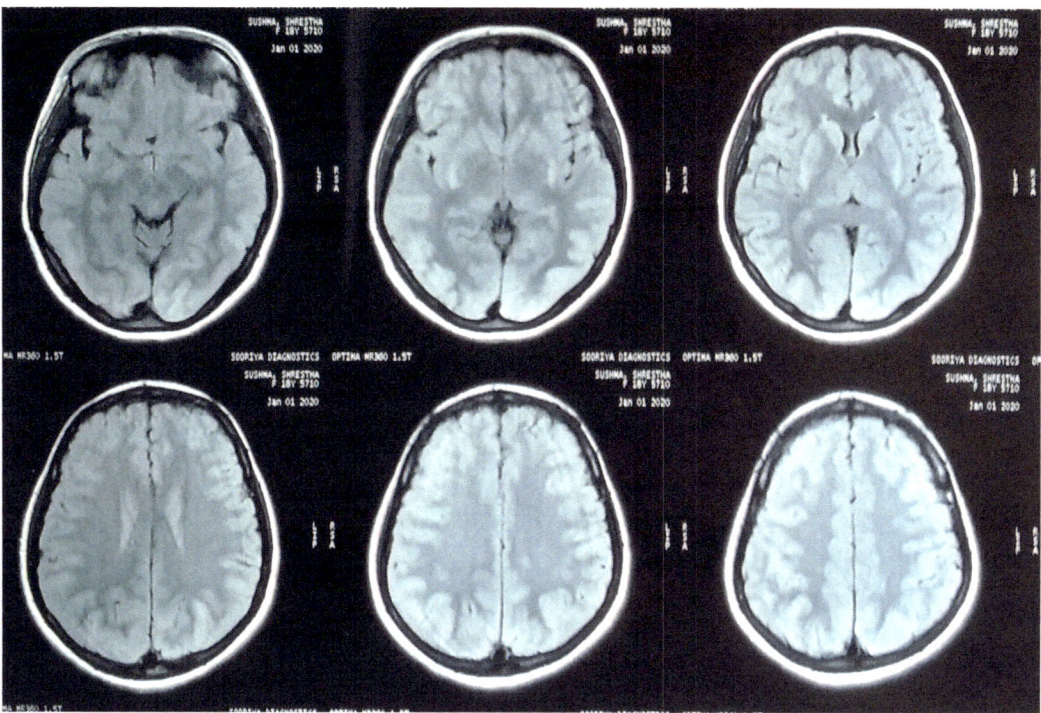

Fig. 33.2 MRI brain T2 FLAIR showed hyperintense posterior putamen and bilateral cerebral cortex, prominent in occipital region

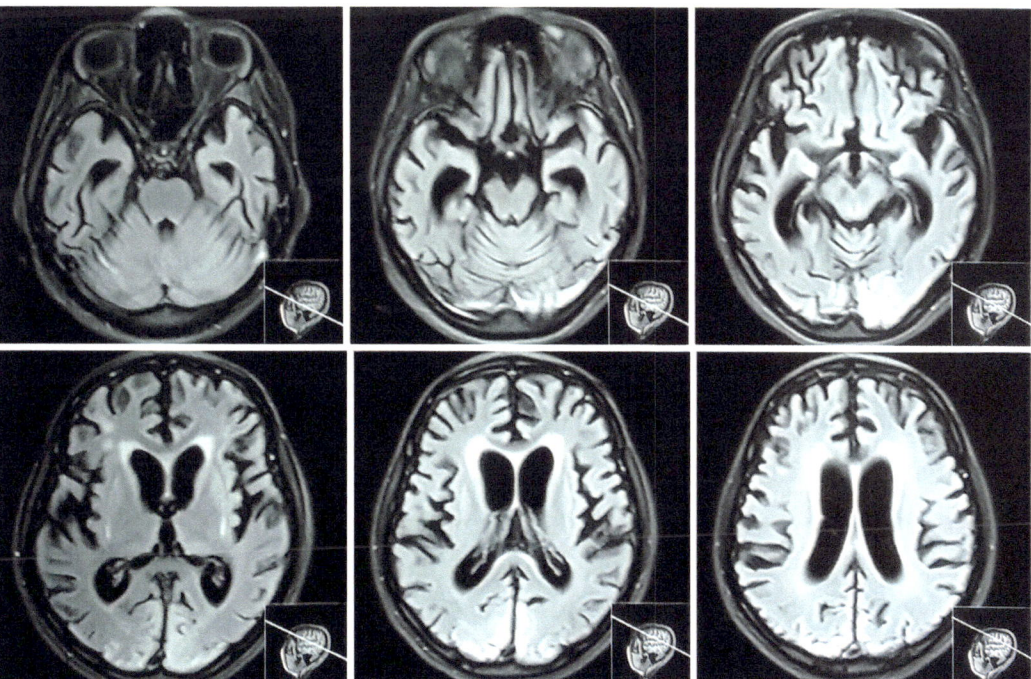

Fig. 33.3 MRI brain T2 FLAIR done 4 months later showed significant cerebral atrophy with gliotic changes over bilateral occipital lobes and hyperintense lesion on bilateral frontal lobe and posterior putamen

33.1 Introduction

Consciousness is the state of awareness of self and surroundings. In contrast, coma is a state of absent responsiveness or prolonged unconsciousness in which the patient lies with the eyes closed, cannot be aroused, and has no awareness of self and surroundings. In comatose patients, noxious stimulation cannot produce spontaneous periods of wakefulness and eye opening, unlike in patients in vegetative state. Hence, coma is characterized by the absence of arousal, awareness, and responsiveness to self and environment lasting for more than 1 h [1].

33.2 Anatomy and Pathophysiological Basis of Coma

The anatomy and pathophysiological cause of coma is either a mechanical destruction of the cerebral cortex or brainstem (anatomic coma) or a global disruption of brain metabolic processes (metabolic coma). Coma of metabolic origin is produced by the interruption of energy substrate delivery (hypoxia, ischemia, hypoglycemia) or by alteration of neurophysiologic responses of neuronal membranes (drug or alcohol intoxication, toxic endogenous metabolites, or epilepsy) [1]. These endogenous metabolic toxins like acetone bodies in diabetes, derivatives of amino acids in uremia, and ammonia in hepatic coma roughly correspond to the level of coma. Similarly, the impairment of consciousness that accompanies pulmonary insufficiency is related mainly to hypercapnia. In acute hyponatremia, neuronal dysfunction results from the intracellular movement of water, leading to neuronal swelling and the loss of potassium chloride from the cells. The coma of toxic and metabolic diseases evolves through the stages of drowsiness, confusion, and stupor.

Physiologically, arousal is the function of ascending reticular activating system (ARAS), and it constitutes a complex pathway from the brainstem, diencephalon, and limbic cortex to the cerebral cortex. This involves cholinergic, noradrenergic, glutaminergic, aminergic, and hypocretinergic neurons that project from the ARAS and terminate in the thalamocortical areas producing cortical activation [2]. In addition, extrathalamic projections from the brainstem reticular neurons terminate in the posterior hypothalamus and the basal forebrain regions. The latter projects to the cerebral cortex (mesocortical projection) causing wakefulness. Together, these pathways maintain the state of alertness to the self and surroundings, inactivation of which may thus lead to an unarousable state.

Therefore, the anatomy and pathophysiological basis of coma are either structural damage or toxic/metabolic disturbances of the brainstem ARAS and its connections.

33.3 Etiology of Coma

Stroke is the leading cause of coma, particularly hemispheric or brainstem infarction, subarachnoidal or parenchymal bleed with ventricular extension, or primary ventricular bleed with ventricular tamponade [3]. Similarly, traumatic brain injury, which can lead to diffuse axonal injury, multiple contusions with multiple bleeds, subarachnoid hemorrhage, subdural hematoma, and epidural hematoma, is another important cause of coma. Brain metastasis of tumors like choriocarcinoma, bronchogenic carcinoma, cholangiocarcinoma, and carcinomatous meningitis are also possible causes. Likewise, infectious encephalitis (Japanese encephalitis and Herpes simplex encephalitis), cerebral malaria, autoimmune encephalitis, brain abscess, and subtle forms of status epilepticus can lead a patient to coma. Further, a cardiac arrest and cardiopulmonary resuscitation can cause a sudden cut-off of blood flow and oxygen into the brain, resulting in edema [4]. Eventually, all structural lesions may lead to edema of the cerebral cortex and brain parenchyma, causing the brain to push down on the brainstem (rostrocaudal deterioration).

Common metabolic causes of coma include status epilepticus; endocrinopathies (e.g., myxedema, hypoadrenalism); systemic neuroinfection; alcohol; exposure to in-house and environmental toxins; anoxic-ischemic encephalopathies; overdose of medications (e.g., sedatives, hypnotics, SSRI); insulin overdose leading to hypoglycemia; and drug abuse with cocaine, amphetamine, and opioids. Toxic encephalopathies resulting from methyl alcohol, ethylene glycol, dyselectrolytemia, carbon monoxide poisoning, and cyanide poisoning are an important cause of coma. Additionally, substances that are normally found in the body could cause toxemia when the body fails to dispose of them properly. An example would be ammonia in liver diseases, urea in kidney failure, and carbon dioxide in a severe asthmatic attack resulting in hepatic encephalopathy, uremic encephalopathy, and anoxic encephalopathy respectively, all of which can lead to coma. Other causes include Wernicke's encephalopathy, hypoglycemia, hypercalcemia, heat stroke, hyperosmolar nonketotic hyperglycemia, diabetic ketoacidosis, and hypercapnia. These often lead to coma via damage to the RAS.

33.4 Immediate Assessment of the Comatose Patients

Immediate assessment of coma requires a quick, sequentially structured history along with relevant physical, systemic, and neurological evaluation so as to discover the etiology and assess the severity of coma, ultimately leading to its timely management. A careful history from the eye witness, especially regarding the onset of coma, is of paramount importance. An abrupt onset with a sudden drop in Glasgow Coma Scale (GCS) is suggestive of a structural lesion, whereas a more insidious onset with prodromal symptoms like confusion and delirium preceding coma is likely due to toxins and derangement of metabolism.

A quick survey to evaluate notable physical findings of the head, neck, chest, abdomen, and extremities should be performed [3]. Airway, breathing, and circulation should be assessed and simultaneously managed during the first minute of evaluation. Similarly, the odor from the patient's body will help to identify the etiology of coma to some extent, i.e., the odor of melena,

spoiled fruit odor, uriniferous odor, fecal fetor, and fetor hepaticus may indicate gastrointestinal bleed, diabetic ketoacidosis, uremia, and hepatic encephalopathy, respectively. Similarly, inspection of the skin can offer clues toward the cause of coma such as spider naevi/jaundice/ascites, hyperpigmentation, pallor/dry/shrunken skin, hypodermic injection scars, cyanosis, and cutaneous bleeding, suggesting hepatic encephalopathy, Addison's disease, hemorrhage, hypoglycemic coma, cyanide/carbon monoxide poisoning, and bleeding disorders, respectively.

Measurement of vital signs including temperature and pulse oximetry is essential to avoid missing complications like hypothermia, hyperthermia, and hypoxemia. Similarly, general, physical, and systemic examinations bear utmost significance. For instance, the presence of murmurs during cardiac auscultation, rhythm disturbances in the ECG, and carotid bruits hint toward thromboembolism as the cause of coma.

33.5 Fundoscopy in a Comatose Patient

Fundoscopy can be used to visualize the features of the retina, optic cup, optic disk, fovea, macula, retinal arteries, and retinal veins. Swelling of the optic disk is a sign of raised intracranial pressure or hypercarbia. Cherry red spot appearance in the fovea is a sign of central retinal artery occlusion. Retinal and subhyaloid hemorrhage is often a sign of subarachnoidal hemorrhage.

33.6 Neurological Assessment in Coma

Neurological assessment of coma is a structured and concise evaluation of the comatose patient. It consists of the assessment of the level of consciousness, brainstem reflexes, motor responses, posturing, appraisal of breathing patterns, meningeal syndrome, rostrocaudal progression due to supratentorial mass, and lateralizing signs, i.e., either deficits or hyperactive signs. Immediate neurological assessment and initiation of treatment enable prevention of the reversible causes of coma and allow timely intervention [5]. It will also offer the localization and the degree of neurological deficit and enable the differentiation of structural vs. nonstructural cause of coma, thereby forecasting the prognosis of the comatose patient.

At first, the neck should be stabilized in all instances if there is a history of trauma to the head and spine until a cervical spine fracture or subluxation of the cervical vertebra is ruled out. This is usually done using a plain x-ray of the cervical spine and a plain computed tomography of the head (CT), in order to prevent cervical cord injury.

Neurological examination of the comatose patient starts primarily with the assessment of the level of consciousness. It is the best measure of brain dysfunction, which also gives the outcome, the predictive value, and assists the initiation of appropriate therapeutic measures. Assessment of the arousal system can be done using the GCS, which is a neurological scale that assesses the level of consciousness or the functional status of the patient's central nervous system. This scale, published in 1974 by Teasdale and Jennett, was initially developed to assess the arousal system in patients who had traumatic head injury but now has become a valuable scale in terms of localization and prognostication of comatose patients of different etiologies. The score is obtained from three different tests assessing eye movements, verbal responses, and motor responses. It varies between 3 (deep coma or death) and 15 (fully awake) [6].

The most suitable time to assess the prognosis of a comatose patient is probably after the vitals are stabilized and the patient is already resuscitated. However, since resuscitated patients are often intubated as well as sedated, it would be difficult to assess the full scale. Motor scores may be useful in these situations. Presence of comorbidities, age of the patient, duration and etiology of the coma, pupillary size and reactivity, ocular responsiveness and its movement, gaze preference, breathing pattern, posturing, and initial neuroimaging findings help sum up the value to predict the outcome of comatose patients.

There is also a good correlation between early GCS scores and outcome [7]. Repeated observations of the coma scale guide us to monitor the changes in the level of consciousness as an index of recovery, deterioration, or complication.

33.7 Pupils in Comatose Patient

Pupillary size, reactivity, and symmetry should be assessed in all cases. Bilateral mid-position to large unreactive pupils may occur in midbrain lesions, anoxic brain injury, and overdose of anticholinergic drugs. Similarly, bilateral pupillary dilatation and unreactive pupils may accompany seizures. On the other hand, fixed and dilated pupils appear after anoxic or ischemic stroke, in hypothermia, and in barbiturate intoxication.

Likewise, bilateral pinpoint and sluggishly reactive pupils are found in extensive pontine lesions (interrupting descending sympathetic pupillodilatator fibers), use of cholinergic eye drops in glaucoma, use of opiates, thalamic hemorrhage, and hydrocephalus. Similarly, anisocoria with unreactive pupils is attributable to ipsilateral temporal lobe compression of the third cranial nerve in uncal herniation and rupture of the aneurysm at the junction of the posterior communicating artery and internal carotid artery. A sympathetic lesion, either intra-parenchymal or extra-parenchymal, causes Horner syndrome with miosis. Toxic and metabolic conditions can cause small and reactive pupil similar to that of thalamic lesions. On the other hand, atropine poisoning causes prominent bilateral fixed and dilated pupils.

33.8 Ocular Movements in a Comatose Patient

Examination of ocular movements in a comatose patient along with the assessment of reflex ocular movements, particularly oculocephalic reflex (Doll's eye phenomenon/maneuver), should not be performed until the stability of the neck has been adequately assessed. Voluntary ocular movement cannot be assessed in comatose patients. So, the assessment can be done by interpreting the resting eye position and reflex eye movements. Normally, the eyes are in midposition and conjugate in movement. Therefore, a careful observation must be paid to the resting position of the eyes [8].

Voluntary ocular movements are generated in the brainstem but are triggered by the cerebral cortex. Patients in coma cannot move their eyes purposefully, and the diagnosis of gaze and cranial nerve palsies is therefore performed by the Doll's head maneuver (once cervical stability is ensured) and by the cold caloric test. Doll's eye maneuver is tested by observing eye movements in response to lateral rotation of head. The eyes move conjugately in the opposite direction at the same time only in the presence of an intact reflex arc, i.e., cervical, vestibular, brainstem (medial longitudinal fasciculus, parapontine reticular formation, and the efferent motor neurons of cranial nerves third and sixth) and eye muscles.

Cold caloric test is positive in patients with an intact brainstem and functioning afferent eighth and efferent third and sixth cranial nerves. In the test, the external auditory canal is irrigated with cold water, which results in a tonic deviation of both the eyes toward the side of cold irrigation in a conscious patient. In patients with brain death, however, there is no movement of eyes. Similarly, there is deviation of both the eyes in downward and upward directions on bilateral irrigation with cold and hot water, respectively, in a conscious patient with an intact reflex arc. A unilateral third nerve palsy causes the affected eye to be displaced downward and laterally, while the sixth nerve palsy produces an inward deviation.

Conjugate deviation of the eyes to one side indicates damage to the pons on the opposite side or a lesion on the frontal lobe on the same side. The eyes deviate toward the hemispheric lesion and away from the brainstem. Disconjugate eyes at rest may indicate intranuclear ophthalmoplegia or paresis of the individual muscles of the eyes in preexisting tropia or phoria. A conjugate downward and inward deviation of the eyes is found in thalamic and subthalamic lesions. A downward deviation of the eyes is found in hepatic coma, brainstem lesion, and tectal compression, whereas an upward deviation hints toward encephalitis, seizure disorder, brainstem ischemia, or normal sleep. A skewed deviation of the eyes, i.e., a maintained deviation of one eye above the other is the sign of a posterior fossa lesion [9].

Ocular bobbing, i.e., rapid conjugate downward movement and slow return to the primary position, is seen when the lateral movements of eyes are lost which is due to the destruction of the pontine tegmentum, transtentorial herniation, or toxic-metabolic effects in a comatose patient. A unilateral dilated unreactive pupil with the eyes abducted at rest and incapable of complete adduction is found in transtentorial herniation in a patient in coma. An unexplained disconjugate eye indicates raised intracranial pressure (ICP) due to sixth nerve palsy or brainstem lesion, and a downward deviation of the eyes occurs in the lesion of the thalamus, post-seizure in metabolic coma, or in barbiturate poisoning.

A repetitive excursion of the eyes from one side to another within 3–4 s, i.e., ping-pong gaze or periodic alternating gaze in a comatose patient is characteristic of cerebellar hemorrhage, cerebellitis, or bilateral cerebral lesions with an intact brainstem. Similarly, ocular dipping refers to a slow downward movement of the eyes followed by a rapid return to the primary position found in diffuse hemispheric lesions.

33.9 Coma and Respiration

Neural centers that control respiratory rhythm and depth are located in the medulla and pons. The medulla, which contains a pacemaker, sets the basic rhythm of breathing, and pontine center assumes the responsibility to smoothen the basic rhythm of inspiration and expiration set by the medulla. Breathing patterns may have localizing value in comatose patients, but they are not always consistent. For example, central neurogenic hyperventilation occurs if the lesion is located just ventral to the aqueduct of Sylvius or in the upper pons ventral to the fourth ventricle, either as primary lesions or as secondary to transtentorial herniation. On the other hand, hyperventilation may occur in metabolic acidosis, shock of different origins, analgesic drugs, hepatic encephalopathy, or pulmonary congestion and pulmonary embolism.

Kussmaul breathing is a deep and regular breathing found in metabolic acidosis, i.e., diabetic ketoacidosis, uremic, hepatic, lactic and alcoholic acidosis, that does not have a localizing value. In contrast, there are certain other breathing patterns which possess a value in the localization of the lesions like ataxic, apneustic, and Cheyne-Stokes breathing patterns. Ataxic breathing refers to the type of breathing which is irregular in rate and rhythm. Ataxic breathing and gasping are signs of lower brainstem damage which may progress to apnea. Similarly, apneustic breathing refers to a breathing pattern characterized by prolonged inspiratory gap and a pause at full inspiration due to lesions of dorsolateral tegmental lesion of the middle and caudal pons. Cheyne-Stokes respiration, which is characterized by periods of hyperventilation and apnea alternating in a crescendo-decrescendo fashion, occurs in bilateral hemispheric lesion and in impending transtentorial herniation.

33.10 Assessment of the Motor Function

Motor function is assessed by observing spontaneous limb movements, posturing, motor response to verbal commands, facial grimacing, and response (or lack thereof) to noxious stimuli. Lack of motor response to noxious stimuli is due to toxins, metabolic derangements, lower brainstem dysfunction, and cervical trauma. Asymmetry of the power of muscles, deep tendon reflexes, tone, somesthetic sensation, or extensor plantar response suggest coma of structural origin.

Posturing of the body is also important to localize the structural lesions. Decorticate posturing, i.e., upper limb flexion and lower limb extension, is due to the lesion in the cerebral hemisphere, internal capsule, and thalamus. Similarly, decerebrate posturing, i.e., where the

head is in an opisthotonus position, the arms are rotated inward, and the feet and toes are bent in the equinovarus position, is found in coma of structural origin, i.e., compression of midbrain, anoxic-ischemic brain injury, metabolic coma, and infections. Generalized and symmetrical posturing point toward the possibility of a toxic-metabolic cause where diencephalic and brainstem ARAS are damaged [10].

Reflex activity of the limb is characterized by the presence of withdrawal or abnormal unilateral/bilateral extension or flexion during noxious stimulation. If the reflex activity is asymmetrical, it suggests the possibility of a structural lesion. Likewise, changes in the position of the body and respiration in response to noxious stimuli are the signs of rostrocaudal deterioration; this should not be confused with seizure or movement disorders like ballistic movements, choreoathetotic movements, or facial grimacing seen in the structural lesions of the subthalamic and basal ganglia. Similarly, gegenhalten or paratonia, i.e., resistance to passive movement that increases with the velocity of movement and is continuous through the full range of motion is attributable to diffuse forebrain dysfunction.

During physical or motor examination, the examiner, by giving the stimuli, finds out the level of responsiveness. If there is no clear reaction to verbal commands, noxious stimuli may be applied to supraorbital ridge, toenail bed, or sternum, or by pinching the soft tissue of the upper arm near the axilla. To rule out the possibility of malingering or functional disorder, a forceful eyelid opening test and arm dropping test are performed. In a conscious patient without motor deficits, there is resistance during arm dropping and eyelid opening.

33.11 Rapid Management of the Comatose Patients

While managing a comatose patient, the neurologist must have an organized strategy so that he/she detects reversible causes of coma, if any, and halts the ongoing cerebral injury by making a sequential and hierarchical plan for the patient's management. Early recognition of the potential for catastrophic deterioration is essential. Immediate support of the airway, breathing, and circulation should be performed before efforts to make a diagnosis or to address the specific cause of coma are undertaken. As mentioned earlier, if there is a history of trauma of cervical spine and head, the cervical spine should be immobilized to prevent spinal cord injury [11].

The principle of emerging management of the comatose patient is the clearance of tracheobronchial tree and maintenance of stable hemodynamics [12]. The patency of the airway is an initial priority to provide adequate ventilation and oxygenation. To maintain blood pressure, vasopressors and inotropes are given so that the patient is hemodynamically stable. Intravenous access should be established during the first minute of evaluation [11].

Laboratory work, i.e., blood gas analysis, basic serum chemistry, and hematological tests (urgent bedside blood for glucose, serum electrolytes, renal function test, liver function test, thyroid function test, complete blood count, and coagulation profile) should be performed within the first minute of coma. If the cause of coma is suspected to be infection, lumbar puncture should be done, unless contraindicated, after performing the CT/MRI and fundoscopic studies. The sample of the cerebrospinal fluid should be sent for microbiological examination [3]. Similarly, toxicological screening including urine toxicology and serum ethanol level should be sent to identify the toxins. If the cause of coma is not identified after performing the CT scan, then an MRI should be obtained to rule out minute structural changes of the central nervous system. If ischemic stroke or subarachnoid hemorrhage is suspected, magnetic resonance angiogram should be performed which can provide information about regional perfusion and vascular patency. Oxygen therapy should be initiated immediately to correct hypoxia-induced coma. If rapid finger testing of glucose is not available, empirical intravenous 50% dextrose should be administered, which will reverse coma secondary to hypoglycemia [13].

If a patient with chronic alcoholism in a malabsorptive state with a risk of nutritional deficiency is suspected, thiamine 100 mg is commonly administered intravenously with dextrose to prevent the precipitation of Wernicke's encephalopathy. If the coma is secondary to excess administration of benzodiazepine, intravenous 0.25 mg flumazenil is given. If there is a suspicion of opioid toxicity, intravenous 0.04–0.4 mg naloxone can be administered, which will rapidly reverse the respiratory depression and coma. The history of ingestion of acetaminophen warrants the use of N-acetylcysteine, an antidote. Similarly, physostigmine may be administered if anticholinergic toxicity is suspected. If there is an index of suspicion of ongoing status epilepticus, intravenous antiepileptic drugs should be initiated. A history of the overdose of antipsychotic drugs and suspicion of neuroleptic malignant syndrome warrants the use of dantrolene. Appropriate antibiotics should be administered if there is suspicion of acute pyogenic meningitis before CT and lumbar puncture to avoid the possibility of delay in treatment.

If the comatose patient has a structural lesion, i.e., subarachnoid parenchymal hemorrhage with intraventricular extension, intra-cerebellar/cerebral hemorrhage with rostrocaudal deterioration, or primary ventricular hemorrhage with ventricular tamponade, urgent life-saving neurosurgical intervention might be warranted.

33.12 Prognosis of Coma

Most of the patients who survive the initial insult recover from coma within 2–4 weeks. The extent of the recovery, however, is variable, ranging from full recovery to a minimally conscious or vegetative state. This is determined by the etiology, the depth, and the duration of coma at presentation [14].

Some patients of traumatic brain injury recover from coma within the first day, some permanently lose all brainstem functions (become brain dead), whereas others progress to wakeful unawareness (vegetative state). The prognosis of coma induced by traumatic brain injury is better than that caused by structural cerebral disease, which carries the worst prognosis, with only 7% of patients achieving moderate or good recovery. If the brain damage is severe, a comatose patient may be permanently disabled or never regain consciousness. A coma that results from drug poisoning has a high rate of recovery if prompt medical attention is provided. In contrast, patients in coma associated with cerebral hypoxia tend to have a poor outcome [15].

The depth of coma at presentation also affects the prognosis; the higher the GCS at presentation, the better the outcome [9]. Patients who receive CPR early (when needed) also tend to have a better outcome than those who received CPR late. Further, survival and outcome in coma are strongly correlated with the duration of coma. The longer a person is in coma, the worse is the prognosis. Those who wake up after a long duration in a coma may have significant physical, psychological, and psychiatric disabilities. Other important prognostic indicators include the age at cardiac arrest and presence of comorbidities. As expected, younger patients with lesser/no comorbidities have better outcomes than their older counterparts. Similarly, comatose patients with nonconvulsive status epilepticus have a better outcome if antiepileptic drugs are started earlier than in those where the drug administration is delayed. Prompt medical attention on noticing the signs of sudden raised intracranial pressure, hypoglycemia, and status epilepticus may lead to improved outcome.

There is no established relation between cerebral metabolic rate of glucose or oxygen (as measured by PET scan) and patient outcome [16]. Comorbidities, age, duration, etiology, breathing patterns, posturing, neuroimaging findings, and EEG findings on the whole help to predict the outcome of comatose patients.

References

1. Plum F, Posner JB. The diagnosis of stupor and coma. Contemp Neurol Ser. 1972;10:1–286.
2. Edlow BL, Takahashi E, Wu O, Benner T, Dai G, Bu L, et al. Neuroanatomic connectivity of the human ascending arousal system critical to consciousness and its disorders. J Neuropathol Exp Neurol. 2012;71(6):531–46.
3. Traub SJ, Wijdicks EF. Initial diagnosis and management of coma. Emerg Med Clin North Am. 2016;34(4):777–93.
4. Geocadin RG, Koenig MA, Jia X, Stevens RD, Peberdy MA. Management of brain injury after resuscitation from cardiac arrest. Neurol Clin. 2008;26(2):487–506, ix
5. Rabinstein AA. Coma and brain death. Continuum (Minneap Minn). 2018;24(6):1708–31.
6. Teasdale G, Jennett B. Assessment of coma and impaired consciousness. A practical scale. Lancet. 1974;2(7872):81–4.
7. Teasdale G, Jennett B. Assessment and prognosis of coma after head injury. Acta Neurochir. 1976;34(1–4):45–55.
8. Berger JR. Stupor and coma. In: Neurology in clinical practice. Philadelphia: Butterworth-Heinemann/Elsevier; 2008. p. 39–58.
9. Stevens RD, Bhardwaj A. Approach to the comatose patient. Crit Care Med. 2006;34(1):31–41.
10. Wijdicks EF. Management of the comatose patient. Handb Clin Neurol. 2017;140:117–29.
11. Huff JS, Stevens RD, Weingart SD, Smith WS. Emergency neurological life support: approach to the patient with coma. Neurocrit Care. 2012;17(Suppl 1):S54–9.
12. Rabinstein AA, Wijdicks EF. Management of the comatose patient. Handb Clin Neurol. 2008;90:353–67.
13. Bates D. The management of medical coma. J Neurol Neurosurg Psychiatry. 1993;56(6):589–98.
14. Firsching R. Coma after acute head injury. Dtsch Arztebl Int. 2017;114(18):313–20.
15. Levy DE, Bates D, Caronna JJ, Cartlidge NE, Knill-Jones RP, Lapinski RH, et al. Prognosis in nontraumatic coma. Ann Intern Med. 1981;94(3):293–301.
16. Jaggi JL, Obrist WD, Gennarelli TA, Langfitt TW. Relationship of early cerebral blood flow and metabolism to outcome in acute head injury. J Neurosurg. 1990;72(2):176–82.

Anirban Ghosal

Case Scenario

A 6-year-old boy presented to the outpatient department for acute-onset visual disturbances. He was born full term with a normal birth weight and normal delivery out of a non-consanguineous marriage. His birth and perinatal history were uneventful, but he had a mild gross motor developmental delay. He started to have recurrent vomiting at 3 years of age, unrelated to feeding. He happened to be sleepy, less interactive and lethargic most of the time since 4 years of age. Recently after a febrile episode, he developed difficulty recognising family members though he could identify them by voice. His speech became slurred and had one episode of generalised tonic-clonic seizure.

MRI brain showed bilateral occipital predominant white matter signal abnormality with sparing of the subcortical U fibres (Fig. 34.1). Despite being a dark-skinned kid, a pigmentation was evident in perioral region, axilla and groin (Fig. 34.2). His 8 a.m. cortisol was low and plasma ACTH was markedly high, indicating a primary adrenal insufficiency. The diagnosis of X-linked adrenoleukodystrophy was made. Elevated plasma levels of very long chain fatty acids confirmed the diagnosis.

Antiepileptics and Lorenzo's oil were added from the neurology side, and hydrocortisone supplementation was done after an endocrinology consultation. Despite all measures he continued to deteriorate and later developed spasticity in the limbs, swallowing difficulty and balance problems.

A. Ghosal (✉)
Institute of Neuroscience, Kolkata, India

© Springer Nature Singapore Pte Ltd. 2024
K. K. Oli et al. (eds.), *Case-based Approach to Common Neurological Disorders*,
https://doi.org/10.1007/978-981-99-8676-7_34

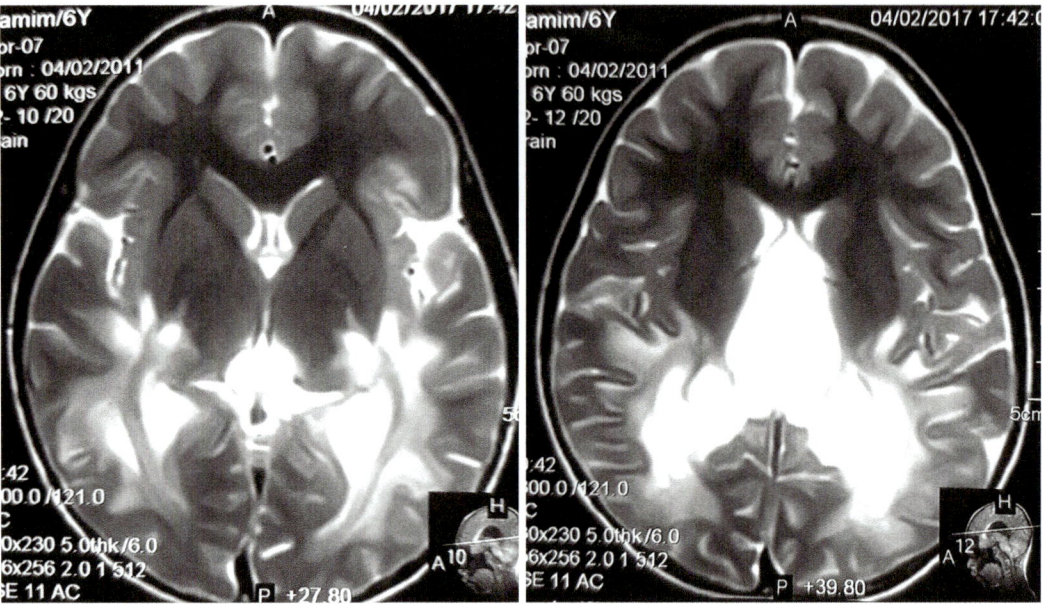

Fig. 34.1 MRI brain T2-weighted axial image showing bilateral parieto-occipital white matter hyperintense signal change sparing subcortical U fibres. Also note the presence of the cyst of cavum vergae

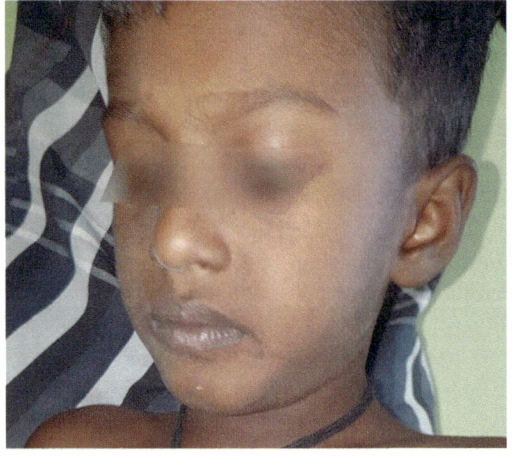

Fig. 34.2 Note the dark pigmentation in perioral and neck region

34.1 Introduction

Inborn errors of metabolism are underlooked, as individually they are rare and considered untreatable by most clinicians. However, they collectively constitute a significant public health burden and directly or indirectly affect the neurological system. Damage is caused by toxins, energy or neurotransmitter deficiency or through blockage of an essential metabolic or biochemical pathway [1].

In a broader way, they may be divided into small- and large-molecule disorders. The former group includes amino and organic acidopathies and urea cycle disorders. Neonates with these disorders lack the necessary enzymes to break the substance loads and suffer when they are exposed for the first time to a normal substance. These disorders flare up in stressful conditions.

Large-molecule disorders, in contrast, are slowly progressive, as the macromolecules gradually accumulate inside cells. Lysosomal, peroxisomal and glycogen storage disorders are amongst them, and depending on predilections of accumulation and damage to particular areas of the nervous system, they lead to leukodystrophy (white matter damage) or poliodystrophy (grey matter damage).

Poor feeding, lethargy, recurrent vomiting on feed initiation, decreasing responsiveness, hypotonia or movement abnormalities should arouse suspicion in a neonate. Parental consanguinity is a clue as many of these disorders are autosomal recessive. Previous neonatal death or stillbirth and recurrent worsening after exposure to a particular dietary substance like cow's milk (galactose) or fruit juice/honey (fructose) demand probing.

34.2 Small-Molecule Disorders

1. *GLUT-1 deficiency syndrome*: infantile seizures, developmental delay, intellectual deficiency, ataxia, dystonia and microcephaly are common clinical features. Seizures begin in early infancy with behavioural arrest, pallor, cyanosis, opsoclonus-like eye movement and apnoea. As they grow up, seizures change into atypical absence, astatic or generalised tonic-clonic seizures.

   D-glucose, an obligate fuel for brain metabolism, is transported through the blood brain barrier by GLUT-1, which normally is in abundance in brain capillaries, astroglial cells and the TBC membrane. GLUT-1 deficiency is the first genetically determined abnormality of the blood brain barrier and may have autosomal recessive inheritance.

   Low CSF glucose and normal-to-low normal lactate are the diagnostic clues. In sequencing of SCLC 2A1 gene, mutation is found in 90% cases. Ketogenic diet controls seizures in early stages but less effective for cognitive problem. Antiepileptics are mostly ineffective. Recently, anaplerotic therapy with triheptanoin is being studied.

2. *Hyperammonaemia*: Hepatic urea cycle is the prime system for mammalian ammonia detoxification, and all six enzymes in this cycle can be defective [2].

   Neonatal hyperammonaemia: Birth asphyxia and prematurity may lead to transient hyperammonaemia, reflecting the immature stage of the liver, and do not need treatment. Sepsis causes elevated ammonia level and needs exclusion. Infants with raised ammonia due to organic acidopathies or urea cycle disorders become symptomatic after 1–3 days of protein feed. In contrast, pyruvate metabolism disorders (pyruvate dehydrogenase or pyruvate carboxylase deficiency) become symptomatic in early 24 h. Respiratory alkalosis and hyperventilation are common in urea cycle disorders. This distinguishes them from organic acidurias, where ketoacidosis (except in Maple syrup urine disease [MSUD]) occurs. All urea cycle genes are autosomal recessive, except ornithine carbamyl transferase, which is X-linked. Hyperammonaemic coma in a new born is an emergency, and rapid peritoneal or haemodialysis is necessary. Intravenous sodium benzoate and sodium phenylbutyrate are other therapy adjuncts. Temporarily protein should be eliminated from the diet, and energy needs to be supplemented by glucose. Valproate therapy is a common cause of hyperammonaemia, especially in children with carnitine deficiency and unrecognised fatty acid oxidation or urea cycle disorder. L-carnitine supplementation helps here.

3. *Aminoacidurias*: Though rare, neurodegeneration in these diseases is preventable if early intervention is done.

   Maple syrup urine disease, a branched-chain amino acid metabolism disorder, produces a characteristic odour in the urine of an infant who develops poor feeding, abnormal respiration, convulsion and opisthotonos at the end of the first week of life. Late-onset form may present with growth and psychomotor delay and ataxia. Lifelong dietary restriction of branched-chain amino acids is needed, and some forms are thiamine responsive. Some of the methyl malonic acidurias respond to vitamin B_{12}.

   Type II glutaric acidurias present with recurrent vomiting and hyperglycaemia in neonates. Structural brain abnormality and cardiomyopathy are noted. Carnitine and riboflavin supplementation helps. Neonatal *nonketotic hyperglycinaemia* present with opisthotonos, disconjugate eye movement, myoclonus and refractory seizures. CSF glycine is several times higher than that in blood, and there is spongy degeneration of brain. It's a disease where dietary protein restriction, high-dose sodium benzoate and dextromethorphan may be helpful. Homocystinuria manifests as tall stature, lens dislocation, intellectual deficiency and thromboembolic events. Some respond to methylcobalamin.

Vitamin-responsive aminoacidurias:

(a) *Pyridoxine-dependent seizures*: an autosomal recessive disorder presenting with jitteriness, convulsions and excessive auditory startle. There is increased excretion of xanthurenic acid in response tryptophan load. Pyridoxine loading suppresses the seizures, and daily supplementation allows normal neurodevelopment.

(b) *Biopterin deficiency*: hypotonia, myoclonus and generalised tonic-clonic seizures in neonates with increased phenylalanine level. Here, tetrahydrobiopterin, which is a cofactor in phenylalanine metabolism, is deficient, and its supplementation allows seizure control.

4. *Organic acidurias*: Propionic, isovaleric and methylmalonic acidurias are three classical forms presenting with encephalopathy, seizures or movement disorders [3]. Treatment involved are dialysis, haemofiltration or dietary modifications.

Type I glutaric aciduria manifests as microcephaly, hypotonia and hyperkinetic movement disorder, which worsen in metabolically stressful conditions. MRI brain shows widened sylvian fissures with large extra-axial vacant spaces over fronto-temporal convexities. Striatal signal change and necrosis occur in untreated cases. A carnitine supplement before basal ganglia injury is of substantial benefit.

Canavan disease is a spongiform leukodystrophy, where N-acetylaspartic acid accumulation leads to progressive macrocephaly, hypotonia, seizures, spasticity and neuroregression.

5. *Disorders of purine and pyrimidine metabolism*: Purine and pyrimidine participate in nucleotide synthesis, i.e. ATP or ADP synthesis. Anaemia, immune deficiency, hyperuricaemia leading to renal stones and even renal failure can occur in these diseases. Developmental delay, autism and sensory neural hearing problem are among other manifestations.

Lesch Nyhan syndrome is an X-linked recessive disorder leading to hyperuricaemia in blood urine and CSF. Urate crystals deposit in joints and kidney. Self-mutilation behaviour, choreoathetosis and spasticity develop in the second year of life. Allopurinol helps with hyperuricaemia, but the child needs to be restrained to prevent self-mutilation. Even therapeutic dental extraction is needed. DBS surgery was even tried in some cases of self-mutilation.

6. *Porphyrias*: They are haem synthesis disorders. Acute intermittent porphyria, the most common type, presents as psychosis, seizures, abdominal pain, autonomic neuropathy and painful peripheral neuropathy [4]. Fasting state, certain drugs and alcohol precipitate decompensation. Urine porphobilinogen assay is needed for diagnosis. Fluid and electrolyte balance maintenance, treatment of neuropathic pain with gabapentin and avoidance of offending drugs are the mainstay of therapy. IV heme arginate and prehematin are needed to block the metabolic pathway, but their availability is a concern.

7. *Disorders of metal metabolism*:

Copper:

Wilson's disease, also known as hepatolenticular degeneration, is due to a defective transport of copper from liver to bile and blood. Mutation in ATP-7B gene causes accumulation of copper in liver, which overflows to blood and then deposited in lentiform nuclei in brain, leading to extrapyramidal disorders [5].

Chronic liver disease, haemolytic anaemia, thrombocytopenia, renal tubular acidosis and neuroregression in cognitive domain appear in young children usually in the first decade. Deteriorating scholastic performance, behavioural issues, bulbar problems like dysphagia, dysarthria and a "vacuous smile" due to facial muscle dystonia guide clinicians towards diagnosis. A coarse wing-beating tremor in outstretched hands, ataxia, myoclonus and seizures (in 6% of cases) are seen.

The presence of KF ring in the cornea due to copper accumulation, increased 24 h urinary copper excretion, low serum ceruloplasmin and genetic testing are needed for diagnosis.

Treatment involves penicillamine, a copper chelator, which is started in very low dose with gradual build-up. Zinc, which impairs copper absorption in gut, trientine and tetra-thiomolybdate are other therapy options. Avoidance of copper-rich food like liver, chocolate, cocoa, mushrooms, nuts and shell-fish is recommended. Liver transplant may stabilise the underlying metabolic problem, and in some cases, sustained neurological improvements can occur.

Menkes disease is caused by mutation in X-linked ATP-7A gene, leading to systemic copper deficiency. It's seen exclusively in boys in the first 2 months of life with development regression, hypotonia, seizures, sparse twisted easily breakable hair, hypoglycaemia and hypothermia. Due to abnormal collagen formation, there is metaphysical damage in bones and dilatation of blood vessels, which rupture easily, leading to intracranial haemorrhage. Most children do not survive beyond 3 years. Subcutaneous copper histidine instituted before permanent damage can give some benefit.

Iron:

Important disorders in this group are NBIA-1 or PKAN and NBIA-2 or PLAN (PLA2G6-associated neurodegeneration).

PKAN presents in the first decade with intellectual disability, progressive ataxia and oromandibular dystonia. Supranuclear gaze palsy, acanthocytes in peripheral blood and retinal pigmentation are seen. Iron deposited in the globus pallidus leads to an area of hypointensity with a central hyperintensity in the MRI brain with "the eyes of the tiger" sign. The treatment is symptomatic. A few studies describe the role of deferiprone, an iron chelator.

PLAN or PARK 14 or NBIA-2 manifests as ataxia, truncal hypotonia, limb spasticity, nystagmus, optic atrophy and peripheral neuropathy. MRI shows cerebellar atrophy and iron in the globus pallidus without hyperintensity.

8. *Nonhereditary neurometabolic disorders*:

Hypocalcaemia— a common cause of neonatal seizures, spasms and tetany. *Fahr's disease* or familial cerebral calcinosis leads to basal ganglia, cerebellar dentate nuclei calcification and movement disorders.

Rapid correction of *hyponatraemia* leads to central pontine and extrapontine myelinolysis from osmotic demyelination in CNS.

Hypoglycaemia – premature neonates and neonates of diabetic mothers are mostly susceptible, leading to seizures.

9. *Neuro-acanthocytosis*: Acanthocytes are irregular-shaped RBCs with spiny projections.

Chorea acanthocytosis presents with hyperkinetic movement disorder, characteristic "feeding dyskinesia" and psychiatric manifestations like obsession, seizures, peripheral neuropathy and proximal weakness [6]. Defect is caused by chorein, an abnormal protein leading to membrane defects in RBCs.

Abetalipoproteinaemia is caused by mutation in microsomal triglyceride transfer protein, leading to diarrhoea and very low blood lipids. Fat-soluble vitamins are low. Vitamin E deficiency leads to a spinocerebellar syndrome with ophthalmoplegia, ataxia and pigmentation in retina. Vitamin K deficiency leads to haemorrhagic disorders.

34.3 Large-Molecule Disorders

They include lysosomal, peroxisomal and glycogen storage disorders.

Metabolic syndromes in neurology are a vast entity, and discussion regarding each is out of the scope of this chapter. We have discussed some of the common, though easily missed, conditions in brief, mainly clinically, for the help of the reader.

References

1. Patterson MC. Inborn errors of metabolism. In: Merritt's neurology. 13th ed. Philadelphia: Wolters Kluwer; 2016. p. 1150–73; chap. 134.
2. Haberle J. Clinical practice: the management of hyperammonemia. Eur J Paediatr. 2011;170:21–34.

3. Killer S, Burgard P, Sauer SW, et al. Current concepts in organic acidurias: understanding intra and extra-cerebral disease manifestation. J Inherit Metab Dis. 2013;36:635–44.

4. Kuo HC, Huang CC, Chu CC, et al. Neurological complications of acute intermittent porphyria. Eur Neurol. 2011;66:247–52.

5. Dusek P, Litwin T. Wilson disease and other neuro-degeneration and metal accumulations. Neurol Clin. 2015;33:175–204.

6. Miquel M, Spampinato U, Latxague C, et al. Short and long term outcome of bilateral pallidal stimulation in chorea-acanthocytosis. PLos One. 2013;8:e79241.

Traumatic Brain Injury

35

Ahmed Abd Elazim and Shraddha Mainali

Case Scenario

A 31-year-old un-helmeted biker presented to our trauma center after a motorbike crash. Patient was unresponsive at the scene and got intubated by paramedics for airway protection. His Glasgow Coma Scale (GCS) at the field was 3T (Table 35.1). Upon arrival to the hospital, his GCS was 8T (opened eye to pain and localized to painful stimulation with right arm). Pupils were equal and reactive. Blood pressure (BP) was 137/87 mm of Hg, pulse was 97/min, respiratory rate was 16/min, temperature was 36.7 °C, and oxygen saturation was 100% on volume control ventilation with minimal settings. Past medical and surgical history was unremarkable. Head Computed Tomography scan (CTH) revealed bilateral traumatic subarachnoid hemorrhage (SAH), bilateral extra-axial hematomas, left occipital contusion, evidence of diffuse axonal injury (DAI), as well as comminuted bilateral parietal and occipital bone fractures with underlying pneumocephalus (Fig. 35.1a, b, c, and d). In addition, he had ruptured right tympanic membrane. CT angiography of head and neck was unremarkable. CT chest showed non-displaced

fracture of posterior tenth rib, but no other significant body trauma was found. Lab parameters on presentation were within normal limits. The patient was admitted to the neurocritical care unit, where a right-sided intraparenchymal intracranial pressure (ICP) monitor was placed. Initial ICP recording was 32 mmHg. At the time, mean arterial pressure (MAP) was 84 mmHg with cerebral perfusion pressure (CPP) of 52 mmHg (goal CPP 60–70 mmHg). Head of bed was elevated to 45°, and he was transiently hyperventilated with $PaCO_2$ goal of 30–35 mm Hg. After initial propofol bolus of 20 mg, propofol and fentanyl were started. Intravenous mannitol 20% at the dose of 1 g/kg was administered, and 3% hypertonic saline was started at 100 cc/h. Combined acute measures improved ICP to 20 mmHg initially. However, the patient had multiple ICP crises in the first 2 weeks, requiring multiple sedatives including pentobarbital coma, recurrent boluses of hyperosmolar therapy, and paralytics. Cerebral blood flow (CBF) and partial pressure of brain tissue oxygenation ($PbtO_2$) were closely monitored using intraparenchymal devices and optimized as needed with a goal CBF of 20–40 mL/100 g/min and a goal $PbtO_2$ of 25–35 mmHg. Left-sided external ventricular drain (EVD) was also placed. Patient remained intermittently on pressors while requiring heavy sedation for ICP management. Video EEG (vEEG) was placed to evaluate for non-convulsive status epilepticus (NCSE) and was negative for seizures. Daily transcranial doppler

A. A. Elazim (✉)
Department of Neurology, University of New Mexico, Albuquerque, NM, USA
e-mail: aabdelazim@salud.unm.edu

S. Mainali
Department of Neurology, Virginia Commonwealth University, Richmond, VA, USA

© Springer Nature Singapore Pte Ltd. 2024
K. K. Oli et al. (eds.), *Case-based Approach to Common Neurological Disorders*,
https://doi.org/10.1007/978-981-99-8676-7_35

Table 35.1 Glasgow Coma Scale

Best eye response	Best motor response	Best verbal response
4 Eye opening spontaneously	6 Obeys commands	5 Oriented
3 Eye opening to commands	5 Localizes to painful stimulation	4 Confused
2 Eye opening to pain	4 Withdraws to painful stimuli	3 Inappropriate words
1 No response	3 Flexion to painful stimuli (decortication)	2 Incomprehensible sounds
	2 Extension to painful stimuli (decerebration)	1 No response
	1 No response	

Fig. 35.1 Initial CTH showing scalp hematoma, bilateral extra-axial hematomas, and left parietal contusion (**a**), SAH and multiple contusions (**b**), multiple skull fractures (**c** and **d**) with associated pneumocephalus (arrow)

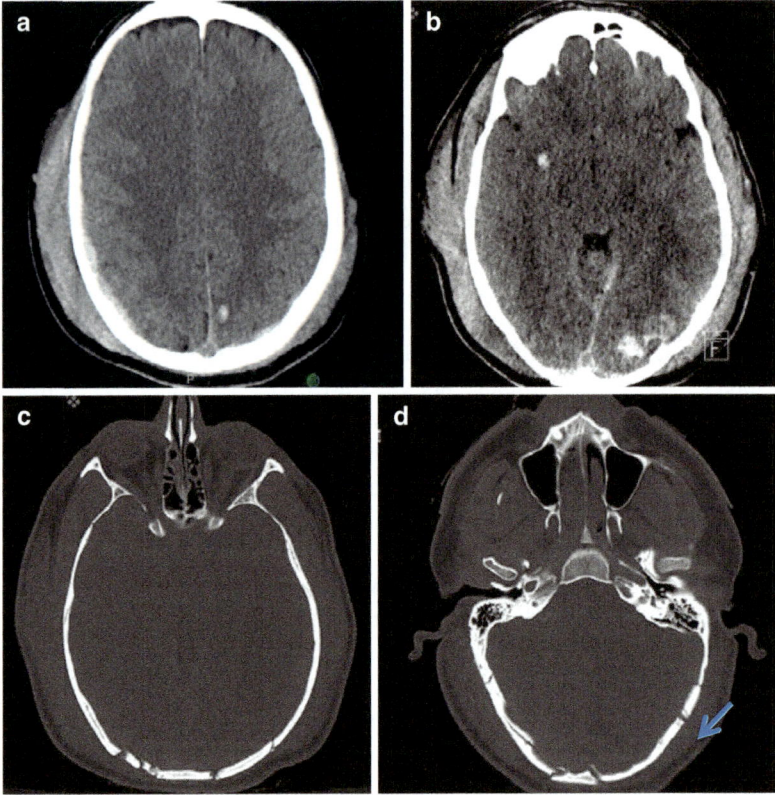

was performed to monitor for vasospasm. On day 11, tracheostomy and percutaneous gastrostomy tubes were placed. During the ICU stay, patient had multiple episodes of paroxysmal sympathetic hyperactivity, and ICU course was further complicated by hospital-acquired pneumonia and grade 3 decubitus ulcer. He was finally discharged to rehabilitation facility after 38 days of hospitalization with a Glasgow Outcome Scale of 13 (Table 35.2). At the time of discharge, he was able to tolerate dysphagia diet with thin consistency. Tracheostomy tube was successfully removed on day 45. He continued to receive aggressive physical, occupational, speech, cognitive, and psychological

Table 35.2 Glasgow Outcome Scale

Glasgow outcome score	Functional status
1	Death
2	Persistent vegetative state. Minimal responsiveness
3	Severe disability. Conscious but disabled. Dependent on others for activities of daily living
4	Moderate disability. Disabled but independent. Able to work in sheltered settings
5	Good recovery. Able to resume normal life despite minor deficits

therapy for 2 weeks in the inpatient rehabilitation facility. He was discharged and sent home with his family and continued outpatient therapy. After 4 months of injury, patient had regained full strength with good cognition (GCS 15) and was able to return to work.

35.1 Introduction

Traumatic brain injury (TBI) is defined as a pathological insult to the brain caused by an external force as a result of a direct blow to the head or impact elsewhere in the body with the transmission of mechanical forces to the brain [1]. Below, we will discuss the epidemiology, pathophysiology, classification, types of injury, management, and outcomes of TBI.

35.2 Epidemiology

Traumatic brain injury is a global health problem, especially among young population. The World Health Organization (WHO) predicts that TBI will transcend several other major causes of death and disability by year 2020, as industrialization and motorization continue to increase globally. It is estimated that TBI affects about ten million people worldwide, leading to either hospitalization or death. Motor vehicle accidents, falls, and violence are the most common causes of TBI globally. Men are significantly more prone to TBI than women worldwide. Overall, the incidence of TBI varies across the world based on urbanization, road traffic conditions, social structure, prevalence of violence, proportion of young population, etc. Outcomes are known to be worse in the low- and middle-income countries due to lack of access to health care as well as lack of advanced management strategies [2–4].

35.3 Pathophysiology

Brain injury in TBI occurs through primary and secondary mechanisms. The primary brain injury is the injury that occurs at the moment of impact.

Common mechanisms of injury include direct impact, rapid acceleration/deceleration injury, penetrating injury, and blast waves. Despite the varied nature of injury, they all result in mechanical forces leading to tissue injury and can present as a combination of scalp injury, skull fracture, surface contusion, penetrating wounds, intracranial hemorrhage, diffuse vascular injury, diffuse axonal injury, cranial nerve (CN) injury, or injury to deep structures like the pituitary stalk. The initial impact causes compression, stretching, distortion, and displacement of brain tissue, leading to cellular injury. Furthermore, mechanical forces can cause axonal damage, leading to impaired neuronal conduction.

Secondary brain injury is triggered by mechanical and biochemical changes that start at the time of injury and continue for hours to days. These changes result in the initiation of a cascade of molecular mechanisms leading to cell injury. Each type of head injury might trigger different pathophysiological mechanisms of secondary injury with variable duration. Mechanistic pathways involved in secondary injury include:

1. Neurotransmitter-mediated injury: biomechanical injury triggers ionic flux leading to glutamate release. Energy-dependent ionic pumps attempt to restore ionic balance creating high metabolic demand and energy crisis.
2. Calcium-mediated cytoskeletal damage and mitochondrial dysfunction: calcium ions accumulate intracellularly, causing cytoskeletal damage, and are sequestered in the mitochondria, resulting in the failure of oxidative metabolism. This mismatch in energy supply and demand worsens energy crisis and poses risk for secondary cellular injury.
3. Free-radical generation: alteration of intracellular redox state leads to free-radical generation.
4. Initiation of inflammatory cascade.
5. Gene activation and initiation of apoptotic cascade.

Various systemic and intracranial factors also worsen secondary brain injury. Such systemic factors include hypoxemia, hypotension or severe hypertension, severe hypocapnia or hypercapnia, hypoglycemia or hyperglycemia, coagulopathy or hypercoagulability, severe anemia, acidosis, severe electrolyte imbalances, fever, and superimposed infections. Intracranial factors contributing to secondary brain injury include high intracranial pressure (ICP), hematoma expansion, cerebral edema, hydrocephalus, seizures, vasospasm, delayed ischemia, brain compression, and brain herniation. The goal of TBI management is to prevent or minimize the effects of secondary brain injury [5–7].

35.4 Classification

Historically, TBI has been classified into three main groups based on clinical severity. Mild, moderate, and severe TBI are briefly discussed below [8–12].

35.4.1 Mild TBI/Concussion

Mild TBI is defined as a brief neurological impairment with spontaneous resolution of symptoms. Criteria for mild TBI include GCS $\geq$ 13, normal CTH, loss of consciousness (LOC) <30 min following the injury, and post-traumatic amnesia (PTA) of <24 h following the injury. Clinically, patients may present with (1) physical symptoms (headache, nausea, vomiting, dizziness, visual changes, fatigue, photophobia, or phonophobia), (2) emotional symptoms (irritability, nervousness, labile mood, etc.), (3) cognitive issues (mental fogginess, memory problems, attention deficit, delayed response, etc.), and (4) sleep-related problems (insomnia, excessive sleepiness, increase sleep latency, etc.). Systematic serial evaluation is important to determine safety regarding return to school, work, or sports and identify individuals with persistent symptoms needing further management.

- Post-concussion syndrome (PCS): It comprises constellations of concussion symptoms that may persist up to 6 weeks. Predisposing factors for PCS include prior concussion, headaches, attention deficit hyperactivity disorder, and other neuropsychiatric conditions.
- Chronic traumatic encephalopathy (CTE): It is a neurodegenerative condition as a result of repeated trauma to the brain. Histopathologically, abnormal deposition of Tau protein is seen. Clinically, patients present with confusion, impulse control issues, aggression, depression, and progressive memory loss.

35.4.2 Moderate and Severe TBI

Patients are classified as moderate TBI if initial GCS is 9–12 and as severe TBI if initial GCS is $\leq$8 in the presence of abnormal brain imaging. Patients with moderate and severe TBI have LOC >30 minutes and PTA >24 hours following the injury.

Although this classification system has been validated, there are several confounding factors leading to false classification of severity of TBI. For example, intoxication or sedation provided by paramedics en route to the hospital can alter the GCS on presentation. Furthermore, the systemic or psychological shock and organ failure with polytrauma can alter GCS and extend the period of post-traumatic amnesia. Brain imaging is not always obtained especially in cases of apparent mild symptoms. Moreover, the initial GCS or length of post-traumatic amnesia is not consistently documented. Given the unreliability of some of the TBI severity indicators and frequency of missed documentation, Malec et al. have developed a classification system called the "Mayo TBI Severity Classification System" based on positive evidence available in the medical record (Table 35.3).

Table 35.3 Mayo TBI severity classification system

A. Classify as Moderate-Severe (Definite) TBI if one or more of the following criteria apply:

1. Death due to this Traumatic brain Injury (TBI)
2. Loss of consciousness of 30 minutes or more
3. Post-traumatic anterograde amnesia of 24 hours or more
4. Worst Glasgow Coma Scale full score in first 24 hours <13 (unless invalidated upon review, e.g., attributable to intoxication, sedation, systemic shock)
5. One or more of the following present:
   • Intracerebral hematoma
   • Subdural hematoma
   • Epidural hematoma
   • Cerebral contusion
   • Hemorrhagic contusion
   • Penetrating TBI (dura penetrated)
   • Subarachnoid hemorrhage
   • Brain Stem Injury

B. If none of Criteria A apply, classify as Mild (Probable) TBI if one or more of the following criteria apply:

1. Loss of consciousness of momentary to less than 30 minutes
2. Post-traumatic anterograde amnesia of momentary to less than 24 hours
3. Depressed, basilar or linear skull fracture (dura intact)

C. If none of Criteria A or B apply, classify as Symptomatic (Possible) TBI if one or more of the following symptoms are present:

1. Blurred vision
2. Confusion (mental state changes)
3. Dazed
4. Dizziness
5. Focal neurologic symptoms
6. Headache
7. Nausea

Table 35.4 Marshall CT scoring system

Grade	Description
Diffuse injury I	No visible pathology on CT
Diffuse injury II	Presence of lesion on CT with midline shift 0–5 mm. Cisterns are present. No high- or mixed-density lesion >25 cm³ including bone fragments or foreign bodies
Diffuse injury III	Abnormal CT with obliteration of cisterns, midline shift 0–5 mm. No high- or mixed-density lesion >25 cm³
Diffuse injury IV	Midline shift >5 mm, no high- or mixed-density lesion >25 cm³
Diffuse injury V	Any surgically evacuated lesion
Diffuse injury VI	Non-evacuated mass lesion, high- or mixed-density lesion >25 cm³

1. Skull Fracture

   Fractures can occur in the Vault or base of the skull. Vault fractures are often linear. It can be open or closed where open fractures communicate with the outside environment and closed fractures don't. It can be simple (only one bone fragment present) or compound (two or more bone fragments present). It can be depressed (inward displacement of the fragments) or non-depressed. Fractures can involve sinuses and are often associated with underlying hematomas. Basilar skull fractures are usually caused by dissipated force and can often result in cranial nerve injury and may present with CSF otorrhea or rhinorrhea. Hematomas may occur around the eye (raccoon sign), behind the ear (battle sign) or behind the ear drum (hemotympanum).

2. Epidural Hematoma (EDH)

   EDH occurs in the potential space between the skull and the dura. It crosses dural attachments but does not cross suture lines. Characteristically, it has a lens-shaped appearance. Over 85% of EDH occurs due to arterial injury. It occurs commonly in the middle cranial fossa due to tear of middle meningeal artery but can occur in anterior cranial fossa due to rupture of anterior meningeal artery or rupture of dural venous sinuses. In ~15% of cases, it can occur due to tear of dural sinuses

35.5 Types of Injury

Traumatic brain injury can lead to various types of injuries, most of which can be found on neuroimaging. Marshall Scale is a widely used CT-based grading scale that helps to classify injuries in six different categories (Table 35.4). It has value in accurately predicting the risk of increased intracranial pressure and outcomes in adults but lacks reproducibility in patients with multiple types of brain injury. Different types of head injury sustained in TBI are discussed below:

or confluence of sinuses in the posterior fossa. EDH can rapidly enlarge, causing a mass effect. Patients can present with varied clinical symptoms from brief LOC to coma. Some patients manifest "triple phase" with initial LOC followed by lucid interval and subsequent worsening of symptoms as hematoma continues to expand. Acute symptomatic EDH is a neurologic emergency that often requires surgical decompression to prevent irreversible brain injury and death caused by hematoma expansion, elevated ICP, and brain herniation. Surgical evacuation is recommended in patients with hematoma volume > 30 cc and in patients with GCS ≤ 8 with anisocoria. Few clinically stable patients may be managed non-operatively. However, close monitoring and follow-up brain imaging are required to ensure the stability of the hematoma.

3. Subdural Hematomas (SDH)

Acute SDH is usually caused by rupture of the bridging veins that drain the cortical surfaces to the dural sinuses. Hematoma forms between the dura and the arachnoid membranes. Slow venous bleeding commonly stops due to the effect of the rising ICP or by direct compression of the vein by the hematoma. In 20–30% patients, SDH results from the rupture of small cortical arteries. SDH can cross suture lines but is limited by dural attachments and typically appears as a crescent-shaped extra-axial collection. Similar to EDH, most patients need surgical evacuation. Surgical evacuation is recommended in SDH with a thickness > 10 mm and a midline shift >5 mm, regardless of the GCS score. In addition, surgery is recommended if GCS ≤8, if GCS has decreased by ≥2 points from initiate assessment, in case of asymmetric and dilated pupil and persistent high ICP >20. Those with small hematomas (<1 cm) and stable clinical symptoms may be managed non-operatively with close monitoring.

4. Contusions and Intraparenchymal Hemorrhage

Patients commonly present with focal cerebral contusions. It is often seen in the basal frontal and temporal areas that are sus-

ceptible to direct impact in acceleration/deceleration injuries. More severe head injury can lead to disruption of intraparenchymal blood vessels causing intraparenchymal hematomas. Posterior fossa hemorrhage with mass effect should be evacuated emergently. For hemispheric frontal and temporal ICH, surgical evacuation is recommended if hematoma volume is >50 cc. Surgery is also recommended for hematoma volume > 20 cc in patients with GCS 6–8 and midline shift ≥5 mm or effacement of basal cisterns.

5. Subarachnoid Hemorrhage (SAH)

It can occur with disruption of small pial vessels and commonly occurs in the cortices, sylvian fissures, and interpeduncular cisterns. SAH can also occur by extension of intraventricular hemorrhage or cortical hemorrhage. Isolated subarachnoid hemorrhage in the setting of mild TBI typically has a benign neurological outcome.

6. Intraventricular Hemorrhage (IVH)

It results from the tearing of subependymal veins or by extension from adjacent intraparenchymal or subarachnoid hemorrhage. It is more commonly seen in severe TBI and leads to the development of hydrocephalus. External ventricular drainage is often needed to avoid worsening hydrocephalus.

7. Diffuse Axonal Injury (DAI)

It is characterized by diffuse injury to the white matter tracts. This shearing injury is caused by rotational movements of the parenchyma within the skull and stretching and bending of fibers at the craniospinal junction. High-velocity acceleration/deceleration of the brain tissue during lateral motions of the head also results in shearing forces, especially against the falx and tentorium, resulting in DAI. MRI is more sensitive than CTH for the detection of DAI and can be seen as multiple small foci of white matter hemorrhages, typically in the cortical gray-white junction, corpus callosum, and midbrain.

8. Coup and Contrecoup Injury

Coup injury occurs at the site of impact, while contrecoup injury occurs opposite to the site of impact. Neuropathological studies suggest that the contrecoup injury is frequently more severe than the coup injury. Various theories have been proposed to describe the mechanism of coup-contrecoup injury. Some more popular theories include positive pressure theory, negative pressure or cavitation theory, rotational shear-stress theory, and angular acceleration theory. Discussions of the mechanistic theories are beyond the scope of this chapter. However, readers are encouraged to refer to the review article by Post et al. for details [11].

9. Brain Herniation

Brain herniation is a result of pressure differential between the intracranial compartments. It leads to brain injury by compression or traction on neural and vascular structures. Below we discuss some common types of herniation syndromes.

- Subfalcine herniation – This occur in the setting of frontal mass effect where the cingulate gyrus is pushed under the falx cerebri. This can lead to compression of anterior cerebral arteries causing infarction of frontal and parietal lobes.
- Transtentorial herniation – It results from downward displacement of supratentorial brain tissue into the infratentorial compartment and is a result of supratentorial mass lesions, edema, or hydrocephalus. This leads to compression of the ipsilateral third CN, stretching of the contralateral third CN, compression of the upper brainstem and the cerebral peduncles, as well as traction of the superior portion of the basilar artery and the posterior cerebral arteries, leading to occipital lobe infarction. Uncal herniation is the most common type of transtentorial herniation, where the medial edge of the uncus and hippocampal gyrus displaces over the ipsilateral edge of the tentorium.
- Cerebellar herniation – The cerebellar tonsils are pushed through the foramen magnum, causing medullary and cervical spinal cord compression, which can lead to bradycardia and respiratory arrest.

35.6 Management of TBI

1. Prehospital Management

Triage of trauma victims is the process of rapidly and accurately evaluating patients to determine the extent of their injuries and the appropriate level of medical care required. Besides the implementation of basic life support measures and triage, the main goals of prehospital management should be focused on preventing hypoxia ($PaO_2 < 60$ mm Hg) and hypotension (systolic blood pressure < 90). Brain is more vulnerable to these insults in the setting of an acute TBI, and hypotension and hypoxia are known to be associated with poor outcomes. Endotracheal intubation at the scene can be performed in the presence of a highly trained paramedic in patients with GCS ≤8. Fluid resuscitation should be started using isotonic crystalloids to avoid hypotension. Rapid transport to the hospital should be the priority, and prehospital providers must do all they can to minimize the amount of time spent on the scene. Patients with TBI are at high risk for concomitant spine injury; hence, appropriate spine stabilization measures should be taken during transport [13].

2. Emergency Department Management

Upon arrival to the emergency department (ED), it is important to re-assess the vitals and send basic labs, including a toxicology screen. A neurological assessment should be performed, and GCS should be documented. Systemic survey should be performed to assess the extent and severity of injury. Noncontrast CT brain should be performed urgently in patients with GCS ≤ 14. CT cervical spine should be performed to evaluate for neck injuries. Signs of elevated ICP should be recognized and treated emergently. Glucose should be optimized and coagulopathy reversed. Neurosurgical consultation is required in patients with abnormal CTH with mass effects and surgical indications, as discussed above [14–16].

In the case of depressed skull fracture, surgery with segment elevation and debridement are recommended for open skull fractures that are depressed greater than the thickness of the cranium or if there is dural injury with ICH, frontal sinus involvement, wound contamination, pneumocephalus, or cosmetic deformity. For penetrating skull injuries, superficial debridement and dural closure are indicated to prevent CSF leaks. Small entry wounds should be treated with simple closure. Prophylactic broad-spectrum antibiotic is indicated in the setting of a penetrating injury.

3. Management in the Critical Care Unit

The goal of critical care management for moderate-severe TBI is to prevent further brain injury and provide optimal condition for recovery. Control of factors that can potentiate secondary brain injury is important. Critical care management strategies are focused on ICP management (goal ICP <22 mmHg), ventilator management and avoidance of hypoxia (goal PaO_2 > 60), maintenance of optimal BP (goal systolic BP ≥100 mmHg for patients 50–69 years and ≥ 110 mmHg for patients 15–49 or > 70 years), sedation and pain control, management of coagulopathy, nutritional support, glucose control (100 mg/dL–160 mg/dL), correction of acid-base and electrolytes abnormalities, fever management, treatment of infections and management of seizures, etc. [17, 18].

35.6.1 ICP Monitoring and Management

Indications for ICP monitoring in TBI include GCS ≤8 and an abnormal CTH showing evidence of mass effect from brain hemorrhage or brain edema. ICP monitoring is also warranted in patients with normal CTH in patients of age > 40 years, motor posturing, and systolic BP <90 mmHg. Treatment of ICP >22 mmHg is necessary as higher ICP levels are associated with high mortality. In patients with EVD, controlled CSF drainage helps lower ICP. Other measures for acute ICP management include head elevation at 30°, optimization of venous drainage by

keeping head in optimum position, and hyperventilation. Hyperventilation if performed should be temporary with a goal of $PaCO_2$ in the 30–35 mmHg range, and hyperventilation with $PaCO_2$ < 25 mmHg should be avoided. Due to concern for vasoconstriction, hypoventilation should be avoided in the first 24 h when cerebral blood flow is critically low. Hyperosmolar therapy using mannitol boluses at the dose of 0.25–1 g/kg every 4–6h can be used while monitoring serum osmolality (maintain <320) and osmolar gap (maintain <20). Continuous or bolus doses of hypertonic saline at various concentrations can also be successfully used for ICP control while closely monitoring serum sodium and serum osmolality. Sedatives like propofol, benzodiazepines, opioids, and barbiturates, as well as paralytics should be used for refractory ICP. It is important to note that the rate of propofol infusion syndrome is relatively high in TBI patients, and hence proper clinical assessment and lab monitoring are necessary. For patients who fail to achieve ICP control despite maximum medical management, a wide frontotemporoparietal decompressive craniectomy should be considered as clinically appropriate [19–23].

35.6.2 Cerebral Perfusion Pressure

Optimization of cerebral blood flow is one of the primary goals of TBI management. Normally, cerebral autoregulation allows maintenance of adequate cerebral blood flow (CBF) across a wide range (50–150 mmHg) of mean arterial blood pressures (MAP). Normal autoregulation is commonly disrupted in patients with moderate-to-severe TBI. CPP (MAP-ICP) can be used as a surrogate marker for cerebral blood flow in TBI. Goal CPP should be maintained between 60 and 70 mmHg [24].

35.6.3 Post-traumatic Seizures

The incidence of post-traumatic seizures ranges from 6 to 30%. Since seizures can worsen secondary brain injury, prophylactic antiepileptic medication is recommended for 7 days post TBI. Phenytoin is commonly used for seizure prophylaxis, but levetiracetam has been used alternatively with reported success. About 15–25% of patients with moderate-to-severe TBI are reported to have subclinical seizures; hence, continuous electroencephalographic monitoring is indicated to detect subclinical seizures [25–27].

In additional to routine ICP measurement using parenchymal or external ventricular drainage system, various advanced monitoring techniques have been developed which allow measurement of cerebral oxygenation, cerebral blood flow, and cerebral microdialysis. It is important to understand that no monitoring technique can improve outcome unless the data acquired is used to drive appropriate intervention. Some of the monitoring techniques are discussed below.

- *Jugular venous oximetry (SjVO₂)*

   This can be achieved by the use of internal jugular (IJ) cannulation in a cephalad manner, which allows monitoring of oxygen saturation in the IJ as it exits the brain. Normal $SjVO_2$ is around 60%. Values <50% are found to be associated with worse outcome.
- *Brain tissue oxygen tension (PbtO₂)*: $PbtO_2$ can be obtained with the use of intraparenchymal monitor place in the white matter of the brain. $PbtO_2$ > 20 mmHg is considered normal and < 15 mmHg suggests tissue ischemia.
- *Cerebral microdialysis*: With the help of intraparenchymal probe, this allows measurement of extracellular glucose, lactate, pyruvate, and glutamate. A lactate:pyruvate ratio > 40 is suggestive of anaerobic metabolism and can worsen secondary brain injury.
- *Thermal diffusion flowmetry*: This intraparenchymal probe allows continuous measurement of CBF. The optimum range of CBF to prevent secondary brain injury remains to be determined. However, values between 20 and 40 mL/100 g/min appear to be a reasonable goal in most patients.

35.6.4 Nutrition

Feeding should be initiated at least by the fifth day and at most by the seventh day post-injury. Transgastric jejunal feeding is preferred to reduce the rate of ventilator-associated pneumonia.

35.7 Rehabilitation and Outcome

Outcome of TBI is dependent on multiple factors including severity of TBI, extent of secondary brain injury, type of intracranial lesions, presence of bleeding diathesis, medical comorbidities, and hospital-related complications, including hospital-acquired infections. In general moderate-to-severe TBI is associated with high morbidity, and mortality has been reported to be somewhere between 30 and 80%. Of the survivors of severe TBI, approximately 25% regain functional independence. Rehabilitation in the form of physical, occupational, cognitive, and speech therapy improves outcome and helps patient obtain functional independence [28].

In addition to physical and cognitive impairments, patients with TBI suffer from psychiatric conditions. Major depressive disorder is a common psychiatric condition in patients with TBI. Patients suffer from poor cognition, anxiety, aggression, and remain at high risk for suicide. Assessment, management, and proper follow-up care for psychological disorders are important for survivors of TBI.

References

1. Menon DK, Schwab K, Wright DW, Maas AI. Position statement: definition of traumatic brain injury. Arch Phys Med Rehabil. 2010;91(11):1637–40.
2. Langlois JA, Rutland-Brown W, Wald MM. The epidemiology and impact of traumatic brain injury: a brief overview. J Head Trauma Rehabil. 2006;21(5):375–8.
3. Langlois JA, Rutland-Brown W, Thomas KE. Traumatic brain injury in the United States: emergency department visits, hospitalizations, and deaths. Atlanta: Centers for Disease Control and Prevention, National Center for Injury Prevention and Control; 2004.

4. Maas AI. Traumatic brain injury: simple data collection will improve the outcome. Wien Klin Wochenschr. 2007;119(1-2):20–2.
5. Greve MW, Zink BJ. Pathophysiology of traumatic brain injury. Mt Sinai J Med. 2009;76(2):97–104.
6. Giza CC, Hovda DA. The new neurometabolic cascade of concussion. Neurosurgery. 2014;75(suppl_4):S24–33.
7. Majdan M, Brazinova A, Rusnak M, Leitgeb J. Outcome prediction after traumatic brain injury: comparison of the performance of routinely used severity scores and multivariable prognostic models. J Neurosci Rural Pract. 2017;8(1):20.
8. Malec JF, Brown AW, Leibson CL, Flaada JT, Mandrekar JN, Diehl NN, Perkins PK. The Mayo classification system for traumatic brain injury severity. J Neurotrauma. 2007;24(9):1417–24.
9. Jones C. Glasgow coma scale. Am J Nurs. 1979;79(9):1551–3.
10. Maas AI, Stocchetti N, Bullock R. Moderate and severe traumatic brain injury in adults. Lancet Neurol. 2008;7(8):728–41.
11. Post A, Hoshizaki TB. Mechanisms of brain impact injuries and their prediction: a review. Trauma. 2012;14(4):327–49.
12. Holly LT, Kelly DF, Counelis GJ, Blinman T, McArthur DL, Cryer HG. Cervical spine trauma associated with moderate and severe head injury: incidence, risk factors, and injury characteristics. J Neurosurg Spine. 2002;96(3):285–91.
13. Badjatia N, Carney N, Crocco TJ, Fallat ME, Hennes HM, Jagoda AS, Jernigan S, Letarte PB, Lerner EB, Moriarty TM, Pons PT. Guidelines for prehospital management of traumatic brain injury 2nd edition. Prehosp Emerg Care. 2008;12:S1.
14. Maas AI, Hukkelhoven CW, Marshall LF, Steyerberg EW. Prediction of outcome in traumatic brain injury with computed tomographic characteristics: a comparison between the computed tomographic classification and combinations of computed tomographic predictors. Neurosurgery. 2005;57(6): 1173–82.
15. Maegele M. Coagulopathy after traumatic brain injury: incidence, pathogenesis, and treatment options. Transfusion. 2013;53(S1):28S.
16. Fong R, Konakondla S, Schirmer CM, Lacroix M. Surgical interventions for severe traumatic brain injury. J Emerg Crit Care Med. 2017;1(10):28.
17. Roberts DJ, Hall RI, Kramer AH, Robertson HL, Gallagher CN, Zygun DA. Sedation for critically ill adults with severe traumatic brain injury: a systematic review of randomized controlled trials. Crit Care Med. 2011;39(12):2743–51.
18. McHugh GS, Engel DC, Butcher I, Steyerberg EW, Lu J, Mushkudiani N, Hernandez AV, Marmarou A, Maas AI, Murray GD. Prognostic value of secondary insults in traumatic brain injury: results from the IMPACT study. J Neurotrauma. 2007;24(2):287–93.
19. Bratton SL, Chestnut RM, Ghajar J, McConnell FH, Harris OA, Hartl R, Manley GT, Nemecek A, Newell DW, Rosenthal G, Schouten J. Guidelines for the management of severe traumatic brain injury. VI. Indications for intracranial pressure monitoring. J Neurotrauma. 2007;24:S37–44.
20. Freeman WD. Management of intracranial pressure. Continuum (Minneap Minn). 2015;21(5 Neurocritical Care):1299–323.
21. Bratton SL, Chestnut RM, Ghajar J, McConnell Hammond FF, Harris OA, Hartl R, Manley GT, Nemecek A, Newell DW, Rosenthal G, Schouten J II. Hyperosmolar therapy. J Neurotrauma. 2007;24(Supplement 1):S14.
22. Ucar T, Akyuz M, Kazan S, Tuncer R. Role of decompressive surgery in the management of severe head injuries: prognostic factors and patient selection. J Neurotrauma. 2005;22(11):1311–8.
23. Carney N, Totten AM, O'Reilly C, Ullman JS, Hawryluk GW, Bell MJ, Bratton SL, Chesnut R, Harris OA, Kissoon N, Rubiano AM. Guidelines for the management of severe traumatic brain injury. Neurosurgery. 2017;80(1):6–15.
24. Juul N, Morris GF, Marshall SB, Marshall LF. Intracranial hypertension and cerebral perfusion pressure: influence on neurological deterioration and outcome in severe head injury. The Executive Committee of the International Selfotel Trial. J Neurosurg. 2000;92(1):1–6.
25. Temkin NR, Dikmen SS, Wilensky AJ, Keihm J, Chabal S, Winn HR. A randomized, double-blind study of phenytoin for the prevention of post-traumatic seizures. N Engl J Med. 1990;323(8):497–502.
26. Vespa PM, Nuwer MR, Nenov V, Ronne-Engstrom E, Hovda DA, Bergsneider M, Kelly DF, Martin NA, Becker DP. Increased incidence and impact of nonconvulsive and convulsive seizures after traumatic brain injury as detected by continuous electroencephalographic monitoring. J Neurosurg. 1999;91(5):750–60.
27. Ronne-Engstrom E, Winkler T. Continuous EEG monitoring in patients with traumatic brain injury reveals a high incidence of epileptiform activity. Acta Neurol Scand. 2006;114(1):47–53.
28. Katz DI, Alexander MP. Traumatic brain injury: predicting course of recovery and outcome for patients admitted to rehabilitation. Arch Neurol. 1994;51(7):661–70.

Spinal Cord Injury

Indranil Ghosh and Subhajit Guha

Case Scenario

A 24-year-old male residing at Barrackpore, West Bengal, had a history of injury of neck following diving in shallow water around 15 h back before he presented to our hospital. Following the injury of the neck, he had lost his consciousness for 10–15 s and developed weakness in all four limbs. The patient was managed conservatively at another hospital outside where MRI of the cervical spine was done which revealed cervical spine injury (C_4–C_5 subluxation and displaced fracture) associated with haematoma and cord compression (Fig. 36.1).

After the patient was brought to our hospital, primary survey was done, which revealed a clear airway and a cervical spine injury. The patient was breathing on his own in a regular, normal pattern, with a respiratory rate of 16/min, at room air, and his oxygen saturation was 98%. The patient had stable haemodynamics with a blood pressure of 120/60 mmHg and a pulse rate of 88 bpm. Disability noted was quadriplegia. No other injuries were noted during exposure. On secondary survey, there was no head injury, and cervical spine was tender. There was no sensation beyond fifth inter-costal space with no tenderness in chest region. There were no visible injuries in abdomen and limbs, and power in all four limbs was 0/5. Focused assessment with sonography in trauma was negative. There was no pelvic, thoracic or limb injury on X-ray.

After admission, the patient was advised to wear a Philadelphia hard cervical collar; deep vein thrombolysis prophylaxis was done by mechanical and drug therapy. Supportive care and medications such as gabapentin, intravenous paracetamol, methylcobalamine and amitriptyline were used. The day after admission, anterior cervical discectomy and fusion surgery were done along with tracheostomy. The patient was given general anaesthesia following awake fibre-optic intubation. After surgery the patient was mechanically ventilated overnight and gradually weaned off and put on a T-piece on oxygen support.

Eight days after the surgery, the patient was put on ventilator as he developed acute respiratory distress syndrome (ARDS), and gradually he became fully ventilator dependent. On about 50th day of admission, patient had sudden cardiac arrest, cardio-pulmonary resuscitation initiated as per advanced cardiac life support protocol but was unsuccessful, and the patient expired.

I. Ghosh (✉) · S. Guha
Department of Neuro-Anaesthesia, Institute of Neurosciences, Kolkata, West Bengal, India

Fig. 36.1 Sagittal section of the cervical spine shows fracture with misalignment of the C4–C5 vertebral bodies and impingement of the C5 vertebral body into the spinal canal, causing canal stenosis, cord compression with surrounding oedema and haematoma

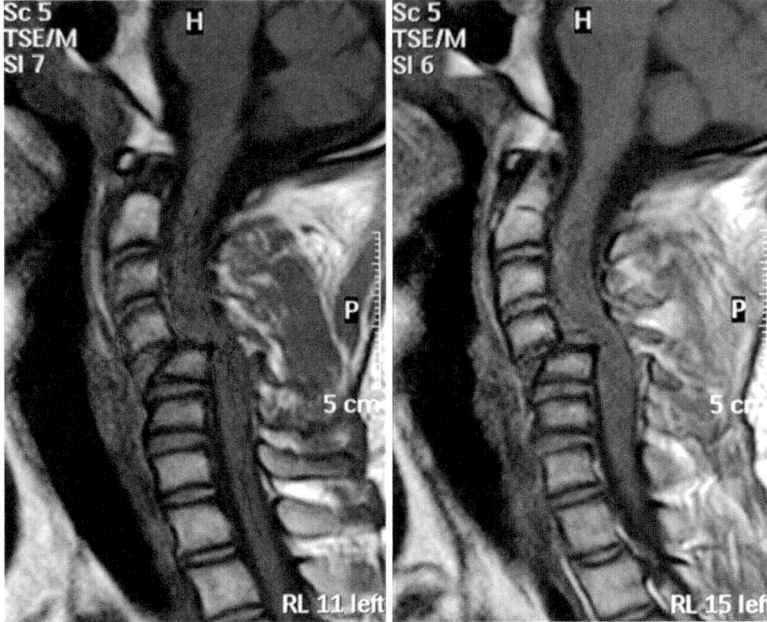

36.1 Introduction

In the US, the incidence of nonfatal spinal cord injury (SCI) per year is approximately 12,000 [1]. The most common (55%) being cervical spinal column injuries. Almost 15% patients suffer from injury involving the thoracolumbar junction [2]. Motor vehicle accidents, fall injuries, gunshot wounds and sporting accidents constitute almost 50% of the SCI (Table 36.1). Tumours, vascular disorder, infections, arthropathy, etc., are the non-traumatic causes of SCIs.

Adequate assessment of the patient, along with appropriate timely decision making, is most important in spine trauma patients. The treatment may vary from patients requiring no intervention at one end to life-threatening spinal column injuries on the other end. All patients with a history of trauma should be assumed to have a cervical spine injury, unless proven otherwise. This is according to Advanced Trauma Life Support (ATLS) protocols.

In this chapter the following points will be discussed: Focused assessment of a patient with spinal cord injury; classification of the skeletal and spinal cord injury; prioritization and decision making; surgical strategy including indication,

Table 36.1 Aetiology of traumatic spinal cord injury [3]

Cause	Percentage of cases (%)
Motor vehicle collision	41.3
Falls	27.3
Violence	15.0
Sports-related injuries	7.9
Others/unknown	8.5

schedule, approach, technique and post-operative care; and the principles of rehabilitation.

36.1.1 Classification

Spinal cord injury is divided into two stages: Initial or primary injury, and later, secondary injury [4–6]. The initial traumatic insult causes the primary injury. The bony fragments (e.g., vertebral body), joint dislocation (e.g., facet joints, intervertebral joints) or arthropathy (spondylosis, spondylolisthesis), ligamentous tears or herniation of intervertebral discs are the sources of the mechanical force [7]. Within minutes following the initial injury the secondary injury starts, and it can evolve over several hours. The pathophysiology mechanisms involved in secondary injury are neuronal ischaemic injury, hypoxia, inflammation, excitotoxicity, lipid peroxidation and

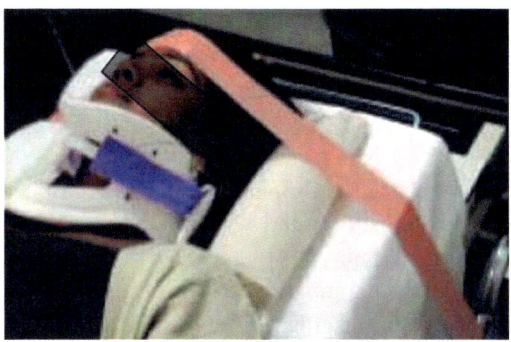

Fig. 36.2 Stabilization of cervical spine before clearance

apoptosis. Ultimately, it leads to further cord oedema, which reaches its severity in about 4 and 6 days post-injury [8, 9].

36.1.2 Initial Stabilization

The patient should be splinted using a cervical spine collar, two sandbags and a forehead tape assuming to have cervical spine injury during the resuscitation and initial assessment phase. A spine board is used for transferring the patient to stabilize the thoracolumbar spine and then on a flat trolley, allowing log rolling with in-line stabilization at the neck only (Fig. 36.2).

36.1.3 Evaluation

The main principles of evaluation are:

1. Assessing and classifying the skeletal injury
2. Assessing and classifying the neurological injury
3. Assessing associated spinal injuries
4. Identifying associated non-spinal injuries
5. Establishing treatment priorities during the assessment phase

36.1.4 Instability

Instability has been defined as 'the loss of the ability of the spine under physiological loads to maintain its pattern of displacement so that there is no initial or additional neurological deficit, no major deformity and no incapacitating pain'. A definitive management and the surgical approach are based on the presence of instability and its grading. Identification of instability aids in the decision making process and also helps to initiate early treatment process and future prognostication.

36.1.5 Neurological Classification

A thorough neurological examination is needed after initial general stabilization. The American Spinal Injury Association (ASIA) standard is used for prognostication. It also has a role in initial assessment and follow-up [10]. The ASIA scale has a sensory and a motor component: 28 dermatomes (from C2 to S4–5) on the right and left sides are tested to assess the sensory component, which includes light touch and pinprick sensation also. A three-point scale, ranging from 0 (absent) to 2 (normal or intact) is used to score each modality separately. Muscle functions corresponding to ten paired myotomes (C5-T1 and L2-S1) are used to assess the motor component. External anal sphincter should also be tested for voluntary contraction. The Medical Research Council grading system (0–5 score) is used to assess the muscle strength.

ASIA Impairment Scale should be determined as follows:

A = complete. No sensory or motor functions in sacral segments S4–S5.
B = sensory incomplete. Sensory but not motor function is preserved below the neurological level of injury, including S4–S5, and no motor function is preserved more than three levels below the motor level on each side of the body.
C = motor complete. Motor function is preserved below the neurological level, and more than half of the muscles below the neurological level of injury have a muscle grade less than 3.
D = motor incomplete. Motor function is preserved below the neurological level, and at least half of the muscles below the neurological level of injury have a muscle grade > 3.

E = Normal. Sensation and motor functions are normal in all segments tested [11].

ASIA Impairment Scale score has a prognostic value. ASIA-A patients will not regain function in 80% of cases. Out of these patients only 15% have a chance to improve; a further lesser number of patients have a chance to regain useful motor function. More than half (54%) of the ASIA-B patients and the majority (86%) of ASIA C–D patients have a chance to regain their sensory and motor functions [12].

36.1.6 Imaging

Trauma patients who have complaints of neck pain, spinal tenderness, symptoms or signs of a neurological deficit related to the spine and patients who cannot be clearly assessed (the ones who are unconscious, uncooperative, incoherent or intoxicated) need radiographic study of the spinal cord [10].

To identify the patients at low risk for cervical fracture/subluxation/dislocation, the National Emergency X-Radiography Utilization Study (NEXUS) protocol was designed. It consists of five criteria:

1. No posterior midline cervical tenderness
2. No intoxication
3. Normal mental status
4. No other painful injuries
5. No neurological deficit

NEXUS protocol has a sensitivity of 99% and a negative predictive value of 99.9% for cervical spinal cord injuries [13]. Imaging of the neck or the spinal cord is not needed in the patients at low risk.

Canadian C-Spine Rule is another protocol to assess the need for radiographic study of spinal cord. It consists of:

1. The presence of a high-risk factor that mandates radiography (age > 65 years, dangerous mechanism of trauma, or paraesthesia in extremities).

2. The presence of low-risk factors allowing for a safe assessment of the range of motion.
3. The ability to actively rotate the neck 45° to the left and right.

The Canadian C-Spine Rule protocol resulted in 100% sensitivity and 42.5% specificity for cervical spinal injury [14].

Computed tomography (CT) is the first choice among the imaging modalities. A three-view spine X-ray is recommended (anteroposterior, odontoid and lateral views) if CT scan is not available, which can be supplemented later by a CT scan [10]. Lesions can be detected by MRI even if the CT scan is normal; thus MRI should be done within the first 48 h after the trauma. Presence of haemorrhage, extent of oedema and severity of the initial compression can be detected by MRI, and thereby outcome can be predicted. Intraspinal haemorrhages (>1 cm long) as well as longitudinal T2 signal changes >3 cm are the predictors of poor prognosis [15].

36.1.7 Airway Management

Respiratory complications are common (36–83% incidence rate) during the acute phase of SCI. Reduced vital capacity, retention of secretions, autonomic dysfunction, atelectasis, pneumonia or respiratory failure that require mechanical ventilation are the common complications [16].

The level of injury and the ASIA classification are the two most important predictors of endotracheal intubation in spinal cord injury patients. Almost all lesiond above C5 require fibre optic intubation preferably in awake condition. Alternatively intubation can be done electively with manual in-line stabilization, avoiding hyperextension, rotation and other movements of the neck [16].

Patients with cervical spine injury at a lower level or incomplete lesions may be managed conservatively with close monitoring of lung function parameters like vital capacity, maximum inspiratory pressure and carbon dioxide partial pressure levels [16]. Weaning from the ventilator and extubation with lesions above C4 are possible in less than half of the patient population. Patients with ASIA-A lesions, a history of smoking and previous lung disease will require tracheostomy at some point in time. Early tracheostomy (within 10 days) may give benefit to reduce the days of mechanical ventilation and ICU stay [17].

36.1.8 Cardiovascular Management

Direct cervical or thoracic spinal trauma leading to neurogenic shock causes hypotension, or it may be due to polytrauma. Disruption in supraspinal control results in a loss of sympathetic tone, and the parasympathetic tone via the vagus nerve remains intact; this causes an imbalance in autonomic control and neurogenic shock. The end result is a loss of peripheral vascular tone and bradycardia [18].

Hypotension leads to a reduction in spinal cord flow and perfusion, and this contributes to secondary injury after acute SCI. Thus, the current recommendation suggests to maintain mean arterial pressure (MAP) at 85–90 mmHg for 7 days after injury (level III evidence) [10]. In order to achieve that goal euvolemic status should be maintained by infusion of crystalloids in association with vasopressors if needed, the mainstay of treatment is to maintain Euvolemic status should be maintained by infusion of crystalloids, if needed in association with vasopressors [19]. Invasive blood pressure monitoring is safer in these patients. Patients with high cervical spine injury and those with complete lesions may need resuscitation. These lesions are poor predictors of cardiovascular status [20]. In 7–10 days post-injury the cardiovascular instability can be either transient and episodic or recurrent. In SCI, determining which vasopressor is better, what the optimal therapy duration is and what the MAP level is below which vasopressor support should be initiated is inconclusive [21].

The choice of vasopressor depends on the level of the SCI and the patient's haemodynamic status. A drug with chronotropic and inotropic effects as well as a vasoconstrictor like noradrenaline (or, alternatively, dopamine) could be a good option in cervical or high thoracic lesions with both hypotension and bradycardia. A pure vasopressor drug such as phenylephrine could be appropriate for low thoracic lesions, where hypotension is usually the result of peripheral vasodilation [22].

Majority of patients (up to 70%) experience at least one of the following: tachycardia, bradycardia, elevated troponin, new-onset atrial fibrillation, atrial flutter or electrocardiogram ST changes consistent with ischaemia after the use of vasoactive drugs. Side effects are more common with the use of dopamine compared to noradrenaline and phenylephrine. Older population (55–60 years) are more prone to side effects [23–25]. Recently, Altaf et al. concluded that noradrenaline is superior to dopamine to maintain MAP with a lower intrathecal pressure and correspondingly higher spinal cord perfusion pressure [26].

36.2 Decompressive Surgery

The main aim of surgical decompression is to reduce secondary hypoxia and ischaemia by relieving the progressive pressure on the microcirculation due to oedema and haemorrhage [19]. Surgery is indicated in the case of (1) progressive neurological impairment due to significant cord compression and (2) a fracture where close reduction is not effective or not amenable, such as unstable vertebral fractures.

36.3 The Surgical Timing

Early surgery (within 24 h) after acute spinal cord injury is more than twice as likely to have a two-grade ASIA Impairment Scale improvement and a similar complication rate compared to patients with late surgery (after 24 h) [27]. The present recommendation is surgical decompression in the first 24 h [10].

36.3.1 Intravenous Methylprednisolone

Since 1984, various clinical trials have been done to demonstrate the beneficial role of methylprednisolone (MP) in humans with SCI. This synthetic corticosteroid exerts its beneficial effect by upregulating anti-inflammatory factors as well as decreasing oxidative stress. In animal model of SCI, this drug enhances endogenous cell survival. It also reduces oedema, prevents intracellular potassium depletion and inhibits lipid peroxidation [28].

In the National Spinal Cord Injury Study I (1984), one group received 1000 mg bolus MP, followed by the same dose daily for 10 days, and the second group received 100 mg bolus and then daily. A difference in motor or sensory neurological recovery was observed between groups, and wound infections were more prevalent in the high-dose group [29].

The National Spinal Cord Injury Study II (1990) compared MP 30 mg/kg intravenously, followed by 5.4 mg/kg/h over 23 h, to naloxone and placebo. At the end of 1 year, no significant difference was noted in neurological function among the groups. Though modest improvement in motor recovery was found in the subset of patients who received the corticosteroid within 8 h, in MP patients wound infections were more frequent [30].

In the National Spinal Cord Injury Study III (1997), three treatment groups were compared: MP for 48 h, the same drug administered for 24 h and tirilazad mesylate. The treatment was given within 8 h of SCI. The results showed that in patients treated between 3 to 8 h after trauma, the 48-h regimen was associated with a greater motor but not functional recovery. In addition, more severe sepsis and pneumonia were noted in patients who had received a longer duration of treatment [31].

Meta-analysis and systematic review do not support the use of methylprednisolone in acute SCI, as evidence from multiple randomized controlled trials and observational studies has shown no long-term benefits. Moreover, MP also increases gastrointestinal haemorrhage [32].

36.3.2 Neuroprotection

Multiple approaches using neuroprotective drugs have been studied, and many drugs are currently under investigation to reduce secondary damage after an SCI. Gangliosides are present in neuronal membranes. These glycolipid molecules can enhance axonal regeneration. They have a variety of neuroprotective effects, such as prevention of apoptosis and anti-excitotoxic activity. However, this drug is no longer recommended in SCI, as randomized controlled trials reported no difference in neurological recovery after 6 months [33, 34].

Naloxone (an opioid antagonist) was compared with MP and placebo in the National Spinal Cord Injury Study II trial, where drugs were given within 12 h in 487 patients with SCI. The result showed no differences in motor scores between groups [30].

Nimodipine (an L-type calcium channel blocker) acts by preventing calcium-dependent apoptotic enzymes and by blocking the release of glutamate from the presynaptic nerve terminal. It has shown no difference in neurological status at 1 year in comparison with placebo in patients with SCI.

Tirilazad mesylate is a drug that attenuates peroxidation of neuronal membranes. The drug was compared with MP in the National Spinal Cord Injury Study III trial. The study showed no difference between groups [31].

Hypothermia has shown multiple benefits in patients with SCI in animal studies. It has shown improvement in patients with SCI by decreasing basal metabolic rate in the central nervous system, reduction in inflammation, apoptosis, excitotoxicity, oedema, gliosis and increased angiogenesis [35]. One pilot study in which spinal cord-injured humans were exposed to hypothermia showed a neurological recovery trend (43% vs. 21%) and no difference in complication rates [36]. In another study, out of 35 ASIA-A hypothermic (33 °C for 48 h) patients who started within 6 h post-injury, 4 patients converted to ASIA-B in the next 24 h, while 35.5% showed an improvement of at least one grade on the ASIA scale at the latest follow-up [37]. Riluzole, a sodium-channel blocker, reduces secondary injury by blocking pathological activation of sodium channels and reducing the release of glutamate in preclinical models of SCI. A phase I/II trial demonstrated a benefit in motor scores in patients treated with the drug [38]. A phase II/III trial, the Riluzole in Spinal Cord Injury Study, has shown favourable results [39].

Minocycline is an antibiotic with anti-inflammatory properties, including inhibition of tumour necrosis factor alpha, interleukin-1 beta, cyclooxygenase-2 and nitric oxide synthase. In a phase II study, the ASIA motor score improved in patients treated with minocycline ($p = 0.05$) [40]. This led to a phase III trial, the Minocycline in Acute Spinal Cord Injury, which has shown improvement in neurological and histological outcomes [41].

In animal model of SCI, fibroblast growth factor has been shown to protect against excitotoxicity and to reduce free radical production. A fibroblast growth factor analogue called SUN 13837 was evaluated in a phase I/II trial completed in 2015 and showed improved functional recovery [42]. The cytokine granulocyte colony-stimulating factor is neuroprotective in SCI by promoting cell survival and inhibiting tumour necrosis factor alpha and interleukin-1 beta. The benefits are demonstrated in two small, non-randomized studies that demonstrated improvements in ASIA motor scores with drug use [43, 44].

36.3.3 Neurodegeneration

SCI patients have demonstrated promising results when subjected to cell-based therapies. A wide number of cell types—embryonic stem cells, induced pluripotent stem cells, olfactory ensheathing cells, Schwann cells, mesenchymal cells and activated autologous macrophages—are being evaluated. Cellular transplantation alone, or in combination with other therapies, demonstrated neurological recovery, but no one type was superior to the other. This observation is true for human studies also, with no major adverse events. However, a lot of patients undergo some spontaneous recovery in the next 6 months after injury without any active intervention [28].

Embryonic and induced pluripotent stem cells are capable of multiple functions in the form of regeneration, axon remyelination, anti-inflammation and so forth. Schwann cells also behave in a similar fashion and have got injury-healing capabilities. Olfactory ensheathing cells and mesenchymal cells are capable of modulating inflammatory response at various levels. Although they decrease inflammatory cell infiltration, increase pro-survival trophic factor levels and promote tissue sparing [19, 28], these therapies are still in the experimental stage.

References

1. National Spinal Cord Injury Statistical Centre [database on the Internet] 2010. [cited 2010 November 01].
2. Goldberg W, Mueller C, Panacek E, Tigges S, Hoffman JR, Mower WR. Distribution and patterns of blunt traumatic cervical spine injury. Ann Emerg Med. 2001;38:17–21.
3. Dooney N, Dagal A. Anesthetic considerations in acute spinal cord trauma. Int J Crit Illn Inj Sci. 2011;1:36–43.
4. Janssen L, Hansebout RR. Pathogenesis of spinal cord injury and newer treatments. A review. Spine (Phila Pa 1976). 1989;14:23–32.
5. Tator CH, Duncan EG, Edmonds VE, Lapczak LI, Andrews DF. Neurological recovery, mortality and length of stay after acute spinal cord injury associated with changes in management. Paraplegia. 1995;33:254–62.
6. Hulsebosch CE. Recent advances in pathophysiology and treatment of spinal cord injury. Adv Physiol Educ. 2002;26:238–55.
7. Sekhon LH, Fehlings MG. Epidemiology, demographics, and pathophysiology of acute spinal cord injury. Spine (Phila Pa 1976). 2001;26:S2–12.
8. Young W. Secondary CNS injury. J Neurotrauma. 1988;5:219–21.
9. Hurlbert RJ. Strategies of medical intervention in the management of acute spinal cord injury. Spine (Phila Pa 1976). 2006;31(Suppl. 11):S16–21.
10. Walters BC, Hadley MN, Hurlbert RJ, Aarabi B, Dhall SS, Gelb DE, et al. Guidelines for the management of acute cervical spine and spinal cord injuries: 2013 update. Neurosurgery. 2013;60(Suppl. 1):82–91.
11. Kirshblum SC, Burns SP, Biering-Sorensen F, Donovan W, Graves DE, Jha A, et al. International standards for neurological classification of spinal cord injury (revised 2011). J Spinal Cord Med. 2011;34(6):535–46.

12. Le CT, Price M. Survival from spinal cord injury. J Chronic Dis. 1982;35(6):487–92.
13. Hoffman JR, Mower WR, Wolfson AB, Todd KH, Zucker MI. Validity of a set of clinical criteria to rule out injury to the cervical spine in patients with blunt trauma. N Engl J Med. 2000;343(2):94–9.
14. Stiell IG, Wells GA, Vandemheen KL, Clement CM, Lesiuk H, De Maio VJ, et al. The Canadian C-spine rule for radiography in alert and stable trauma patients. JAMA. 2001;286(15):1841–8.
15. Krishna V, Andrews H, Varma A, Mintzer J, Kindy MS, Guest J. Spinal cord injury: how can we improve the classification and quantification of its severity and prognosis? J Neurotrauma. 2014;31(3):215–27.
16. Vazquez RG, Sedes PR, Farina MM, Marques AM, Velasco EF. Respiratory management in the patient with spinal cord injury. Biomed Res Int. 2013;2013:168757. https://doi.org/10.1155/2013/168757.
17. Choi HJ, Paeng SH, Kim ST, Lee KS, Kim MS, Jung YT. The effectiveness of early tracheostomy in cervical spinal cord injury patients. J Korean Neurosurg Soc. 2013;54:220–4.
18. Hagen EM. Acute complications of spinal cord injuries. World J Orthop. 2015;6(1):17–23.
19. Ahuja CS, Martin AR, Fehlings MG. Recent advances in managing spinal cord injury secondary to trauma. F1000 Res. 2016;5(F1000 Faculty Rev):1017.
20. Casha S, Christie S. A systematic review of intensive cardiopulmonary management after spinal cord injury. J Neurotrauma. 2011;28(8):1479–95.
21. Ploumis A, Yadlapalli N, Fehlings MG, Kwon BK, Vaccaro AR. A systematic review of the evidence supporting a role for vasopressor support in acute SCI. Spinal Cord. 2010;48(5):356–62.
22. Consortium for Spinal Cord Medicine. Early acute management in adults with spinal cord injury: a clinical practice guideline for health-care professionals. J Spinal Cord Med. 2008;31(4):403–79.
23. Readdy WJ, Whetstone WD, Ferguson AR, Talbott JF, Inoue T, Saigal R. Complications and outcomes of vasopressor usage in acute traumatic central cord syndrome. J Neurosurg Spine. 2015;23(5):574–80.
24. Readdy WJ, Dhall SS. Vasopressor administration in spinal cord injury: should we apply a universal standard to all injury patterns? Neural Regen Res. 2016;11(3):420–1.
25. Inoue T, Manley GT, Patel N, Whetstone WD. Medical and surgical management after spinal cord injury: vasopressor usage, early surgeries and complications. J Neurotrauma. 2014;31(3):284–91.
26. Altaf F, Griesdale DE, Belanger L, Ritchie L, Markez J, Ailon T, et al. The differential effects of norepinephrine and dopamine on cerebrospinal fluid pressure and spinal cord perfusion pressure after acute human spinal cord injury. Spinal Cord. 2017;55(1):33–8.
27. Fehlings MG, Vaccaro A, Wilson JR, Singh A, Cadotte DW, Harrop JS, et al. Early versus delayed decompression for traumatic cervical spinal cord injury: results of the Surgical Timing in Acute Spinal Cord Injury Study (STASCIS). PLoS One. 2012;7(1):e320.
28. Wilson JR, Forgione N, Fehlings MG. Emerging therapies for acute traumatic spinal cord injury. CMAJ. 2013;185(6):485–92.
29. Bracken MB, Collins WF, Freeman DF, Shepard MJ, Wagner FW, Silten RM, et al. Efficacy of methylprednisolone in acute spinal cord injury. JAMA. 1984;251(1):45–52.
30. Bracken MB, Shepard MJ, Collins WF, Holford TR, Young W, Baskin DS, et al. A randomized, controlled trial of methylprednisolone or naloxone in the treatment of acute spinal cord injury: results of the Second National Acute Spinal Cord Injury Study. N Engl J Med. 1990;322(20):1405–11.
31. Bracken MB, Shepard MJ, Holford TR, Leo-Summers L, Aldrich EF, Fazl M, et al. Administration of methylprednisolone for 24 or 48 h or tirilazad mesylate for 48 h in the treatment of acute spinal cord injury: results of the Third National Acute Spinal Cord Injury Randomized Controlled Trial. JAMA. 1997;277(20):1597–604.
32. Evaniew N, Belley-Côté EP, Fallah N, Noonan VK, Rivers CS, Dvorak MF. Methylprednisolone for the treatment of patients with acute spinal cord injuries: a systematic review and meta-analysis. J Neurotrauma. 2016;33(5):468–81.
33. Geisler FH, Coleman WP, Grieco G, Poonian D. The Sygen multicenter acute spinal cord injury study. Spine. 2001;26(Suppl. 24):87–98.
34. Petitjean ME, Pointillart V, Dixmerias F, Wiart L, Sztark F, Lassié P, et al. Medical treatment of spinal cord injury in the acute stage. Ann Fr Anesth Reanim. 1998;17(2):115–22.
35. Wang J, Pearse DD. Therapeutic hypothermia in spinal cord injury: the status of its use and open questions. Int J Mol Sci. 2015;16(8):16848–79.
36. Levi AD, Green BA, Wang MY, Dietrich WD, Brindle T, Vanni S, et al. Clinical application of modest hypothermia after spinal cord injury. J Neurotrauma. 2009;26(3):407–15.
37. Dididze M, Green BA, Dietrich WD, Vanni S, Wang MY, Levi AD. Systemic hypothermia in acute cervical spinal cord injury: a case-controlled study. Spinal Cord. 2013;51(5):395–400.
38. Grossman RG, Fehlings MG, Frankowski RF, Burau KD, Chow DS, Tator C, et al. A prospective, multicenter, phase I matched-comparison group trial of safety, pharmacokinetics, and preliminary efficacy of riluzole in patients with traumatic spinal cord injury. J Neurotrauma. 2014;31(3):239–55.
39. AOSpine North America Research Network. Riluzole in spinal cord injury study. (RISCIS). 2016 [cited 2016 Jul 13]. Clinical Trials.gov.
40. Casha S, Zygun D, McGowan MD, Bains I, Yong VW, Hurlbert RJ. Results of phase II placebo-controlled randomized trial of minocycline in acute spinal cord injury. Brain. 2012;135(4):1224–36.

41. Rick Hansen Institute. Minocycline in acute spinal cord injury (MASC). Clinical Trials.gov. NCT 01828203. 2014 [cited 2014 Oct 16].

42. Daiichi Sankyo Inc. Study to evaluate the efficacy, safety, and pharmacokinetics of SUN13837 injection in adult subjects with Acute Spinal Cord Injury (ASCI). Clinical Trials.gov. NCT01502631.

43. Kamiya K, Koda M, Furuya T, Kato K, Takahashi H, Sakuma T, et al. Neuroprotective therapy with granulocyte colony-stimulating factor in acute spinal cord injury: a comparison with high-dose with methylprednisolone as a historical control. Eur Spine J. 2015;24(5):963–7.

44. Takahashi H, Yamazaki M, Okawa A, Sakuma T, Kato K, Hashimoto M, et al. Neuroprotective therapy using granulocyte colony-stimulating factor for acute spinal cord injury: a phase I/IIa clinical trial. Eur Spine J. 2012;21(12):2580–7.

Alzheimer's Disease

37

Krishna Dhungana

Case Scenario

A 72-year-old male who had completed his education up to bachelor level presented to Neurology outpatient clinic with a 2-year history of progressive memory decline. His memory deficit was more noticeable when he was asked to recall recent events than events in the remote past. He had no problems in finding his way back home. His attention, language, and judgment were normal. The patient did not have a family history of dementia. On examination, Mini-Mental Score Examination (MMSE) score was 22. He had problems with the recollection of recent events and poor performance on categorical fluency. His delayed recall was impaired. His language and visuospatial skills were normal.

Complete blood count, random blood sugar, renal function test, and liver function test were within normal limits. Calcium and magnesium levels were normal. Serological tests including HIV and VDRL were non-reactive. Thyroid function test was normal, and vitamin B_{12} level was 525. MRI of brain revealed global cerebral atrophy with predominant involvement of bilateral medial temporal lobe and hippocampus. The patient was started on donepezil 5 mg once a day and increased to 10 mg per day over a period of 2 months. The family was counseled regarding the nature of disease and the precautions to be taken. On follow-up after 6 months, his MMSE score was 24 out of 30.

37.1 Introduction

Alzheimer's disease (AD) is the most common cause of dementia. It is a neurodegenerative disease characterized by progressive cognitive decline as well as behavioral changes and is associated with amyloid and tau deposition in the brain. It is the leading cause of mortality and morbidity in older age groups. Cognitive dysfunction includes deficits in short-term memory, executive function, visuospatial function, and praxis.

37.2 Epidemiology

Alzheimer's disease (AD) is the most common neurodegenerative disorder and the sixth most common cause of death in the United States [1]. The onset is usually after the age of 65 years. It is increasingly prevalent with advancing age. Major risk factors for the development of Alzheimer's disease are the presence of apolipoprotein gene E4 alleles (APOE4), low educational status, family history of AD, traumatic brain injuries, and cardiovascular risk factors such as diabetes, hypertension, and dyslipid-

K. Dhungana (✉)
Department of Neurology, Kathmandu Medical College Teaching Hospital, Sinamangal, Kathmandu, Nepal

© Springer Nature Singapore Pte Ltd. 2024
K. K. Oli et al. (eds.), *Case-based Approach to Common Neurological Disorders*,
https://doi.org/10.1007/978-981-99-8676-7_37

emia. Around two-thirds of patients diagnosed with AD are women [2].

37.3 Clinical Features

AD usually occurs in older age, but can also occur before the age of 60 [3]. With increasing age, the incidence and prevalence of AD increase exponentially. The most common initial symptom of AD is memory impairment [4]. Recent episodic memories are affected early in the disease. Memories from the distant past and immediate memories are usually spared. The hippocampus, entorhinal cortex, and related structures in the medial temporal lobe are responsible for memory of recent events [5]. Memory deficits increase insidiously, later in the disease process, further involving deficits of semantic memory and immediate recall. In patients with AD, there is impaired ability to recall objects with selective cues [6].

Later in the disease process, deficits in language often manifest. In the early stage of the disease, subtle decline in visuospatial skills is seen. An impairment in executive function may be mild or prominent in the early stages of the disease. Occasionally, all these three domains—language, visuospatial skills, and executive functions—may be present as the prominent initial symptom [7].

In the middle and late stages of the disease, neuropsychiatric symptoms are common. However, these symptoms can present earlier as abnormal behavior, anosognosia, apathy, anxiety, and irritability. Other neuropsychiatric manifestations such as psychosis and agitation are often difficult to manage. Early in the disease, mild-to-moderate depressive symptoms are also frequently present. Later in the disease, disturbances of appetite and sleep, disinhibition, and alterations in perception or thought commonly occur. Insight is often absent in the early stages of the disease, which is also difficult to manage.

Apraxia usually occurs later in the disease course, usually after involvement of memory and language [8]. Apraxia can be elicited by asking the patient to perform ideomotor tasks. Due to apraxia, patient has difficulty with dressing, using utensils, and doing household tasks. Hyposmia is common in patients with AD. In AD, sleep disturbances are common in which patients have decreased sleep time with fragmented pattern [9]. In the later stages of disease, seizures can occur in 10–20% of patients with AD, and the predominant seizure type is focal dyscognitive seizure.

In the early stages of the disease, patients have a normal neurologic examination. Parkinsonian symptoms, such as bradykinesia and rigidity, can be seen in the later stages of AD. Pyramidal signs and myoclonus are also seen in the later stage of AD [10]. Similarly, pathologic reflexes such as grasp, root, and suck reflexes may be prominent in the late course. Patients are ultimately mute, incontinent, and bedridden in the advanced stage of the disease. Ultimately, multiple complications arise, such as choking, malnutrition, bedsores, deep venous thrombosis, and urinary tract infections, in the advanced stage. These complications are also the major cause of mortality in patients with AD.

37.3.1 Diagnostic Criteria

The Diagnostic and Statistical Manual of Mental Disorders, Fifth Edition (DSM-5), is currently the diagnostic standard for dementia, which is categorized as neurocognitive disorder (NCD) [11]. NCD is further subdivided into major and minor NCD. The diagnosis of major (loss of ability to do daily activities) and minor (independent and able to do daily activities) neurocognitive impairment requires objective cognitive decline, which is not caused by delirium or another neurologic, medical, or psychiatric disorder.

37.3.2 Role of Biomarkers in the Diagnosis of AD

The most established AD fluid biomarkers are CSF Aβ and tau protein levels. In the early stage, pathologic Aβ deposition occurs in the brain and is associated with reduction in CSF Aβ [12]. The levels of CSF total and phosphorylated tau levels increase in AD [13–16]. The CSF tau changes occur in the late course and are linked with cognitive impairment in patients with AD [17–20].

37.4 Genetics

The major genetic risk factor for sporadic AD is APOE4 gene variant. One copy of APOE4 gene variant increases the odds for developing AD 3 times, and two copies increase the odds 15-fold [21]. Autosomal dominant variants of AD have also been reported. In this variant, first symptoms are usually noticed in patients of age group 30–40 years. In cases of autosomal dominant AD, genetic mutations in amyloid precursor protein (APP), presenilin 1(PSEN1), and presenilin 2 (PSEN2) genes are seen. Early-onset autosomal dominant AD accounts for less than 2% of all patients with AD.

37.4.1 Pathology

There are both overproduction and reduced clearance of amyloid in AD. The downstream events are tau hyperphosphorylation and neuronal toxicity. There are regional neuronal and synaptic loss, extracellular β-amyloid deposition in the form of neuritic plaques, and intraneuronal tau protein deposition in the form of intraneuronal neurofibrillary tangles causing brain atrophy. β-Amyloid deposition is also seen in the cerebral blood vessels, which range from small amounts to major deposits, causing varieties of distortion in cerebral arteries.

37.4.2 Differential Diagnosis

Vascular dementia, dementia with Lewy body, and frontotemporal dementia should be considered as the various differential diagnoses of AD. Ischemic stroke, hemorrhagic stroke, and small vessel disease can lead to vascular dementia. Dementia with Lewy body is characterized by the presence of visual hallucinations, parkin-

sonism, autonomic dysfunction, sleep disorders, cognitive fluctuations, and neuroleptic hypersensitivity. In frontotemporal dementia, there are manifestations such as personality changes, social and emotional behavior abnormalities, and impairment of executive functioning in the behavioral variant. In the primary progressive form of frontotemporal dementia, there is gradual progressive language impairment.

37.4.3 Treatment

Patients with AD have reduced cerebral content of choline acetyltransferase, which leads to a decrease in acetylcholine synthesis. The medications that have been approved for use in AD are the acetylcholinesterase inhibitors (AChEIs) and the N-methyl-D-aspartate (NMDA) receptor antagonist memantine. Use of AChEIs should be considered in patients with mild-to-moderate AD [22]. AChEIs inhibit cholinesterase at the synaptic cleft and increase cholinergic transmission (Table 37.1).

The AChEIs that are currently approved for use in AD are donepezil, rivastigmine, and galantamine. These agents show some improvement in cognitive domains, including memory and concentration, as well as global and functional outcome measures. However, their therapeutic cognitive and functional effects seem to be modest and purely symptomatic. The most common side effects are nausea, vomiting, and diarrhea, and gradual dose escalation may be needed. Patient may also develop bradycardia or hypotension with these agents. One AChEI can be substituted with another if side effect occurs with one of the agents. If a patient is not benefiting or develops significant side effects, the therapy should be stopped.

Memantine is an NMDA receptor antagonist with low-to-moderate affinity. It is used as an add-on to ongoing AChEI therapy. Memantine has a beneficial effect on cognitive function, behavior, global function, and activities of daily living [23]. Memantine can be used for moderate-to-severe AD in combination with other AChEIs or even as monotherapy. Confusion and dizziness

Table 37.1 The commonly used drugs, mechanisms of action, and common side effects

Drug	Target dosage	Class	Mechanism of action	Common side effects
Donepezil	10 mg/day	Cholinesterase inhibitor	Prevents the breakdown of acetylcholine in the brain	Nausea, vomiting, diarrhea
Rivastigmine	6 mg twice daily	Cholinesterase inhibitor	Prevents the breakdown of acetylcholine in the brain	Anorexia, weight loss, bradycardia
Galantamine	12 mg twice daily	Cholinesterase inhibitor	Prevents the breakdown of acetylcholine in the brain	
Memantine	10 mg twice daily	NMDA receptor antagonist	Inhibits stimulation at the NMDA receptor	Dizziness, confusion

are the common adverse effects but occur less frequently.

Aducanumab is a recombinant monoclonal antibody directed against amyloid beta. Using the accelerated approval pathway, the US Food and Drug Administration has approved aducanumab for the treatment of mild AD. Post-approval trials are required to verify the clinical benefit.

Initially non-pharmacologic techniques are employed for the behavioral symptoms of AD. A quiet, familiar environment should be provided. Doors should be labeled, and sufficient lighting should be provided in all rooms. Positive and clear language should be used to reassure and distract the patient to address aggressive behavior. Selective serotonin reuptake inhibitors (SSRIs) are used to treat depression, which also alleviates agitation, anxiety, and irritability. Atypical neuroleptics are used to treat agitation or disruptive behavior. However, they should be used cautiously to avoid the toxicity at higher doses.

References

1. Alzheimer's Association. 2015 Alzheimer's disease facts and figures. Alzheimers Dement. 2015;11(3):322–84.
2. Gurland BJ, Wilder DE, Lantigua R, Stern Y, Chen J, Killeffer EH, et al. Rates of dementia in three ethnoracial groups. Int J Geriatr Psychiatry. 1999;14(6):481–93.
3. Braak H, Braak E. Frequency of stages of Alzheimer-related lesions in different age categories. Neurobiol Aging. 1997;18(4):351.
4. Markowitsch HJ, Staniloiu A. Amnestic disorders. Lancet. 2012;380(9851):1429–40.
5. Scoville WB, Milner B. Loss of recent memory after bilateral hippocampal lesions. J Neurol Neurosurg Psychiatry. 1957;20(1):11.
6. Wagner M, Wolf S, Reischies FM, Daerr M, Wolfsgruber S, Jessen F, et al. Biomarker validation of a cued recall memory deficit in prodromal Alzheimer disease. Neurology. 2012;78(6):379–86.
7. McKhann GM, Knopman DS, Chertkow H, Hyman BT, Jack CR Jr, Kawas CH, et al. The diagnosis of dementia due to Alzheimer's disease: recommendations from the National Institute on Aging-Alzheimer's Association workgroups on diagnostic guidelines for Alzheimer's disease. Alzheimers Dement. 2011;7(3):263.
8. Parakh R, Roy E, Koo E, Black S. Pantomime and imitation of limb gestures in relation to the severity of Alzheimer's disease. Brain Cogn. 2004;55(2):272.
9. Ju YE, Lucey BP, Holtzman DM. Sleep and Alzheimer disease pathology—a bidirectional relationship. Nat Rev Neurol. 2014;10(2):115.
10. Portet F, Scarmeas N, Cosentino S, Helzner EP, Stern Y. Extrapyramidal signs before and after diagnosis of incident Alzheimer disease in a prospective population study. Arch Neurol. 2009;66(9):1120.
11. American Psychiatric Association. Diagnostic and statistical manual of mental disorders. 5th ed. Washington, DC: American Psychiatric Publishing; 2013.
12. Blennow K, Hampe LH. CSF markers for incipient Alzheimer's disease. Lancet Neurol. 2003;2(10):605–13.
13. Andreasen N, Minthon L, Davidsson P, Vanmechelen E, Vanderstichele H, Winblad B, et al. Evaluation of CSF-tau and CSF-Abeta42 as diagnostic markers for

Alzheimer disease in clinical practice. Arch Neurol. 2001;58(3):373–9.

14. Blennow K, Wallin A, Agren H, Spenger C, Siegfried J, Vanmechelen E. Tau protein in cerebrospinal fluid: a biochemical marker for axonal degeneration in Alzheimer disease? Mol Chem Neuropathol. 1995;26(3):231–45.

15. Clark CM, Xie S, Chittams J, Ewbank D, Peskind E, Galasko D, et al. Cerebrospinal fluid tau and beta-amyloid: how well do these biomarkers reflect autopsy-confirmed dementia diagnoses? Arch Neurol. 2003;60(12):1696–702.

16. Galasko D, Chang L, Motter R, Clark CM, Kaye J, Knopman D, et al. High cerebrospinal fluid tau and low amyloid beta42 levels in the clinical diagnosis of Alzheimer disease and relation to apolipoprotein E genotype. Arch Neurol. 1998;55(7):937–45.

17. Buerger K, Ewers M, Andreasen N, Zinkowski R, Ishiguro K, Vanmechelen E, et al. Phosphorylated tau predicts rate of cognitive decline in MCI subjects: a comparative CSF study. Neurology. 2005;65(9):1502–3.

18. Buerger K, Teipel SJ, Zinkowski R, Blennow K, Arai H, Engel R, et al. CSF tau protein phosphorylated at threonine 231 correlates with cognitive decline in MCI subjects. Neurology. 2002;59(4):627–9.

19. Riemenschneider M, Lautenschlager N, Wagenpfeil S, Diehl J, Drzezga A, Kurz A. Cerebrospinal fluid tau and beta-amyloid 42 proteins identify Alzheimer disease in subjects with mild cognitive impairment. Arch Neurol. 2002;59(11):1729–34.

20. Wallin AK, Blennow K, Andreasen N, Minthon L. CSF biomarkers for Alzheimer's Disease: levels of beta-amyloid, tau, phosphorylated tau relate to clinical symptoms and survival. Dement Geriatr Cogn Disord. 2006;21(3):131–8.

21. Farrer LA, Cupples LA, Haines JL, Hyman B, Kukull WA, Mayeux R, et al. Effects of age, sex, and ethnicity on the association between apolipoprotein E genotype and Alzheimer disease. A meta-analysis. APOE and Alzheimer Disease Meta Analysis Consortium. JAMA. 1997;278(16):1349–56.

22. Doody RS, Stevens JC, Beck C, Dubinsky RM, Kaye JA, Gwyther L, et al. Practice parameter: management of dementia report of the Quality Standards Subcommittee of the American Academy of Neurology. Neurology. 2001;56(9):1154–66.

23. Matsunaga S, Kishi T, Iwata N. Memantine monotherapy for Alzheimer's disease: a systematic review and meta-analysis. PLoS One. 2015;10(4):e0123289.

Intracranial Hypertension

38

Gentle Sunder Shrestha and Saurabh Pradhan

Intracranial hypertension (ICH) occurs when there is an increase in intracranial pressure (ICP) and is a common pathway for all acute neurological insults. ICH is the leading cause of morbidity and mortality in such patients [1, 2], with a clear association between the severity of ICH and poor outcomes [3]. ICH may be caused by a primary disorder of the central nervous system or may be secondary to other systemic disorders.

38.1 Pathophysiology of Intracranial Hypertension

The brain resides in an enclosed space protected by a bony vault called the cranium. The pressure within, or intracranial pressure (ICP), is normally less than 10–15 mmHg, with minor variations with age, position, and certain actions such as coughing and straining (Table 38.1).

The intracranial space is occupied by the brain parenchyma (80%), blood (12%), and cerebrospinal fluid (CSF) (8%) (Fig. 38.1). The cranium, being a relatively rigid structure, provides excellent protection to these contents but allows very little room for expansion. Therefore, an increase in volume of any one of the components needs to be compensated by a decrease in another so that the ICP remains within the normal limits.

This has been described by Monro-Kellie hypothesis, which states that "the sum of the intracranial volumes of blood, brain and CSF is constant, and that an increase in any one of these must be offset by an equal decrease in another, or else pressure increases" (Table 38.2).

Compensatory mechanisms involved in maintaining ICP include displacement of CSF, an increase in the absorption of CSF, a decrease in the production of CSF, and a reduction in total cerebral blood volume (CBV). Once these mechanisms fail to compensate for the increases in intracranial volume, precipitous rises in ICP occur, as can be described by the intracranial compliance curve, which is not linear. The dangerous increase in ICP can cause a decrease in cerebral blood flow as well as brain distortion, which, if not controlled, will lead to cerebral ischemia and herniation of the brain.

Cerebral perfusion depends upon cerebral perfusion pressure, which is a pressure gradient

G. S. Shrestha (✉)
Department of Critical Care Medicine, Tribhuvan University Teaching Hospital, Maharajgunj, Kathmandu, Nepal

S. Pradhan
Department of Anaesthesiology, Nepal Medical College, Jorpati, Kathmandu, Nepal

Table 38.1 Normal ICP in various age groups

Age group	ICP (mmHg)
Adults	<10–15
Children	3–7
Infants	1.5–6
Newborns	Subatmospheric

© Springer Nature Singapore Pte Ltd. 2024
K. K. Oli et al. (eds.), *Case-based Approach to Common Neurological Disorders*,
https://doi.org/10.1007/978-981-99-8676-7_38

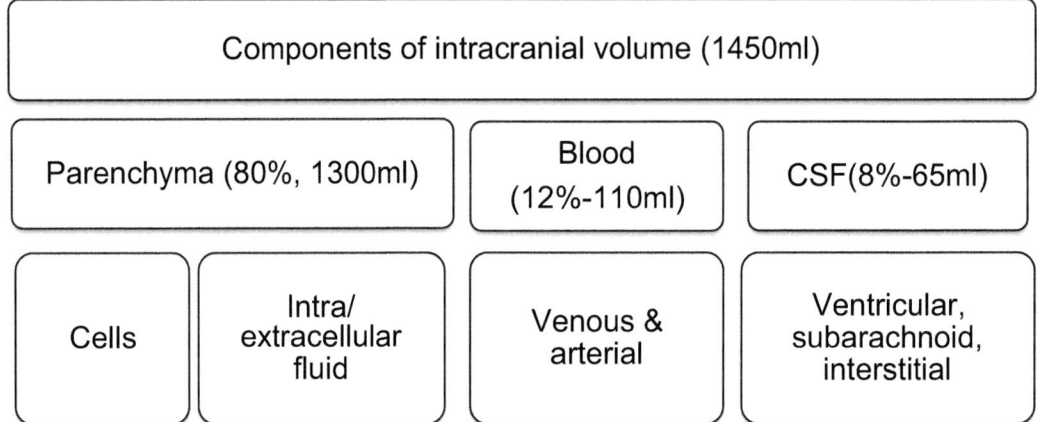

Fig. 38.1 Components of intracranial contents

Table 38.2 Causes of raised ICP

Parenchyma	Blood	CSF
Cellular	*Venous*	*Decreased drainage*
• Tumors	Venous obstruction secondary to	• Obstructive hydrocephalus
• Abscess	• PEEP	*Increased production*
• Contusions/hematomas	• coughing, straining	• Meningeal diseases
Intra/intercellular fluid	• CHF	• Choroid plexus tumors
• Cerebral edema- vasogenic or cytotoxic	• venous sinus thrombosis	
	• head-down tilt, tight neck ties	
	Arterial	
	Arterial dilatation secondary to	
	• ↓PaO_2, ↑$PaCO_2$	
	• Drugs: anesthetic/vasodilators	
	• Fever/seizures	
	• hypertension	

between the mean arterial blood pressure (MAP) and ICP that drives the blood flow.

$$CPP = MAP - ICP$$

However, despite the large variations in MAP and ICP, cerebral blood flow remains relatively constant as a consequence of the alteration of cerebral vascular resistance. This phenomenon is called cerebral auto-regulation, and this relation can be depicted by the mathematical equation:

$$CBF = CPP / CVR$$

where CVR is cerebral vascular resistance and CBF is cerebral blood flow.

However, during disease process, autoregulation becomes disrupted, and any change in MAP or ICP is directly translated to cerebral perfusion. Therefore, any rise in ICP above its compensatory limits can severely compromise CBF.

Another danger of raised ICP is the development of herniation syndromes. The intracranial vault is compartmentalized. The tentorium cerebelli divides it into supratentorial and infratentorial spaces, whereas the falx cerebri creates a partial division of supratentorial space into two. When pressure gradients overcome the resistance of brain tissue, intracranial contents tend to shift from one compartment to another and in the process compressing the adjacent brain parenchyma.

38.2 Clinical Features

Patients may present with a variety of clinical features that may be directly related to intracranial hypertension or to the primary disease causing it. Headache, nausea and vomiting, blurred vision, and somnolence are common. A further rise in ICP may be associated with a gradual decrease in the level of consciousness, ultimately leading to coma. Unilateral pupillary changes and the Cushing reflex, which is hypertension associated with bradycardia and abnormal breathing, herald impending herniation. Fundoscopy may reveal papilledema. However, these clinical features can be observer dependent and are neither sensitive nor specific to raised ICP [4].

38.3 Monitoring of ICP

As the clinical signs and symptoms are not reliable, other modalities are required to monitor ICP. Imaging such as computed tomography (CT) scan or magnetic resonance imaging (MRI) may show the underlying primary disease (e.g., hemorrhage, infarct) along with midline shift, obliteration of basal cisterns, loss of sulci, ventricular effacement, or enlarged ventricles in the event of hydrocephalus and cerebral edema. However, imaging, especially MRI, is costly, time consuming, and carries the risks of

transportation of an unstable critically ill patient [5]. So, repeated imaging is also not possible.

ICP can be monitored invasively by inserting catheters subdurally, intraparenchymally, and in the subarachnoid space (Fig. 38.2). However, the gold standard method is measurement using an intraventricular catheter, through which CSF drainage can also be performed in order to reduce ICP. Due to the invasiveness of these catheters, they are associated with various complications such as infection, hemorrhage, catheter-associated problems like obstruction, malposition, malfunction, air leakage into the ventricle or subarachnoid space, and CSF leakage. This has also led to the development and acceptance of ultrasonic measurement of optic nerve sheath diameter, which is non-invasive, can be done at the bedside, and is relatively accurate [6].

The Brain Trauma Foundation guidelines recommend monitoring ICP in all salvageable patients with a severe traumatic brain injury (TBI) and an abnormal CT scan (hematomas, contusions, swelling, herniation, or compressed basal cisterns) [7]. Even in patients with severe TBI and a normal CT scan, ICP monitoring may be indicated if two or more of the factors are present, which include age over 40 years, unilateral or bilateral motor posturing, and systolic blood pressure < 90 mmHg [6]. Indications for ICP monitoring are less established for other neurological emergencies.

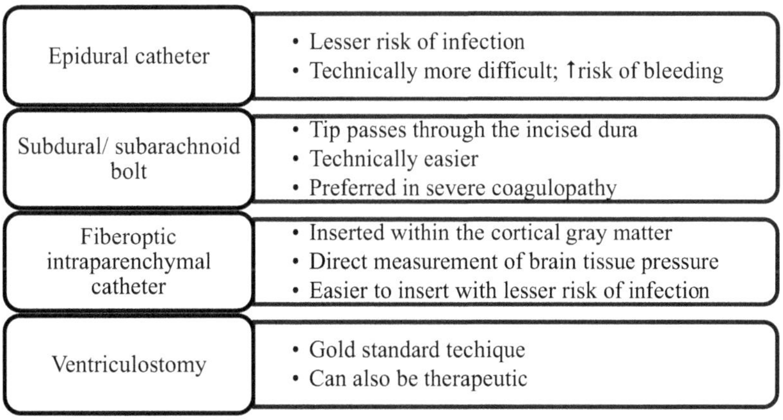

Fig. 38.2 Various modalities for monitoring ICP

Epidural catheter	• Lesser risk of infection • Technically more difficult; ↑risk of bleeding
Subdural/ subarachnoid bolt	• Tip passes through the incised dura • Technically easier • Preferred in severe coagulopathy
Fiberoptic intraparenchymal catheter	• Inserted within the cortical gray matter • Direct measurement of brain tissue pressure • Easier to insert with lesser risk of infection
Ventriculostomy	• Gold standard techique • Can also be therapeutic

38.4 Management of Raised ICP

The definitive therapy for ICH is the treatment of the primary neurological condition. However, more detrimental are the secondary changes that occur because of raised ICP, and regardless of the cause, certain principles are generally applicable. Several methods have been described and studied, with some having better evidence than others, and these treatment strategies can be stratified into tiers (Table 38.3).

From a pathophysiological point of view, raised ICP can be managed by targeting each of the intracranial components, that is, parenchyma, cerebral blood volume (CBV), and CSF (Table 38.4). There are few interventions that are helpful in lowering the tissue and CSF compartment apart from surgical removal of intracranial tissue or CSF drainage by ventriculostomy. However, CBV can be reduced by a vast number of ways, principally by either enhancing venous drainage or decreasing arterial blood flow.

Venous drainage can be enhanced by using maneuvers such as maintaining certain postures like head-up and neutral neck positioning, avoiding circumferential neck pressure (e.g., Philadelphia collars, endotracheal tube ties), and avoiding increases in central venous pressure by minimizing coughing or bucking, keeping positive end-expiratory pressure as low as necessary, and managing cardiac failure or tension pneumothorax. These interventions, although are simple, are often overlooked.

Decreasing arterial blood flow mainly consists of decreasing cerebral metabolic rate of oxygen consumption ($CMRO_2$), as arterial blood flow to the brain is tightly coupled to $CMRO_2$. Sedation and analgesia in a patient with ICH exert specific cerebral protective effects primarily by reducing $CMRO_2$ and secondarily by preventing rises in blood pressure, coughing, and bucking. Sedation and analgesia are also particularly helpful during targeted temperature management [8], management of refractory status epilepticus [9], and paroxysmal sympathetic activity [10].

Seizures can occur in 15–20% of patients with severe TBI [11] and can cause extreme rises in $CMRO_2$. Thus, seizure prophylaxis for such

Table 38.3 A proposed treatment strategy with different tiers of intervention for the management of raised ICP and their inherent pitfalls

Tiers	Treatment	Pitfalls
1.	Maintain airway, ventilation, circulation, head end elevation of at least 30°	Coughing, ventilator asynchrony, ventilator-associated pneumonia
2.	Sedation and analgesia, prevent fever, seizure prophylaxis	Hypotension
3.	CSF drainage from ventricles	Ventriculostomy-related infection
4.	Hyperosmolar therapy	Negative fluid balance, acute kidney injury, hypernatremia
5.	Hyperventilation	Excessive vasoconstriction and cerebral ischemia
6.	Hypothermia	Fluid and electrolyte disturbance, infection
7.	Metabolic suppression (barbiturates)	Hypotension, infection
8.	Decompressive craniectomy	Infection, poor Glasgow Outcome Scale

Table 38.4 A summary of the various interventions that can be applied to control raised ICP

Parenchyma	Blood volume	CSF
Cellular • Removal of tumor, abscess, decompressive craniectomy *Fluid* • Steroids • Diuretics • Hypertonic saline • Fluid mx	*Venous*: • Avoiding causes of high central venous pressure *Arterial* • Avoid/treat causes increasing cerebral blood flow	*Increase drainage* • External drain • Internal shunting *Decrease production* • Acetazolamide

patients for the first 7 days after injury is crucial [12]. Treatment beyond 7 days should be reserved for patients who develop late seizures [6].

$CMRO_2$ has shown a decrease of 6–7% per degree Celsius in temperature reduction, with temperatures in the range of 18–20 °C causing complete suppression of the EEG [13]. Increases in temperature can thus cause increases in CBV and is associated with poor neurologic outcome [14]. Therefore, fever should be strictly controlled with methods such as cooling and antipyretics while also targeting its cause. However, evidences supporting prophylactic induction of hypothermia are lacking and therefore are not recommended [6].

Hypocapnia causes cerebral vasoconstriction and decreases CBV. CBF changes approximately by 3% for each mmHg in $PaCO_2$ [15]. However, as CSF pH rapidly equilibrates to the new $PaCO_2$ level, its effect on ICP is time limited, and as such, prolonged periods of hyperventilation are unsuccessful. Furthermore, it carries a risk of brain ischemia, and hence it is avoided in the first 24 hours after TBI. For these reasons, the use of hyperventilation has been limited to situations where herniation is imminent, and if used, jugular venous oxygen saturation or brain tissue oxygen partial pressure monitoring should be done [6].

High doses of barbiturates have been used to control $CMRO_2$ and even target a complete suppression of EEG, referred to as barbiturate coma. However, it should only be considered for patients with refractory ICH because of the serious complications associated with it. These include hypotension, hypokalemia, respiratory complications, infectious complications, hepatic dysfunction, and renal dysfunction [16]. A loading dose of 10 mg/kg of pentobarbital over 30 min, then 5 mg/kg every hour for three doses, followed by a maintenance dose of 1 mg/kg/h is a commonly used regimen [17].

Apart from controlling CBV, the interstitial fluid portion of the brain parenchyma is also amenable to therapy. Brain volume is highly responsive to changes in water content, and as such, hyperosmolar agents have remained one of the most effective therapies for reducing ICP,

with their use dating back as early as 1919 [18]. Various substances, including urea, glycerol, sorbitol, mannitol, and, more recently, hypertonic saline formulations, have been investigated. Urea, glycerol, and sorbitol are not commonly used due to their moderate efficacy or high side-effect profile. They also have low reflection coefficients, raising concern about their accumulation inside the brain [19]. Hypertonic saline, however, has the highest reflection co-efficient, and several studies have shown it to be equal or even more efficacious than mannitol [20–25]. Nevertheless, due to a lack of large randomized trials, and the long history of its use, mannitol is still recommended by international guidelines [6].

The typical dose of mannitol is 0.25–1.0 g/kg body weight. Major concern with mannitol use is the development of acute renal failure [26]. Therefore, monitoring serum osmolarity, or even better, the osmolar gap (the difference between the calculated serum osmolarity and the measured serum osmolarity), is important during its use. A serum osmolarity of less than 320 mOsm/kg or an osmolar gap less than <55 mOsmol/kg should be maintained to avoid renal toxicity [27].

For ICH refractory to medical therapy, surgical decompression can be performed. This is done by removing a large area of the skull or decompressive craniectomy. This increases the potential volume of the cranial cavity and allows tissue to expand outside the cranium, normalizing ICP and preventing secondary tissue damage. There has always been much controversy regarding the indication and the outcome after surgery, but it is still commonly performed to effectively control ICP. What can be inferred from various evidence is that there is definite mortality benefit, but a favorable neurological outcome depends on various factors [28–31].

References

1. Miller JD, Butterworth JF, Gudeman SK, Faulkner JE, Choi SC, Selhorst JB, et al. Further experience in the management of severe head injury. J Neurosurg. 1981;54:289–99.
2. Myburgh JA, Cooper DJ, Finfer SR, Venkatesh B, Jones D, Higgins A, Bishop N, et al. Epidemiology

and 12-month outcomes from traumatic brain injury in Australia and New Zealand. J Trauma. 2008;64:854–62.

3. Miller JD, Becker DP, Ward JD, Sullivan HG, Adams WE, Rosner MJ. Significance of intracranial hypertension in severe head injury. J Neurosurg. 1977;47:503–16.

4. Shrestha G, Pradhan S. Management of intracranial hypertension: recent advances and future directions. Bangladesh Crit Care J. 2017;5(1):53–62.

5. Rosenberg JB, Shiloh AL, Savel RH, Eisen LA. Noninvasive methods of estimating intracranial pressure. Neurocrit Care. 2011;15:599–608.

6. Dubourg J, Javouhey E, Geeraerts T, Messerer M, Kassai B. Ultrasonography of optic nerve sheath diameter for detection of raised intracranial pressure: a systematic review and meta-analysis. Intensive Care Med. 2011;37:1059–68.

7. Carney N, Totten AM, O'Reilly C, Ullman J, Hawyluk GWJ, Bell MJ, et al. Guidelines for the management of severe traumatic brain injury. Neurosurgery. 2017;80(1):6–15.

8. Dell'Anna AM, Taccone FS, Halenarova K, Citerio G. Sedation after cardiac arrest and during therapeutic hypothermia. Minerva Anestesiol. 2014;80: 954–62.

9. Rossetti AO, Bleck TP. What's new in status epilepticus? Intensive Care Med. 2014;40:1359–62.

10. Perkes I, Baguley IJ, Nott MT, Menon DK. A review of paroxysmal sympathetic hyperactivity after acquired brain injury. Ann Neurol. 2010;68:126–35.

11. Lee ST, Lui TN, Wong CW, Yeh YS, Tzuan WC, Chen TY, et al. Early seizures after severe closed head injury. Can J Neurol Sci. 1997;24:40–3.

12. Temkin NR, Dikmen SS, Wilensky AJ, Keihm J, Chabal S, Winn HR. A randomized, double-blind study of phenytoin for the prevention of posttraumatic seizures. N Engl J Med. 1990;323:497–502.

13. Yan TD, Bannon PG, Bavaria J, Coselli JS, Elefteriades JA, Griepp RB, et al. Consensus on hypothermia in aortic arch surgery. Ann Cardiothorac Surg. 2013;2:163–8.

14. Dietrich WD, Alonso O, Halley M, Busto R. Delayed posttraumatic brain hyperthermia worsens outcome after fluid percussion brain injury: a light and electron microscopic study in rats. Neurosurgery. 1996;38:533–41.

15. Stocchetti N, Maas AI, Chieregato A, van der Plas AA. Hyperventilation in head injury. Chest. 2005;127:1812–27.

16. Schalén W, Sonesson B, Messeter K, Nordström G, Nordström CH. Clinical outcome and cognitive impairment in patients with severe head injuries treated with barbiturate coma. Acta Neurochir (Wien). 1992;117:153–9.

17. Eisenberg HM, Frankowski RF, Contant CF, Marshall LF, Walker MD. High-dose barbiturate control of elevated intracranial pressure in patients with severe head injury. J Neurosurg. 1988;69:15–23.

18. Weed LH, McKibben PS. Pressure changes in the cerebrospinal fluid following intravenous injection of solutions of various concentrations. Am J Physiol. 1919;48:512–30.

19. Marshall LF. Head injury. Recent past, present, and future. Neurosurgery. 2000;47:546.

20. Battison C, Andrews PJ, Graham C, Petty T. Randomized, controlled trial on the effect of a 20% mannitol solution and a 7.5% saline/6% dextran solution on increased intracranial pressure after brain injury. Crit Care Med. 2005;33:196–202.

21. Francony G, Fauvage B, Falcon D, Canet C, Dilou H, Lavagne P, et al. Equimolar doses of mannitol and hypertonic saline in the treatment of increased intracranial pressure. Crit Care Med. 2008;36:795–800.

22. Mortazavi MM, Romeo AK, Deep A, Griessenauer CJ, Shoja MM, Tubbs RS, et al. Hypertonic saline for treating raised intracranial pressure: literature review with meta-analysis. J Neurosurg. 2012;116:210–21.

23. Prabhakar H, Singh GP, Anand V, Kalaivani M. Mannitol versus hypertonic saline for brain relaxation in patients undergoing craniotomy. Cochrane Database Syst Rev. 2014;(7):CD010026.

24. da Silva JC, de Lima FM, Valença MM, de Azevedo Filho HR. Hypertonic saline more efficacious than mannitol in lethal intracranial hypertension model. Neurol Res. 2010;32:139–43.

25. Torre-Healy A, Marko NF, Weil RJ. Hyperosmolar therapy for intracranial hypertension. Neurocrit Care. 2012;17:117–30.

26. Gadallah MF, Lynn M, Work J. Case report: mannitol nephrotoxicity syndrome: role of hemodialysis and postulate of mechanisms. Am J Med Sci. 1995;309:219–22.

27. Dziedzic T, Szczudlik A, Klimkowicz A, Rog TM, Slowik A. Is mannitol safe for patients with intracerebral hemorrhages? Renal considerations. Clin Neurol Neurosurg. 2003;105:87–9.

28. Hofmeijer J, Kappelle LJ, Algra A, Amelink GJ, van Gijn J, van der Worp HB, HAMLET investigators. Surgical decompression for space-occupying cerebral infarction (the Hemicraniectomy After Middle Cerebral Artery infarction with Life-threatening Edema Trial [HAMLET]): a multicentre, open, randomised trial. Lancet Neurol. 2009;8:326–33.

29. Jüttler E, Bösel J, Amiri H, Schiller P, Limprecht R, Hacke W, et al. DESTINY II Study Group. DESTINY II: Decompressive surgery for the treatment of malignant INfarction of the middle cerebral arterY II. Int J Stroke. 2011;6:79–86.

30. Cooper DJ, Rosenfeld JV, Murray L, Arabi YM, Davies AR, D'Urso P, et al. Decompressive craniectomy in diffuse traumatic brain injury. N Engl J Med. 2011;364:1493–502.

31. Hutchinson PJ, Corteen E, Czosnyka M, Mendelow AD, Menon DK, Mitchell P, et al. Decompressive craniectomy in traumatic brain injury: the randomized multicenter RESCUEicp study. Acta Neurochir Suppl. 2006;96:17–20.